T0210160

PHARMACOLOGY HANDBOOK FOR PHYSIOTHERAPISTS

PHARMACOLOGY HANDBOOK FOR PHYSIOTHERAPISTS

JACQUELINE REZNIK   OFER KEREN   JOANNE MORRIS   IFTAH BIRAN

ELSEVIER

ELSEVIER

Elsevier Australia. ACN 001 002 357
(a division of Reed International Books Australia Pty Ltd)
Tower 1, 475 Victoria Avenue, Chatswood, NSW 2067

Copyright 2017 Elsevier Australia

All rights reserved. No part of this publication may be reproduced or transmitted in any form or by any means, electronic or mechanical, including photocopying, recording, or any information storage and retrieval system, without permission in writing from the publisher. Details on how to seek permission, further information about the Publisher's permissions policies and our arrangements with organisations such as the Copyright Clearance Center and the Copyright Licensing Agency, can be found at our website: www.elsevier.com/permissions.

This book and the individual contributions contained in it are protected under copyright by the Publisher (other than as may be noted herein).

Notice

This publication has been carefully reviewed and checked to ensure that the content is as accurate and current as possible at time of publication. We would recommend, however, that the reader verify any procedures, treatments, drug dosages or legal content described in this book. Neither the author, the contributors, nor the publisher assume any liability for injury and/or damage to persons or property arising from any error in or omission from this publication.

National Library of Australia Cataloguing-in-Publication entry

Reznik, Jacqueline, author.

Pharmacology handbook for physiotherapists / Jacqueline
Reznik, Ofer Keren, Joanne Morris,
Iftah Biran.
9780729542142 (paperback)
Pharmacology–Australia–Handbooks, manuals, etc.
Physical therapy–Practice.
Physical therapy–Handbooks, manuals, etc.
Keren, Ofer, author.
Morris, Joanne, author.
Biran, Iftah, author.

615.82

Senior Content Strategist: Melinda McEvoy
Senior Content Development Specialist: Natalie Hunt/Elizabeth Coady
Senior Project Manager: Anitha Rajarathnam
Cover and Internals Design by Natalie Bowra
Edited by Linda Littlemore
Proofread by Forsyth Publishing Services
Index by Robert Swanson
Typeset by Toppan Best-set Premedia Limited
Printed in Singapore by Markono Print Media Pte Ltd

This book is dedicated with love to my late father Charles Goldman, MPS, PhC, who taught me how to 'dance as though no-one is watching you, love as though you've never been hurt, sing as though no-one is listening and to live as though heaven is on earth' (William W Purkey).

Jacqueline Reznik

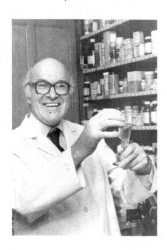

Contents

Foreword

I am honoured to have been asked to write the foreword for this timely and valuable handbook for physiotherapists currently practising in Australia.

Modern physiotherapy has been evolving for more than 100 years in response to the many challenges presented by the past century. Physiotherapists in Australia have been able to practise as primary contact practitioners since 1976, which in turn has challenged the profession to widen its scope of practice to include the possibility of prescribing medicines where indicated.

Prescribing is currently limited to very few jurisdictions, most notably the UK, but I consider that the practice will expand as other countries follow suit. The benefits to patients of streamlined physiotherapy care thus provided, which does not always require them to be shunted between various health practitioners, is something to be welcomed. Currently, Australian physiotherapists are unable to prescribe medicines by law but it is hoped that this legislation will be changed in the near future.

However, ethical practice currently demands that all physiotherapists should understand the importance of managing physiotherapy and pharmacology in the care of their patients. How medicines, including 'over-the-counter' products, affect patients and their physiotherapy outcomes is an important consideration in clinical decision making. Safety coupled with the best of care is paramount.

The authors of *Pharmacology Handbook for Physiotherapists* have risen to the challenge of providing this basic knowledge and produced a very readable, thorough and original work that will enable all Australian physiotherapists to fulfil this ethical responsibility to their patients. The handbook is clearly written with the clinician in mind and reflects the broad spectrum of conditions encountered in practice. In my opinion it is a seminal work that could act as a template for similar publications in other countries, which obviously would have to take into account the regulation of medicines in those jurisdictions.

I trust that this handbook will be well received by physiotherapists in Australia and elsewhere. I just wish that it had been part of the physiotherapy literature when I commenced my career over 50 years ago!

Prue Galley BPhty (Hons), MEdSt, FCSP (Hon.)

Preface/How to use this book

This book is not designed to be read 'cover to cover' but rather as a handbook that allows easy access to information on disease processes, their signs and symptoms and the medications that are being prescribed for your patients to alleviate those signs and symptoms. The text incorporates many tables that are designed to allow the reader to quickly retrieve useful information regarding a patient's drug regimen including possible side effects and duration of action, which may be particularly relevant to physiotherapists, both undergraduate and postgraduate. The book is divided into 11 chapters based on body systems, with a background chapter that includes basic pharmacology and legal implications at the beginning and a chapter for age-related implications of medications at the end. Chapters 2 through 10 deal with medications prescribed for various conditions by body system: cardiovascular, respiratory, women's and men's health, orthopaedic and musculoskeletal, neurological, pain and analgesia, endocrinological, haematological and mental health. This allows the reader to quickly access the information they require by searching via body system for the desired condition or medication.

This handbook is also not intended to compete with the larger and more concise pharmacotherapeutic textbooks or physiotherapeutic textbooks and, for that reason, more detail regarding the medications and physiotherapeutic interventions has not been included. The physiotherapy practice points outlined in each chapter are designed to explain to the reader the effects that the drugs may have on their treatment and provide valuable information on the actions of medications and when and how this interacts with physiotherapy treatment.

The book is not intended to be a 'do as I say book'. It tries, albeit on a limited scale, to describe the 'bigger picture'. Each chapter has been coauthored by a pharmacist, doctor and physiotherapist specialising in that particular area and, where possible, medications used to alleviate signs and symptoms have been described rather than those used for specific conditions. In those cases where exclusive drugs are designed for particular conditions, they have been referred to specifically. All drugs have been referred to by their generic (not brand) names.

At the time of going to print all of the information provided in this book is up to date.

About the editors

Jacqueline Reznik

Jacqueline Reznik, PhD, has a long clinical history in neurological physiotherapy and undergraduate and postgraduate teaching, both in Australia and internationally. Her main clinical and research interests lie in the investigation and treatment of the control of movement following acquired brain and spinal cord injury and in the prevalence and treatment of neurogenic heterotopic ossification. Dr Reznik has held academic positions at universities in the UK, Israel and Australia and currently works as a freelance Consultant Physiotherapist.

Ofer Keren

Ofer Keren, MD, is a physical and rehabilitation medicine specialist. As Director of the Department of Acquired Brain Injury Rehabilitation at Sheba Medical Center at Tel Hashomer, Israel, his main interests include neurophysiology (formerly Director of the Clinical Neurophysiological Unit at Loewenstein Rehabilitation Hospital, Ra'anana, Israel), monitoring of the recovery processes, brain injury and paediatric rehabilitation (formerly Director of the Department of Rehabilitation, Alyn Pediatric and Adolescent Rehabilitation Center, Jerusalem Israel). Dr Keren holds an academic position as Clinical Senior Lecturer, Sackler School of Medicine, Tel Aviv University.

Joanne Morris

Joanne Morris, BSc (Hons) Physiotherapy, MClin Biomech, is an experienced clinical physiotherapist currently undertaking her PhD in Extended Scope Physiotherapy. Jo was the project lead of Australia's first Extended Scope Physiotherapy Program for ACT Health, including the development of the world's first Extended Scope Physiotherapy Graduate Diploma in collaboration with the University of Canberra. Jo completed the Graduate Diploma in Extended Scope Physiotherapy in 2014, which included pharmacology and injecting modules. She is currently employed as an Extended Scope Physiotherapist at the Canberra Hospital in Orthopaedic Outpatients and the Emergency Department.

Iftah Biran

Iftah Biran, MD, is a behavioural neurologist, psychiatrist and psychotherapist. He specialises in the borderline zones of neurology and psychiatry in general, and somatic symptom disorders and functional neurological disorders in particular. He is the liaison psychiatrist to the Department of Neurology at Tel Aviv Medical Center, working with a multidisciplinary team composed of neurologists, physiotherapists, occupational therapists, neurological nurses and social workers.

Contributors

Technical editor

Gregory Kyle BPharm, MClinPharm, PhD, MPS
Professor of Pharmacy (Head of Discipline), Faculty of Health,
Queensland University of Technology
Brisbane, Queensland, Australia

Chapter contributors

Bryan Ashman MBBS, FRACS
Clinical Director, Department of Surgery, Canberra Hospital
Canberra, Australian Capital Territory, Australia

Heather Benson BSc(Hons), PhD
Associate Professor, School of Pharmacy, Curtin Health Innovation Research Institute,
Curtin University
Perth, Western Australia, Australia

Iftah Biran MD
Neurologist and Psychiatrist, Psychotherapist and Behavioural Neurologist;
Working as a Psychiatrist Consult (Liaison Psychiatry) to the Department of Neurology,
Tel Aviv Medical Center, Tel Aviv;
Psychoanalytic candidate, Max Eitingon Institute of Psychoanalysis, Jerusalem, Israel

Bernie Bissett BAppSc(Hons1) Physiotherapy, PhD
Clinical Assistant Professor, Physiotherapy, Discipline of Physiotherapy,
Faculty of Health, University of Canberra;
Senior Physiotherapist, Canberra Hospital and Health Services
Canberra, Australian Capital Territory, Australia

Anthony Hall FSHP, BPharm(Hons), AdvDipClinPharmTeach, DipMedSci(Pall Care)
Senior Lecturer, School of Clinical Sciences, Faculty of Health,
Queensland University of Technology;
Advanced Pharmacist, Persistent Pain, Queensland Health
Brisbane, Queensland, Australia

Ian Heslop BSc(Hons), MSc, DrPH, GradCertBT
Associate Professor Pharmacy, College of Medicine and Dentistry,
James Cook University
Cairns, Queensland, Australia

Karlee Johnston BPharm, MClinPharm
Lead Pharmacist, Division of Critical Care, Canberra Hospital and Health Services
Canberra, Australian Capital Territory, Australia

Ofer Keren MD
Director of Acquired Brain Injury Rehabilitation Department, Sheba Medical Center,
Tel Hashomer;
Clinical Senior Lecturer, Sackler School of Medicine, Tel Aviv University
Tel Aviv, Israel

Miriam Lawrence BPharm(Hons), MClinPharm
Lead Pharmacist for Surgery and Oral Health, Pharmacy Department,
Canberra Hospital and Health Services
Canberra, Australian Capital Territory, Australia

Pam Megaw BAppSc(Hons), PhD
Senior Lecturer in Physiology Biomedicine, James Cook University
Cairns, Queensland, Australia

Imogen Mitchell BsC(Hons), MBBS, PhD, FRCP, FRACP, FCICM
Deputy Dean, Medical School, Australian National University
Canberra, Australian Capital Territory, Australia

Joanne Morris BSc(Hons) Physiotherapy, MSc(Hons) Clinical Biomechanics,
GradDip Extended Scope Physiotherapy, Doctoral Candidate
Extended Scope Physiotherapist, Canberra Hospital and Health Services
Canberra, Australian Capital Territory, Australia

Roberto Orefice MBBS, BApplied Science(Physiotherapy)
Obstetrics and Gynaeology Registrar, Centenary Hospital for Women and Children
Garran, Australian Capital Territory, Australia

Chandima Perera MBBS, MPH, FRACP
Director of Rheumatology Unit and Network Director of Physician Education,
Rheumatology Unit, Canberra Hospital and Health Services
Canberra, Australian Capital Territory, Australia

Jacqueline E Reznik BAppSci, MAPA, MCSP, GradDip(Teaching),
GradDip(Neurology), PhD
International Physiotherapy Consultant
Kfar Yona, Israel;
Townsville, Queensland, Australia

Ilana Schumacher BPharm, MSc, MHA, PhD
Health Care Management & Rational Use of Pharmaceuticals Advisor;
Pharmaceuticals, Disposable Medical Devices and Combination Products Strategic
Consultant (R&D, QA/QC, Analytics, Stability & RA issues)
Beit Arie, Israel

Richard Talbot BPhys, GradCertHighEd
Senior Physiotherapist, Canberra Hospital and Health Services
Canberra, Australian Capital Territory, Australia

Kathryn Vine APAM, BPty, MPty (Sports), GradDip (Extended Scope of Practice
Physiotherapy)
Physiotherapist, Physiotherapy Department, Canberra Hospital and Health Services
Canberra, Australian Capital Territory, Australia

Robert Will BSc(Hons), MBBS, FRACP, EMBA
Consultant Rheumatologist;
Clinical Associate Professor of Medicine, University of Western Australia
Perth, Western Australia, Australia

Anthony Wright BSc(Hons), GradCertEduc, MPhtySt, PhD
Professor, School of Physiotherapy and Exercise Science, Curtin University
Perth, Western Australia, Australia

Reviewers

Carlos Bello Musculoskeletal Physiotherapist APA
Physiotherapist, Physical Spinal and Physiotherapy Clinic, Dynamic Pain Care, Boronia;
Big Hands Australia, Chirnside Park
Victoria, Australia

Courtney Clark BPhty, MHSc
Lecturer, School of Allied Health Sciences, Griffith University
Southport, Queensland, Australia

Seamus E Dalton MBBS, FAFRM (RACP), FACSP
Consultant Physician in Rehabilitation and Sports and Exercise Medicine,
North Sydney Sports Medicine Centre
St Leonards, New South Wales, Australia

Phil Doley BAppSc (Physio), Cert (Ortho) APAM
Principal Physiotherapist, Victor Harbor Physiotherapy Clinic
Victor Harbor, South Australia, Australia

Patricia Filby BPhty
Senior Physiotherapist, Royal Hobart Hospital
Hobart, Tasmania, Australia

Phoebe Freeman BPhty(Hons)
Physiotherapist, Regent St Physiotherapy
New Lambton, New South Wales, Australia

Nicole Reinke BSc(Hons), GradCert (Ed), MEd, PhD
Lecturer in Pathophysiology, School of Health and Sport Sciences,
University of the Sunshine Coast
Sippy Downs, Queensland, Australia

Jennie Scarvell BAppSc (Physio), GCHE, PhD
Professor and Head of Discipline, Physiotherapy, Faculty of Health,
University of Canberra
Canberra, Australian Capital Territory, Australia

Peter Suffolk BPhty, MSc
Coordinator, Student Led Physiotherapy and Physiotherapy Clinical Educator
Faculty of Health Clinics, Health Hub, University of Canberra
Canberra, Australian Capital Territory, Australia

Acknowledgements

We would like to thank all of our contributors to this project and, in particular, Professor Greg Kyle, without whose technical advice and amazing pharmacological knowledge this book would not have been possible.

We would also like to thank our wonderful team at Elsevier, Melinda McEvoy, Natalie Hunt, Elizabeth Coady, Anitha Rajarathnam and Linda Littlemore.

Introduction and background concepts

Gregory Kyle, Jacqueline Reznik, Joanne Morris, Ofer Keren, Pam Megaw

OVERVIEW

Legal and ethical issues
National and state legislation
Registration
Continuing professional development
Funding and the Pharmaceutical Benefits Scheme
Grey areas in physiotherapy prescribing in Australia
Provision of information in relation to medicines
Quality Use of Medicines (QUM)

Basic pharmacology and pharmacokinetic concepts
Pharmacology concepts
Pharmacokinetic concepts

Administration and monitoring of medications
Injection therapies
Polypharmacy
Monitoring of medications

Physiology of the autonomic nervous system

■ Introduction

This chapter is designed to present to the reader the raison d'être for this handbook, including the legal and ethical issues underlying prescription and monitoring of medications for the physiotherapist. It also introduces some basic pharmacology and pharmacokinetic concepts, and discusses some of the common methods of administration and monitoring of medications. Since the autonomic nervous system (ANS) plays an important role in the activity of all body systems, and as such in all pharmacotherapeutic interventions, an introduction to the basic physiology of this system has also been included in this chapter.

This handbook has not been designed as a pharmaceutical textbook or a physiotherapy textbook for interventions for specific conditions. Rather, it is a quick guide to enable physiotherapists to have a better understanding of the medications that their patients may be prescribed and how they (the medications) may impact upon the treatment given by the physiotherapist, and vice versa.

Traditionally, only medical practitioners and dentists were permitted to prescribe medications for reducing or preventing negative symptoms and/or slowing the progress of disease.

Physiotherapists and other allied health professionals in some countries[1] are now being authorised to prescribe certain medications as part of their clinical practice.

The rationale behind extending the pharmacological knowledge and responsibilities of physiotherapists is that, in the modern multidisciplinary approach of modern care, it is crucial that all members of the team are aware and knowledgeable about the disease process and possible programs, options and implications. The physiotherapist, as a member of the team, should be able to fully understand the therapeutic process including its pharmacological ramifications. In addition, physiotherapists have regular contact with patients within their traditional role, and may therefore be in a unique position to identify issues with medications, monitor the patient's reaction to medications and possibly highlight the need for a review of a patient's current medications. Physiotherapists should also be aware of the growing rise of over-the-counter (OTC) medications and food supplements that patients may be taking without informing their caregivers. In this regard they can help the prescribing agent to decide how to continue with a specific medication. If and when physiotherapists have prescribing authority, they can undertake this process and communicate recommendations and decisions to other team members.

This handbook is primarily written as a guide to drug usage, dosage, side effects and possible interactions with other medications for Australian physiotherapists, both undergraduate and postgraduate. It is anticipated that this handbook will be useful to physiotherapists today and possibly in the future if physiotherapy prescribing rights are broadly adopted within Australia.

As in many countries, healthcare in Australia is under increasing pressure to meet patient needs, including access to medication; one potential avenue is to expand non-medical prescribing, which at the time of printing is under governmental consideration. In the event that physiotherapists with appropriate training are licensed to prescribe, it is essential that they have an understanding of the effects of drugs relating to the symptoms they treat or manage and any potential effects on patients' other medications. In order to monitor these effects the physiotherapist needs to know the intended outcomes of the pharmacotherapy and use specific objective measures in order to determine the effectiveness of the drug regimens.

The chapters dealing with medications as applied to specific body systems[2] will be approached from a symptomatic viewpoint, listing potential drugs for specific symptoms. In order to allow the reader to achieve a better understanding of the way in which the drugs work, these chapters, when appropriate, are written from the anatomical/morphological aspect to the pathological/lesions (impairment) and from function to dysfunction (disability).

The major focus of this handbook is on pharmacotherapy as it applies to conditions assessed and treated by physiotherapists, and therefore only very brief descriptions of the anatomy/physiology and relevant physiotherapeutic interventions will be given. We hope this will be sufficient to allow understanding

---

[1] See the section 'Legal and ethical issues' for the Australian context.
[2] See the 'Contents' section.

of the disease process and the drug interactions. Since similar signs and symptoms may exist for differing pathologies, in the main, drug administration for the signs and symptoms rather than the pathologies will be discussed. In some cases, however, where disease-specific medications exist, they will be considered. Full references will be given at the end of each chapter to allow the reader to further explore the concepts briefly discussed.

Legal and ethical issues

Physiotherapists require a range of structures to safely and effectively prescribe medications. These include a legal framework, relevant training, registration in relation to prescribing, oversight of practices in relation to medication and a means of monitored continuous training/professional development (Morris & Grimmer 2014; Nissen et al. 2010). At the time of printing no such structures exist in Australia. This places physiotherapists, who may already be prescribing on a formal or ad hoc basis, at significant clinical and legal risk and presents a risk to the profession as a whole. This section on the legal and ethical issues briefly addresses these concerns in the context of physiotherapy practice in Australia at the time of printing.

For the purposes of this book the definition of 'prescribing' in relation to medications is:

an iterative process involving the steps of information gathering, clinical decision making, communication and evaluation, which results in the initiation, continuation or cessation of a medicine (National Prescribing Service Ltd 2012).

National and state legislation

The prescription, supply, management and administration of medication in Australia are controlled by the state and territory Medicines, Poisons and Therapeutic Goods Acts/Regulations (of various names). These laws determine:

- who can prescribe, supply and administer
- which medicines
- in what circumstances and manner
- for what purpose.

At the time of printing each state and territory within Australia has its own independent legislation in relation to medicines[3], although the general principles of these are similar. This means that there is state-by-state variability as to how physiotherapists are legally able (or unable) to incorporate the use of medicines in their clinical practice. There is capacity in some states for physiotherapists to administer and/or prescribe a limited range of medications or to trial prescribing under a 'standing order', 'research framework' or 'permit' provided by the state's chief medical officer or in certain practice settings, such as state government hospitals. In other states physiotherapists are not legally permitted to prescribe or administer any medications.

---

[3]For further information contact state and/or territory health departments.

Registration

National registration and accreditation for health professionals in Australia is governed by the Australian Health Practitioner Regulation Agency (AHPRA). AHPRA works with the 14 health practitioner boards to implement national registration and accreditation.

In addition to general registration, some national boards offer endorsements of registration for health practitioners who are deemed to have the qualifications, knowledge and skills to operate in a defined or an extended scope of practice. While the specific registration standards for endorsement of these tasks vary between the professions, there are some common key eligibility criteria that are required prior to granting (and maintaining) endorsed registrations.[4] In addition to these eligibility criteria, professional references, practice portfolios detailing a range of relevant experiences and employment histories may be required for endorsement. Prescribing and administering medications are included by the relevant national boards and AHPRA as endorsed tasks for nurse practitioners, podiatrists, optometrists and midwives.

There are variations across the professions regarding how endorsements are obtained and monitored; they may be determined on an individual basis for each practitioner, dependent upon their relevant qualifications, experience and training at each National Board's discretion. At the time of printing there are no provisions for endorsements for physiotherapists through AHPRA and the Physiotherapy Board of Australia.

In the case of nursing, when professionals demonstrate that they have met the appropriate additional requirements for an endorsement to their registration, it may lead to a change in the title a professional is permitted to use. The national law has clear restrictions on the use of protected titles – only people who have met the requirements of the national law can use a protected title. For example, the protected titles that apply to nurses and midwives are (Nursing and Midwifery Board of Australia 2014):

+ Nurse
+ Registered Nurse
+ Enrolled Nurse
+ Nurse Practitioner
+ Midwife
+ Midwife Practitioner.

It is an offence for anyone either knowingly or recklessly to use any of the protected titles to convince another person that they are registered under the Act unless they are registered and have therefore met the registration requirement to adopt a title. The titles 'Physiotherapist' and 'Physical Therapist' are protected titles under national law. In relation to registration there are strict criteria that apply to each registered professional's scope of practice, the notations that appear on the Register of Practitioners and the permitted use of protected titling. These criteria are set for each profession by the national board and are essential standards for registration and re-registration by each professional with AHPRA.

---

[4]See the AHPRA website (https://www.ahpra.gov.au) for further information.

Continuing professional development

Under the national law, which governs the operations of the national boards and AHPRA, all registered health practitioners must undertake continuing professional development (CPD). The national boards for each profession are responsible for setting CPD requirements within the 12-month registration period:

> All practising physiotherapists are required to participate in CPD activities that contribute directly to maintaining and improving their competence in their chosen scope of practice. Practising physiotherapists must complete at least 20 hours of CPD per year (Physiotherapy Board of Australia 2010, p. 1).

For those professions with endorsed registrations there are additional CPD requirements that relate directly to their 'extended scope' role in order for them to maintain their 'endorsed' status.

Funding and the Pharmaceutical Benefits Scheme

The Pharmaceutical Benefits Scheme (PBS) is a national government program that subsidises a schedule of medications for all Australian residents and citizens who have a Medicare card and international visitors who are eligible for immediate treatment through reciprocal healthcare arrangements. Current countries with reciprocal arrangements are Belgium, Finland, Italy, Malta, the Netherlands, New Zealand, Norway, Ireland (Republic), Slovenia, Sweden and the United Kingdom (Department of Human Services 2016). The PBS schedule is available online and is updated on the first day of every month. Currently, medicines covered by the PBS can only be prescribed by medical practitioners, dentists, optometrists, eligible midwives and nurse practitioners who are approved to prescribe PBS medicines under the *National Health Act 1953* (Cth). Prescription benefits, which occur in the form of a reduced cost for medications, supplied under the PBS are administered by Medicare under the *Health Insurance Act 1973* (Cth). Therefore, a possible limiting factor in the prescription of medications by physiotherapists in Australia is the lack of access to the PBS and the associated access and cost implications for patients.

Further information regarding the PBS can be accessed via the PBS website (www.pbs.gov.au).

Grey areas in physiotherapy prescribing in Australia

Grey areas for physiotherapists in relation to prescribing are in the provision of advice regarding OTC medications and/or advising changes to medications already in use by patients (Grimmer et al. 2002; Kumar & Grimmer 2005; Sullivan & Lansbury 1999). Physiotherapists have been known to provide advice regarding non-steroidal anti-inflammatory drugs (NSAIDs) and pain medication (Braund & Haxby Abbott 2011; Grimmer et al. 2002; Sullivan & Lansbury 1999). There is evidence of inconsistent training in relation to pharmacology in undergraduate and postgraduate physiotherapy programs in Australia and, therefore, it is likely that there is variation in the advice provided (Denehy 2014). This raises ethical and legal issues for physiotherapists who provide advice when they may have limited knowledge or training in relation to medications, a factor which may have implications for their professional indemnity insurance.

BOX 1.1 Principles of non-medical prescribing	
Principle 1	Patient safety and access to high-quality care is of paramount importance
Principle 2	Prescribing rights will be granted in a way that will help enhance timely access to medicines and be safe and cost-effective for the consumer
Principle 3	Health professionals must have an understanding of and a commitment to the principles of Quality Use of Medicines
Principle 4	Prescribing and dispensing functions should be clearly delineated
Principle 5	Priority will be given to clarify and agree all inter-professional issues which will impact on continuity of care for the patient
Principle 6	Prescribing as an activity should complement and value-add to the spectrum of other core services provided by that health profession
Principle 7	A credentialling process should be implemented to ensure practitioners possess the appropriate competencies
Principle 8	Outcomes of any trials or pilot programs on prescribing by non-medical health professionals will be used to inform the framework

Principle for a National Framework for Prescribing by Non-medical Health Professionals, 2010 © Pharmaceutical Society of Australia. Reproduced with permission 2016.

The Pharmaceutical Society of Australia has developed a set of principles in relation to non-medical prescribing (Box 1.1)[5] (Pharmaceutical Society of Australia 2010).

These principles should be utilised by physiotherapists in the future or by physiotherapists currently prescribing or administering medications under a standing order (see the section 'National and state legislation' above). They should, however, be adopted by all physiotherapists in their interactions with medicines, regardless of whether they prescribe or administer medicines.

Provision of information in relation to medicines

Recommendations by the Australian Pharmacy Council are that all health professionals who administer or supply medications be trained to provide the correct verbal and written information to consumers for all medicines supplied. A valuable resource of written information is the Consumer Medicine Information (CMI) leaflet, which is written and provided by the pharmaceutical company responsible for the medication (Therapeutic Goods Administration 2014). CMIs are required for all prescription medications and some OTC medications, and their purpose is to provide up-to-date information relating to the safe and effective use of the medication. The following advice should be provided:

♦ name of the medicine
♦ names of the active and inactive ingredients

---

[5]A link to the full document is included under 'References'.

- dosage of the medicine
- what the medicine is used for and how it works
- warnings and precautions, such as when the medicine should not be taken
- interactions the medicine might have with food or other medicines
- how to use the medicine properly
- side effects
- what to do in the case of an overdose
- how to store the medicine properly.

Quality Use of Medicines

The Quality Use of Medicines (QUM) is one of the central objectives of Australia's *National Medicines Policy* (Department of Health and Ageing 1999) and therefore directly applicable to physiotherapists involved in medication management.

QUM requires the careful evaluation of management options, selecting a suitable medicine, if a medicine is indicated, and ongoing monitoring and re-evaluation to ensure the safe and effective use of medicines. The term 'medicine' in the context of QUM includes prescription, non-prescription and complementary medicines and as such is highly applicable to all physiotherapists in their daily clinical practice.

On an individual patient level, the application of QUM to the daily management of medical conditions aims to assist in selecting and communicating the most appropriate medicine or non-medicine prevention and treatment options and to provide the individual with optimal and cost-effective outcomes. QUM also encompasses monitoring treatment outcomes in order to allow rapid modification of management depending on patient response.

CAVEAT: The information/education within this manual **does not** permit a Physiotherapist to prescribe or administer **any** medications[6].

■ Basic pharmacology and pharmacokinetic concepts

Drugs (or medications or medicines) are chemical molecules that require a molecular target. Drugs act at the molecular level and the major principle behind understanding drug actions is to know the target molecule (or receptor) and its place in normal physiology and homeostasis. Once this is known, the action (and indeed many side effects) of a given drug can be determined or predicted.

Pharmacology concepts

Most drugs can have one of three main ways of achieving a therapeutic result. They can:
1 stimulate a receptor site (agonist)
2 block a receptor site (antagonist)
3 weakly stimulate a receptor site while blocking it to a pure agonist (partial antagonist) (Figure 1.1).

---

[6]Please refer to the state or territory legislation in your jurisdiction to ascertain your rights in relation to prescribing.

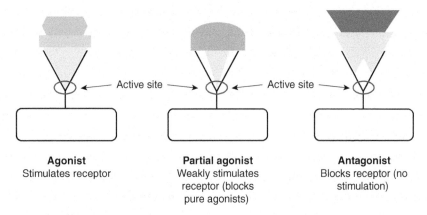

Agonist
Stimulates receptor

Partial agonist
Weakly stimulates
receptor (blocks
pure agonists)

Antagonist
Blocks receptor (no
stimulation)

Figure 1.1 Agonists and antagonists.
Adapted with permission from: WIKI Noticia, Agonist/antagonist. <http://en.wikinoticia.com/lifestyle/
beauty/74711-agonist--antagonist>.

Most drugs have a measurable receptor binding affinity. This is a measure of how well the drug binds to its receptor. If a drug were to bind permanently to its receptor, its action would continue until the body disassembled that receptor and built a new one. For an agonist or partial agonist, this would result in constant stimulation of the receptor to varying degrees. For this reason alone, all agonists are reversible (or competitive) – that is, they bind to their target receptor like Velcro and can jump on and off the receptor site (e.g. salbutamol – a beta-2 receptor agonist). This is the case for most antagonists also; however, there are a few drugs that are irreversible (or non-competitive) antagonists that bind like super-glue, rather than Velcro (e.g. aspirin at the cyclo-oxygenase (COX) enzyme). The 'competitive' term comes from the fact that the drug, natural ligand (i.e. the compound that normally stimulates the receptor in the body) and any antagonists diffuse around the receptor and couple (bind) and de-couple with it (e.g. propranolol, a beta-receptor antagonist or beta-blocker). This generates competition for the receptor site and relative concentrations and binding affinities determine which substance has the greater effect.

The effect produced by a drug either amplifies the natural process (agonist) or reduces it by blocking endogenous stimulation of the receptor (pre- or postsynaptic). For example, salbutamol (a short-acting beta-agonist or SABA) causes bronchodilation by stimulating beta-2 receptors in the lungs. This is an important factor for physiotherapists treating patients with chronic obstructive airways disease (COAD) since the physiotherapy treatment designed to clear the airways physically may be enhanced by prior use of the medication. Conversely, in a patient prescribed atenolol (a beta-blocker), a drug that reduces the heart rate by blocking beta-1 receptors in the heart and as such reduces the action of endogenous adrenaline and noradrenaline (which both stimulate beta receptors), the physiotherapist might observe a reduction in physical capacity directly related to the medication.

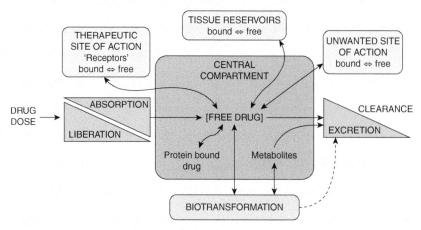

Figure 1.2 Schematic diagram of ADME processes.
Adapted with permission from: Brunton, L.L., Chabner, B.A., Knollmann, B.C., 2010. Goodman and Gilman's The Pharmacological Basis of Therapeutics, twelfth ed. McGraw-Hill, New York.

There are some other mechanisms of action that will be discussed in subsequent chapters as appropriate, but the concept of drugs and receptors described above accounts for the vast majority of drug actions. The action or outcome produced by a drug is known as pharmacodynamics, or what the drug does to the body.

Pharmacokinetic concepts

Pharmacokinetics focuses on what the body does to the drug. It is broken down into four main areas, known as ADME (Figure 1.2):

Absorption – how the drug gets into the body (unless injected intravenously)

Distribution – once absorbed into the blood, where the drug goes

Metabolism – how the body breaks the drug down into other compounds that are more easily excreted

Elimination – how the drug is excreted and eliminated from the body.

In this chapter we deal with the general pharmacokinetic concepts; for more specific detail relating to paediatric and geriatric populations, please see Chapter 11.

Absorption

The majority of drug doses are administered orally; indeed, this is the preferred administration route due to ease and patient comfort. Other major routes of administration include injection (intravenous, intramuscular, subcutaneous, intradermal, intraarticular), topical (skin, eye, nose), inhalation (lung), topical (vaginal, rectal, buccal), rectal (for systemic absorption) and sublingual (under the tongue – for systemic absorption). The route is selected based on the known

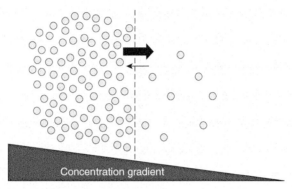

Figure 1.3 Concentration gradient drives passive diffusion.

properties of the drug: its site of action, urgency of treatment, patient's status (e.g. unconscious), the purpose of drug action and for metabolic reasons.

All routes for a systemic action (via the blood) except intravenous injection require the drug to be absorbed. Most non-injection routes and some injections also require the drug to be liberated from its vehicle or carrier (e.g. tablet matrix). Once absorbed, the drug is in the central compartment, or the blood. The blood carries the drug around the body to its site of action, other sites where the drug may act (producing side effects), the liver (metabolism and excretion), kidneys (excretion) and other tissues where the drug may be stored (e.g. adipose tissue for some lipid soluble drugs). Only drugs that are free in the blood are available to be metabolised or excreted.

Distribution

Any drug molecules distributed in other tissues, or bound to proteins in the blood, are essentially 'hidden' from these processes; however, relative concentration gradients ensure that the distribution (and redistribution) is a dynamic process. As concentrations rise (or fall) on one side of a semi-permeable membrane (e.g. the membrane of a tissue), a concentration gradient is established (Figure 1.3). Drug molecules will move along this concentration gradient by passive diffusion to even out the concentrations on both sides of the membrane. Some drugs are involved in active transport mechanisms and this can complicate these mechanisms; however, the vast majority of drugs are controlled via passive diffusion.

When the concentrations on each side of the membrane are equal, equilibrium will be established with equal diffusion in both directions. When the concentration of a drug in the blood begins to fall, due to metabolism and excretion, the concentration gradient will reverse and the drug will diffuse out of the tissue to maintain the equilibrium of equal concentrations.

Metabolism

The liver is the primary organ that metabolises drugs to make them more water soluble so that they can be more readily excreted by the kidneys. It achieves this through a range of oxidative chemical reactions catalysed by enzymes. The main drug-metabolising enzymes in the body are the cytochrome P450 (or CYP) enzyme families. These enzymes can be induced to increase the rate at which drugs are broken down or inhibited. Induction and inhibition of the CYP enzymes may be triggered by other drugs, and this is a major source of drug interactions. CYP enzyme activity may be different in specific populations (women, Asians). These variations in metabolic activity may cause significant changes in drug concentrations.

Elimination

Drugs can be eliminated from the body by excretion or metabolism. Metabolism changes a drug into a different chemical entity. Metabolic changes are usually only minor and, sometimes, the metabolite is an active drug itself – usually through the same mechanism as the parent compound. These are known as 'active metabolites' and are a new drug entity in their own right. In practical terms, an active metabolite will extend the action of a drug. Regardless of whether the metabolite is active or inactive, the drug has been eliminated from the body because the metabolite (a new chemical entity) is different to its parent compound (Figure 1.4).

Excretion can occur through many paths to the outside world, such as renal (via the urine), hepatic (via the bile), via the breath (the basis for roadside breath analysis for alcohol) or via the skin (sweat and sebum). The major pathway is renal, with bile excretion having a minor, but still important, role. Once excreted, the drug (or its metabolite) is removed from the body and is no longer able to perform any pharmacological action (if active).

Pharmacokinetic parameters

The main pharmacokinetic parameters have been summarised below.

◆ **Half-life** ($t_{1/2}$) is the time taken for the drug concentration in the blood to fall by half. Mathematically, it is identical to the half-life concept for radioactivity. Because the decline in drug levels follows an exponential decay, the half-life remains a constant, regardless of the initial concentration.

◆ **Volume of distribution** (V_D – also known as apparent volume of distribution) is the theoretical volume that would be necessary to contain the total amount of an administered drug at the same concentration at which it is observed in the blood plasma. It is defined as the distribution of a medication between plasma and the rest of the body after oral or parenteral dosing. The V_D of a drug represents the degree to which a drug is distributed in body tissue rather than the plasma. V_D is directly correlated with the amount of drug distributed into tissue; a higher V_D indicates a greater proportion of tissue distribution. A V_D greater than the total volume of body water (approximately 42 litres in humans) is possible, and would indicate that the drug is highly distributed into tissue. Volume of distribution may be increased by renal failure (due to fluid retention) and liver failure (due to altered body fluid and plasma protein binding). Conversely, it may be decreased in dehydration.

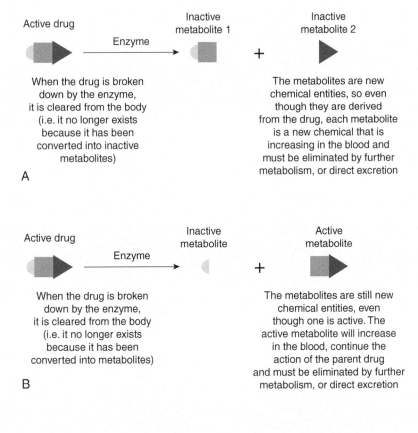

A When the drug is broken down by the enzyme, it is cleared from the body (i.e. it no longer exists because it has been converted into inactive metabolites)

The metabolites are new chemical entities, so even though they are derived from the drug, each metabolite is a new chemical that is increasing in the blood and must be eliminated by further metabolism, or direct excretion

B When the drug is broken down by the enzyme, it is cleared from the body (i.e. it no longer exists because it has been converted into metabolites)

The metabolites are still new chemical entities, even though one is active. The active metabolite will increase in the blood, continue the action of the parent drug and must be eliminated by further metabolism, or direct excretion

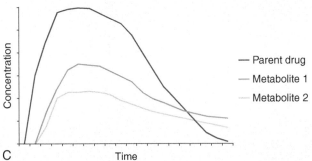

— Parent drug
— Metabolite 1
— Metabolite 2

Figure 1.4 Diagrammatic representation of clearance via metabolism. **A** Metabolism to inactive metabolites. **B** Metabolism to active metabolite. **C** Concentration–time plot of parent drug and metabolite levels.

♦ **Clearance** (C) is the term for elimination where the drug is cleared from the body. There are many sub-terms for clearance: urinary, hepatic, intrinsic etc. Total clearance is the sum of all the various mechanisms used to clear the drug. If a drug has been metabolised, it is deemed to have been 'cleared'. The metabolite is considered to be another chemical entity with its own clearance parameters.

♦ **First-pass effect** is the effect whereby oral administration of a drug produces quite low concentrations in the blood. Drugs with a high first-pass effect are often metabolised in the gut wall before getting into the blood, or because most intestinal circulation is shunted through the liver before circulating to the rest of the body. Ways to reduce this effect are administration methods that avoid swallowing the drug (e.g. injection, rectal, sublingual administration).

♦ **Bioavailability** is the percentage of drug available to the body (measured in the blood) compared to the dose swallowed. For example, if 10 mg of a 50-mg dose was detected through blood tests, the bioavailability would be 20%. This concept takes into account absorption and the first-pass effect.

■ Administration and monitoring of medications

The manner in which a medicine is administered will determine to some extent whether or not the patient gains any clinical benefit, and whether they suffer any adverse effect from the medicine.

Two main factors determine whether or not a drug will reach its intended site of action in the body:

1 the bioavailability of the drug
2 how the drug is given (route of administration).

Bioavailability

♦ Bioavailability is the proportion of an administered drug that reaches the systemic circulation.

♦ Drugs that are given by direct IV injection are said to have 100% bioavailability. Some drugs that are particularly well absorbed by the gastrointestinal mucosa may also have 100% bioavailability. Most drugs, however, do not have this availability by the oral route so that a higher dose of the drug may be required if given orally. The route of administration and its formulation (tablet, capsule, liquid) can clearly influence the bioavailability of a drug.

Routes of administration[7]

Administration of medications may be directed via several routes:

1 the gastrointestinal (GI) system – orally[8]
2 the GI system rectally – using suppositories or enemas

---

[7]For further information on routes of administration please refer to the basic pharmacology and pharmacokinetics concepts sections, cross-referencing where necessary with the relevant drug tables in specific chapters.

[8]This is the commonest route.

3 the respiratory system – through breathing, sniffing or inhalation

4 sublingual (SL) [under the tongue] – by putting the drug near the mucous membrane beneath the tongue; the medication is absorbed in the capillaries of the epithelium; drugs that may be administered by this route include cardiovascular drugs, vitamins and minerals

5 topical (applied on body surfaces – skin or mucous membranes [e.g. inside mouth]) – through the application of creams, foams, gels, lotions, ointments or use of patches; topical administration includes the use of transdermal patches that enable prolonged release; drugs administered by this route include contraceptives, nicotine and capsaicin for pain relief; the active drug for some formulations, such as patches, is released from a polymer matrix

6 injection

  a intravenous – continuous or dose injection

  b intrathecal – pump

  c subcutaneous

  d intradermal

  e intraarticular, synovial

  f intramuscular – for delayed absorption

  g nerve and/or nerve/muscle block.

Dose and timing of medications

The dose is the amount of drug taken at any one time. It may be expressed as the weight of drug (e.g. 250 mg), volume of drug solution (e.g. 10 mL), the number of dosage forms (e.g. 1 capsule, 1 suppository) or some other quantity (e.g. 2 puffs).

The dosage regimen is the dose and the frequency at which the drug doses are given. Examples include 2.5 mL twice a day, one tablet three times a day, one intramuscular (IM) injection every four weeks. The total daily dose is calculated from the dose and the number of times per day the dose is taken.

The dose form is the physical form of a dose of drug. Common dose forms include tablets, capsules, creams, ointments, aerosols and patches. Each dose form may also have a number of specialised forms such as extended-release, buccal, dispersible and chewable tablets. The strength is the amount of drug in the dose form or a unit of the dose form (e.g. 500-mg capsule, 250 mg/5 mL suspension). The optimal dosage is the dosage that gives the desired effect with minimum side effects.

Many factors must be taken into consideration when deciding a dose of drug, including age of the patient, weight, sex, ethnicity, liver and kidney function and whether the patient is a smoker or non-smoker. Other medicines may also affect the drug dose.

Dose and timing of medications are important considerations for physiotherapists when considering the timing of their therapeutic intervention – fuller details will be supplied for individual medications in subsequent chapters of this handbook. Refer to Table 1.1 for the meanings of standard Latin abbreviations used in prescriptions.

TABLE 1.1 Standardised Latin abbreviations used in prescribing medications					
Standard abbreviation	Meaning	Standard abbreviation	Meaning	Standard abbreviation	Meaning
p.c.	after meals	Q4h	every 4 hours	nocte	at night
a.c.	before meals	mane	in the morning	gtt	drops
b.d.	twice a day	h.s.	at bedtime	tab	tablet
t.d.s.	three times a day	Prn	when necessary	cap	capsule
q.i.d.	four times a day	ad.lib.	as desired	ung	ointment

Injection therapies

Injections are usually systemic, although some injections administer the medication locally, i.e. directly to the site of action. Common medications administered locally include local anaesthetics, nerve block and intraarticular/soft-tissue injections. A sterile technique should be used (i.e. the technique includes hand washing, use of a sterile field, use of sterile gloves for application of a sterile dressing and use of sterile instruments).

Joint and soft-tissue injection

The main indications for injection therapy are: inflammatory arthritis (rheumatoid arthritis); synovitis; severe osteoarthritis; bursitis; tendonitis; painful trigger points.

The main contraindications and precautions for injection therapy include: septic arthritis; osteomyelitis; soft-tissue infection; general infection; immune-depression state; bleeding disorders.

Therapeutic injections

These include local anaesthetics (lignocaine) and/or corticosteroid and can be used for therapeutic and/or diagnostic questions. The effects may be seen immediately or within a few days and can last for weeks or months. Non-responsiveness to therapeutic injections might be due to technical difficulties, such as not entering the joint, or incorrect diagnosis and as such this would be an incorrect treatment modality.

Nerve blocks (neurolysis)

A nerve block can be performed by the application of chemical agents to a nerve to impair its function (conduction). It may be performed into the nerve itself and/or at the nerve/muscle junction (synapse) and its effect may be temporary or permanent. The main clinical indications for nerve blocks are for pain treatment and reducing muscle tonus (spasticity or dystonia).

Chemical neurolysis is a nerve block that impairs conduction by means of destruction of a portion of the nerve. The agents most frequently used are phenol, alcohol and local anaesthetics. Chemical neurolysis can be induced at different levels of the peripheral nervous system from the root to the motor end plate.

Local neurolysis can be used to reduce the spasticity effect in specific muscles; the effect of chemical neurolysis is immediate. The effect on spasticity can be localised to the specific muscle or group of muscles that are causing a problem. The duration of the effect is variable, lasting from weeks to months and occasionally even years.

Today the most common biological nerve/muscle junction block is botulinum toxin, the effects of which are not immediate but may last weeks, months or even years.

Nerve blocks are usually performed using a sterile needle that is Teflon-coated, which serves as both a needle for injection as well as an electrode. The needle is connected to a stimulator and/or electromyography (EMG) recording for guiding the place for injection.

*   **Phenol nerve block** – phenol (carbolic acid) – is a derivative of benzene with one hydroxyl group.
*   **Botulinum toxin (BTX)** is a neurotoxic protein produced by the bacterium *Clostridium botulinum* and related species. It can be produced commercially by bacteria of the genus *Clostridium*. It acts by preventing the neurotransmitter acetylcholine, sited at the pre-synaptic vesicles, from being released.[9]

The success of the injection depends upon:

*   choice of the specific sites
*   the appropriate dose
*   the technique of performing the injection
*   the goals for injection and prior discussion of the aims with the patient, therapist and/or caregiver.

Polypharmacy

Polypharmacy is a term that has been in the medical literature for more than 150 years (see www.thekingsfund.org.uk) and is defined here as five or more regular prescription medications (Hubbard et al. 2015). A recent report on polypharmacy by the Kings Fund UK (2013), *Polypharmacy and Medicines Optimisation: Making It Safe and Sound*, has described polypharmacy as being sometimes appropriate and sometimes problematic. Appropriate polypharmacy, when use of medicines has been optimised and they are prescribed for a specific updated condition or illness, according to best evidence, can extend life expectancy and improve a patient's quality of life. Problematic polypharmacy, however, increases the risk of interactions and adverse drug reactions as well as affecting patient compliance and quality of life. Steinman et al. (2014) suggest that the number of drugs that a patient is taking is the single best predictor of harm. Factors that must be taken into consideration when deciding whether or not a drug, or combination of drugs, may be harmful include: the patient's age, medication treatment updated criteria, cross-activity, interference, effect on metabolism

---

[9]For further details regarding BTX injection therapy see Chapter 6.

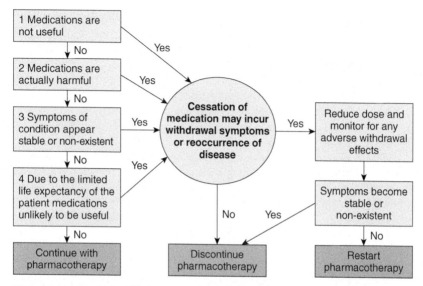

Figure 1.5 Algorithm for deciding the order and mode in which a drug may be discontinued. Adapted from: Scott, I.A., Hilmer, S.N., Reeve, E., et al., 2015. Reducing inappropriate polypharmacy: the process of deprescribing. JAMA Internal Medicine 175 (5), 827–834.

(length of effect), toxicity (therapeutic level), allergic reactions, patient's ability to adhere to treatment and drug intolerance. A recent report by Scott et al. (2015) presents an algorithm for deciding the order and mode in which a drug could be discontinued (Figure 1.5).

The rise in polypharmacy has been attributed to the growth of an ageing and increasingly frail population, many of whom have multiple long-term conditions (Wise 2013). For a more detailed description of polypharmacy in the geriatric population see Chapter 11. Better training in managing multi-morbidity and polypharmacy for all healthcare professionals is required. Since the traditional role of physiotherapists is to assess and treat or manage the patient's quality of life and functional activities, the treating physiotherapist may be in the ideal position to review whether each drug has been prescribed appropriately or inappropriately, both individually and in the context of the other drugs being prescribed.

Monitoring of medications

Therapeutic drug monitoring (TDM) (Birkett 1997) refers to the individualisation of dosage by maintaining plasma, serum or blood drug concentrations within a target range (therapeutic range, therapeutic window). It includes ensuring that:

♦ the patient is taking the proper medication – does the patient need all the drugs/all the medical conditions treated?
♦ the medication is safe – no significant adverse effects

◆ the healthcare professional has knowledge of all the medications the patient takes

◆ the patient adheres to the medication treatment regimen – is the patient really taking all the drugs prescribed?

There are two major sources of variability between individual patients in drug response. These are variations in the relationship between:

1 dose and plasma concentration (pharmacokinetic variability)

2 drug concentration at the receptor and the response (pharmacodynamic variability).

TDM involves not only measuring drug concentrations but also the clinical interpretation of the result (Ghiculescu 2008). When an effect (objective measurable parameter), such as changes in blood pressure, pain or serum cholesterol, is readily measured, the dose of a drug should be adjusted according to the response. The selection of drugs for TDM is important because the concentrations of many drugs are not clearly related to their effects, although TDM may be conducted for these drugs to measure compliance with therapy. TDM may be costly and should only be performed when there are marked advantages to be gained. The timing of TDM is important and, unless it is being used to forecast a dose or there are concerns about its toxicity, samples should be taken when the drug concentration has reached a steady state (which may take several months, depending upon the half-life of the drug). Correct sample timing should also take into account absorption and distribution of the drug. Interpretation of the findings is of paramount importance and needs to consider the context of the individual patient.

Drug monitoring and interpretation services help to improve the safety, efficacy and cost-effectiveness of medications. They promote the principles of rational prescribing and Quality Use of Medicines (QUM) (Gross 1998).

There are a number of limitations associated with TDM; these include the possible scientific inaccuracy of the drug assays, laboratory variability in reporting, limited accessibility in rural Australia and the validity of suggested target ranges (Birkett 1997; Gross 1998).

Unwanted medications

The Australian Government funds a program to dispose of unwanted, expired or no longer needed medications in an environmentally responsible manner. This program is known as the Return of Unwanted Medicines (RUM) program. Medications that are no longer required for whatever reason can be returned to a community pharmacy for appropriate disposal. The pharmacy will place the unwanted medicines into a special RUM bin that is returned through pharmacy wholesaler networks to the RUM facility for appropriate disposal in a specialised high temperature incinerator.

Physiotherapists can encourage any patients who mention that they have unwanted medicines, or who have had dosage changes, to take their old medicines to their pharmacy for disposal. This program is also a good way to remove medicines that are no longer needed from the home to minimise the risk of young children accessing the medicines.

TABLE 1.2 Effect of autonomic nervous system inputs on organ systems

Organ system	Sympathetic input effect	Parasympathetic input effect
Eye	Dilates pupils, reduces accommodation	Constricts pupils, increases accommodation
Blood vessels	Constricts most vessels, dilates skeletal muscle vessels	No effect
Salivary glands	Decreases secretion	Increases secretion
Heart	Increases heart rate and force	Decreases heart rate and force
Respiratory system	Dilates bronchioles	Constricts bronchioles
Gastrointestinal tract	Decreases secretions and motility	Increases secretions and motility
Renal system	Increases renin release	No effect
Reproductive system	Causes ejaculation	Causes erection

Physiology of the autonomic nervous system

Since the autonomic nervous system (ANS) plays an integral role in the actions of most medications as discussed earlier, a brief introduction to it is provided here.

The autonomic nervous system has two branches: the sympathetic nervous system and the parasympathetic nervous system (see Figure 1.6 on pages 20 and 21). The sympathetic nervous system is often considered the 'fight or flight' system, while the parasympathetic nervous system is often considered the 'rest and digest' or 'feed and breed' system. In many cases, these dual systems have 'opposite' actions where one system activates a physiological response and the other inhibits it (see Table 1.2).

The autonomic nervous system has a two-neuron pathway in the peripheral nerves serving the organs (Figure 1.7). The first neuron, the pre-ganglionic neuron, extends from the spinal cord and is a motor neuron, analogous to the motor neurons serving skeletal muscle, and it produces acetylcholine as its neurotransmitter. These motor neurons synapse with the cell bodies of the second or visceral motor neuron, the post-ganglionic neuron, in the autonomic ganglia. The cholinergic receptors in the autonomic ganglia are of the nicotinic family, such as those found at the neuromuscular junction. These receptors gate sodium ion channels and, when acetylcholine binds to them, the visceral motor neuron is depolarised and activated. The visceral motor neurons synapse directly with the target organs, and the neurotransmitter produced varies, depending upon which division of the autonomic nervous system it serves.

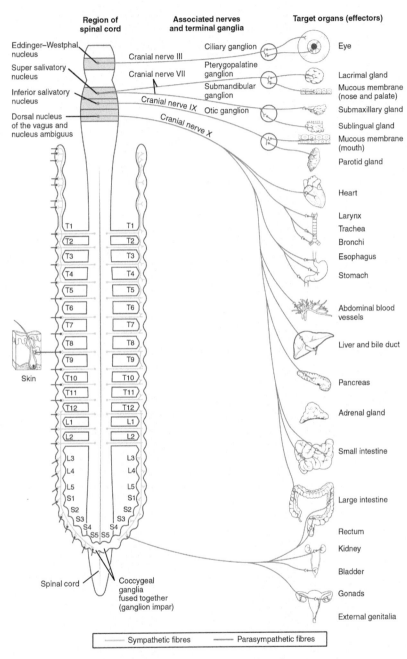

Figure 1.6 Connections of the parasympathetic and sympathetic nervous systems.
Adapted from: OpenStax College, Anatomy & physiology, Figs. 1 and 3, OpenStax Connections. <http://
cnx.org/contents/14fb4ad7-39a1-4eee-ab6e-3ef2482e3e22@8.24>. © Feb 26, 2016 OpenStax. Textbook
content produced by OpenStax is licensed under a Creative Commons Attribution License 4.0.

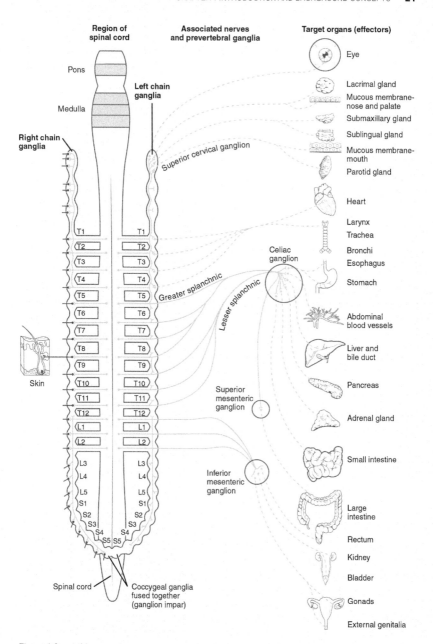

Figure 1.6, cont'd

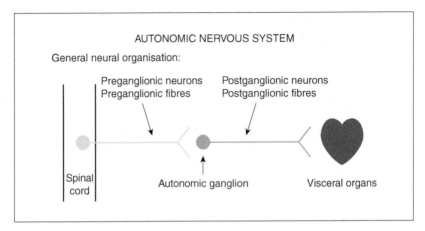

Figure 1.7 General neural organisation.

The preganglionic neurons of the sympathetic division arise from the thoracic and lumbar spinal segments, while those of the parasympathetic system arise from the cranial nerves and sacral spinal segments. The post-ganglionic neurons differ, depending on which division of the autonomic nervous system they serve. If they are part of the parasympathetic division they produce and use acetylcholine as their neurotransmitter, whereas if they are part of the sympathetic division they produce and use noradrenalin as their neurotransmitter. The cholinergic receptors on the organs receiving parasympathetic input are of the muscarinic family. There are at least three types of muscarinic cholinergic receptor. They are all metabotropic receptors and their activation by acetylcholine results in the recruitment of second messenger systems and a variety of cellular responses. The adrenergic receptors on the organs receiving sympathetic input may be of either the α- or β-adrenergic family. There are five types of adrenergic receptor, each with an organ specific distribution. They too are all metabotropic receptors and their activation results in the activation of second messenger systems and a variety of cellular responses.

In addition to directly supplying target organs, the sympathetic division features the adrenal medulla, which is in effect a specialised autonomic ganglion (Figure 1.8). When activated, the adrenal medulla releases adrenalin into the blood stream, which acts hormonally on target organs with the appropriate receptor. These are the same α- and β-adrenergic receptors that mediate the effects of noradrenalin. The activity of the adrenal medulla explains why sympathetic effects are more widespread than parasympathetic effects: there is no hormonally acting equivalent of the adrenal medulla in the parasympathetic division (Figure 1.9).

The modes of action of many drugs administered to patients mimic the actions of neurotransmitters or neuromodulators or prevent the neurotransmitter or neuromodulator from interacting with its receptor (see Table 1.3).

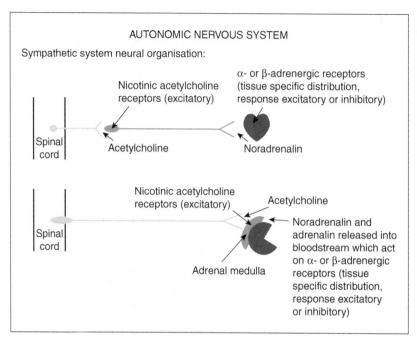

Figure 1.8 Sympathetic system neural organisation.

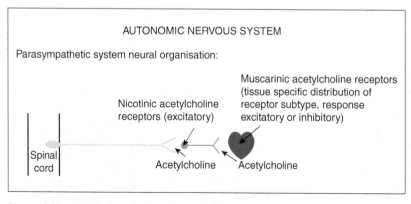

Figure 1.9 Parasympathetic system neural organisation.

TABLE 1.3 Common neurotransmitters and neuromodulators

Category	Transmitter/ modulator	Receptor action on postsynaptic cell	Main anatomical site of action	
			CNS or PNS	Muscle or nerve
Cholinergic	Acetylcholine (ACh) [2 types of receptors: nicotinic receptor and muscarinic receptor]	Inhibitory or excitatory depending upon the receptor: • nicotinic receptors – excitatory • muscarinic receptors – inhibitory or excitatory depending upon receptor subtype	PNS	Muscle (nicotinic and muscarinic) Autonomic ganglia (nicotinic) Visceral organs receiving parasympathetic innervation (muscarinic)
			CNS	Nerves (muscarinic and nicotinic)
Amino acid	Gamma-aminobutyric acid (GABA)	Inhibitory	CNS	Nerve
	Glutamate (Glu)	Excitatory		
	Glycine (Gly)	Inhibitory, primarily in the brain stem and spinal cord	PNS	
	Aspartate	Excitatory	CNS	
Amine	Dopamine (DA)	Inhibitory or excitatory depending upon the receptor	CNS	Nerve
	Histamine	Inhibitory or excitatory depending upon the receptor: • H1 and H2 receptors – excitatory • H3 receptors – inhibitory	CNS	
	Noradrenaline (NA)/ Norepinephrine	Inhibitory or excitatory depending upon the receptor	PNS and CNS	Visceral organs receiving sympathetic innervation
	Seratonin (5-HT)	Usually inhibitory	CNS	Nerve
Peptide	Endorphins	Usually inhibitory	CNS	Nerve
	Enkephalins	Usually inhibitory		
	Substance P	Usually excitatory; mostly peripheral	PNS	Nerve endings
	Galanin	Usually inhibitory	CNS and PNS	Nerve
Gas	Nitric oxide	Excitatory	CNS	Gaseous transmitter, acting on nerves as well as blood vessels

ANS, autonomic nervous system; CNS, central nervous system; PNS, peripheral nervous system.

■ References

Birkett, D., 1997. Therapeutic drug monitoring. Australian Prescriber 20 (1), 9–11.

Braund, R., Haxby Abbott, J., 2011. Recommending NSAIDs and paracetamol: a survey of New Zealand physiotherapists' knowledge and behaviours. Physiotherapy Research International 16, 43–49.

Denehy, L., 2014. *Proceedings of the 2014 APA Symposium, 'Physiotherapy on the pathway to prescribing'; 31 Oct - 2 Nov; Cairns, Australia.* <https://cpd4physios.com.au/enrol/index.php?id=141> (accessed 06.03.15.).

Department of Health and Ageing, Australian Government, 1999. *National Medicines Policy.* <http://www.health.gov.au/internet/main/publishing.nsf/Content/B2FFBF72029EEAC8CA257BF0001BAF3F/$File/NMP2000.pdf> (accessed 11.03.15.).

Department of Human Services, Australian Government, 2016. *Reciprocal Health Care Agreements.* <http://www.humanservices.gov.au/customer/enablers/medicare/reciprocal-health-care-agreements/participating-rhca-countries> (accessed 10.04.15.).

Ghiculescu, R., 2008. Therapeutic drug monitoring: which drugs, why, when and how to do it. Australian Prescriber 31 (2), 42–44.

Grimmer, K., Kumar, S., Gilbert, A., et al., 2002. Non-steroidal anti-inflammatory drugs (NSAIDs): physiotherapists use, knowledge and attitudes. The Australian Journal of Physiotherapy 48, 82–92.

Gross, A.S., 1998. Best practice in therapeutic drug monitoring. British Journal of Clinical Pharmacology 46 (2), 95–99.

Hubbard, R.E., Peel, N.M., Scott, I.A., et al., 2015. Polypharmacy among inpatients aged 70 years or older in Australia. The Medical Journal of Australia 202 (7), 373–377.

Kumar, S., Grimmer, K., 2005. Non-steroidal anti-inflammatory drugs (NSAIDs) and physiotherapy management of musculoskeletal conditions: a professional minefield? Therapeutics and Clinical Risk Management 1, 69–76.

Morris, J., Grimmer, K., 2014. Non-medical prescribing by physiotherapists: issues reported in the current evidence. Manual Therapy 19 (1), 82–86. doi:10.1016/j.math.2013.04.003.

National Prescribing Service Ltd, 2012. Better choices, Better health. Competencies required to prescribe medicines: putting quality use of medicines into practice. National Prescribing Service Ltd, Sydney, p. 8. <https://www.nps.org.au/__data/assets/pdf_file/0004/149719/Prescribing_Competencies_Framework.pdf> (accessed 05.07.16).

Nissen, L., Kyle, G., Stowasser, D., et al., 2010. *Non-medical Prescribing.* <http://www.ahwo.gov.au/documents/NHWT/Non%20Medical%20Prescribing%20Final%20Report.pdf> (accessed 02.15.).

Nursing and Midwifery Board of Australia, 2014. *Fact sheet: The use of health practitioner protected titles.* <http://www.nursingmidwiferyboard.gov.au/documents/default.aspx?record=WD15%2F16164&dbid=AP&chksum=I%2B13CLoIR%2Fv%2FLjR4Oqnp%2Bg%3D%3D> (accessed 23.02.15.).

Pharmaceutical Society of Australia, 2010. *Principles for a National Framework for Prescribing by Non-medical Health Professionals.* <http://www.psa.org.au/download/policies/Prescribing-by-non-medical-health-professionals.pdf> (accessed 23.02.15.).

Physiotherapy Board of Australia, 2010. *Continuing Professional Development Registration Standard.* <http://www.physiotherapyboard.gov.au/documents/default.aspx?record=WD14%2F13673&dbid=AP&chksum=9xWEnE%2BUGQkmmh4w1Zjzmg%3D%3D> (accessed 23.02.15.).

Scott, I.A., Hilmer, S.N., Reeve, E., et al., 2015. Reducing inappropriate polypharmacy: the process of deprescribing. JAMA Internal Medicine 175 (5), 827–834.

Steinman, M., Miao, Y., Boscardin, W., et al., 2014. Prescribing quality in older veterans: a multifocal approach. Journal of General Internal Medicine 29 (10), 1379–1386.

Sullivan, G., Lansbury, G., 1999. Physiotherapists' knowledge of their clients' medication: a survey of practising physiotherapists in New South Wales, Australia. Physiotherapy Theory and Practice 15, 191–198.

Therapeutic Goods Administration, Department of Health, Australian Government, 2014. *Consumer Medicines Information.* <https://www.tga.gov.au/consumer-medicines-information-cmi> (accessed 06.03.15.).

Therapeutic Guidelines Limited, 2010. *eTG complete* [Internet]. Therapeutic Guidelines Limited, Melbourne.

Wise, J., 2013. Polypharmacy: a necessary evil. British Medical Journal 347, f7033. doi:10.1136/bmj.f7033.

Cardiovascular system

Bernie Bissett, Imogen Mitchell, Karlee Johnston, Gregory Kyle

OBJECTIVES

This chapter will discuss the role that medications have in the supplementary management of the most common cardiovascular conditions encountered by physiotherapists. By the end of this chapter (including cross-referencing with other relevant chapters) the reader should have an understanding of:

+ pharmacotherapy options for the major cardiovascular disorders
+ usual dosages, routes of administration and major contraindications and precautions of these medications
+ any potential impact of these medications on physiotherapeutic management.

OVERVIEW

Heart disease

Coronary artery disease and angina (stable and unstable)

Dyslipidaemia

Dysrhythmias

Heart failure

Abnormal blood pressure

Hypertension

Pulmonary hypertension

Hypotension

■ Introduction

Cardiovascular disease is the most common cause of death globally, accounting for 31% of deaths in 2012 (World Health Organization 2016). Many of the risk factors for cardiovascular disease are lifestyle-related and modifiable. Most patients with cardiovascular disease will have their risks managed through a combination of drug therapy and lifestyle modification, including dietary changes. Physical exercise is a key strategy for reducing the impact of cardiovascular disease. Exercise has been demonstrated to improve cardiovascular fitness, improve cardiovascular symptoms and reduce future cardiovascular events (Leon et al. 2005).

Physiotherapists are likely to be directly involved in the care of patients with cardiovascular pathologies in an inpatient setting (e.g. following cardiac surgery or myocardial infarction) or in the community (e.g. cardiac rehabilitation, or in private practice). Effective exercise prescription for these patients requires not only clear understanding of the underlying pathophysiology, but also knowledge of the likely impact of drug therapy on exercise tolerance and other side effects.

Overview of general factors affecting choice of medication

The chapter follows the Australian approved indications as specified on the MIMS registry. Emphasis will be placed on those signs and symptoms and conditions most frequently treated by physiotherapists, and where the physiotherapist's input is vital in monitoring the effects of the prescribed medications in both acute and chronic clinical presentations. The focus of this chapter will be on the major drugs prescribed for specific cardiovascular disorders and their relevance for the physiotherapist (Table 2.1).

TABLE 2.1 Drugs used in cardiovascular disorders

General category	Specific group	Relevance for physiotherapist	Where addressed
Drugs used for cardiovascular disorders – acute decompensation	Chest pain	+++	This chapter
	Arrhythmias	+++	This chapter
	Heart failure	+++	This chapter
	Blood pressure	++	This chapter
	Pulmonary hypertension	++	This chapter
Drugs used for cardiovascular disorders – prevention orientated (primary and secondary)	Coronary artery disease (CAD)	++	This chapter
	Arrhythmias	++	This chapter
	Stroke prevention	++	This chapter
	Heart failure	++	This chapter
	Pulmonary hypertension	+++	This chapter

Each category and the specific subgroup of drugs will be reviewed in terms of mechanism of action, route(s) of administration, effects and adverse effects. Treatment of cardiovascular conditions is complex and variable. The physiotherapist is well placed to advise on the appropriateness of medications that affect the patient's mobility such as those that cause hypotension, bradycardia or tachycardia and may impact on the patient's ability to mobilise optimally. It is important that physiotherapists have an understanding of the mechanism of action of the cardiovascular medications.

Table 2.2 describes the structure, location and signs and symptoms of cardiovascular disorders in terms of the sites of action for associated medication – disease specific information and detailed clinical characteristics are described in Table 2.3.

Table 2.3 provides information on the clinical characteristics of the cardiovascular conditions most commonly encountered by physiotherapists where medication also plays a role. They have been divided into the different characteristics that a patient may be provided medication for (which may be relevant to the treating physiotherapist).

TABLE 2.2 Structure, location, signs and symptoms

Structure	Location	Signs and symptoms (S & S)[a]
Cardiac muscle	Heart	Abnormal blood pressure, heart rate, rhythm and heart failure
Vasculature system	Peripheral, pulmonary, renal, hepatic veins and arteries	Abnormal blood pressure and tissue perfusion, pooling (heart failure)

[a]See Table 2.3 for descriptions of the various signs and symptoms.

TABLE 2.3 Definitions and clinical features of major signs and symptoms seen in cardiovascular disorders

Condition	Signs/symptoms	Clinical characteristics
Coronary artery disease (CAD)	Chest pain, sweating	In CAD chest pain is a result of inadequate blood supply to the myocardium In stable angina pain is typically triggered by physical effort or stress, is reproducible for a given trigger, subsides within 5–15 minutes with cessation of exercise and medication Unstable angina can occur in the absence of a reliable trigger (i.e. can occur at rest), is typically more frequent, more intense, lasts longer than 15 minutes and may require hospitalisation if the symptoms persist (Hammon & Dean 2006a)
	Breathlessness	Due to reduced oxygen supply to the cardiac muscle and increased oxygen demand
	Fatigue	Due to reduced oxygen supply to the cardiac muscle

Continued

TABLE 2.3 Definitions and clinical features of major signs and symptoms seen in cardiovascular disorders—cont'd

Condition	Signs/symptoms	Clinical characteristics
Arrhythmias	Hypotension	Body adapting to new compromised cardiac output
	Palpitations	Abnormal cardiac beats
Heart failure	Breathlessness	Decreased cardiac output, increased pulmonary oedema and increased oxygen demand
	Fatigue	Decreased cardiac output and consequent decreased oxygen delivery and increased oxygen demand
Abnormal blood pressure (hypertension and hypotension)	Headaches (also may be associated with visual disturbances)	Increased blood pressure in the veins and arteries
	Dizziness (also may be associated with visual disturbances)	Decreased blood pressure in the veins and arteries
Pulmonary hypertension	Dyspnoea and fatigue	Poor perfusion of the right ventricle
	Dizziness	
	Palpitations	

■ Heart disease

Coronary artery disease and angina (stable and unstable)

Angina pectoris ('angina') refers to chest pain resulting from inadequate blood supply to the myocardium. It is often a symptom of underlying coronary artery disease, and can be classified as stable or unstable. Stable angina is typically triggered by physical effort or stress, is fairly reproducible for a given trigger but usually subsides within 5–15 minutes following cessation of exercise and administration of medication. In contrast, unstable angina may occur in the absence of a reliable trigger (i.e. can occur at rest), is typically more frequent, more intense, lasts longer than 15 minutes and may require hospitalisation if the symptoms persist (Hammon & Dean 2006a). Patients with coronary artery disease (CAD) are at risk of non-ST-elevation myocardial infarction (NSTEMI) and ST-elevation[1] myocardial infarction (STEMI). Patients with CAD are commonly prescribed multiple medications for symptom control as well as primary and secondary prevention of NSTEMI or STEMI that may include (but is not limited to) antiplatelet medications, medications for dyslipidaemia and beta-blockers.

---

[1]ST elevations refer to a finding on an electrocardiogram wherein the trace in the ST segment is abnormally high above the isoelectric baseline. For further information the reader is directed to a cardiovascular textbook.

> ## PHYSIOTHERAPY PRACTICE POINTS:
> ## CORONARY ARTERY DISEASE AND ANGINA
>
> Physiotherapists may prescribe activities or exercise that can aggravate patients' symptoms of angina, particularly in patients following myocardial infarction, or known coronary heart disease. Importantly, angina pain may not only be felt in the classical central chest area but may also radiate to the neck, jaw or arms. It can also be accompanied by breathlessness, fatigue and sweating. Although angina may be reasonably well managed with medication, physiotherapists should closely monitor any symptoms of new-onset chest pain, particularly during exercise, and offer patients the opportunity to cease activity and rest if this occurs. Glyceryl trinitrate (GTN) (a vasodilator, see Table 2.4) may be readily available in the hospital or community setting. Patients may be reluctant to take GTN due to side effects of headaches or light-headedness caused by the hypotension resulting from widespread vasodilation. Ideally, patients should be seated when GTN is administered to the sublingual mucosa as a dramatic reduction of blood pressure may ensue. Sitting is the preferred posture (on a chair, or on the ground) to minimise the chance of the patient fainting/falling after administration. However, the majority of patients with stable angina should be able to safely participate in physiotherapy with supervision and encouragement.

Pharmacological management for CAD and angina

Nitrates

Nitrates are potent vasodilators that act as nitric oxide donors. They are predominantly used to treat angina, although they can be used as adjunct therapy in heart failure.

A combination of exercise and a low fat diet has been shown to slow the progress of coronary atherosclerosis while increasing physical capacity (Niebauer et al. 1996). Since exercise is a key component of cardiac rehabilitation, the task of the treating physiotherapist is to assist patients find

TABLE 2.4 Nitrate drugs[a]

Drug name	Oral activity	Administration	Onset (minutes)	Duration (hours)
Glyceryl trinitrate (GTN)	N	Sublingual spray/tablet	<5	<1
		Patch	30–60	Until removed
		IV infusion	<10	Length of infusion
Isosorbide dinitrate	Low	Oral tablet	15–40	4–6
		Sublingual tablet	<10	1–2
Isosorbide mononitrate	Y	Controlled release tablet	60–120	8–10

[a]For further information see Table 2.9 at the end of the chapter.
N = no; Y = yes.
Adapted from: Australian Medicines Handbook Pty Ltd, 2015. Australian Medicines Handbook (online). Adelaide: Australian Medicines Handbook Pty Ltd <http:amhonline.amh.net.au/>.

the balance between challenging exercise and the onset of angina symptoms, and this will likely require a patient's judicious administration of appropriate anti-angina medications. If patients continue to struggle with exercise due to the onset of angina, a medical review by their cardiologist or primary care doctor for more intensive management of their angina symptoms is required.

Any unremitting, constant and/or worsening chest pain, during exercise, that does not subside using standard nitrate protocol over 15 minutes requires urgent medical review. These symptoms are likely to signal unstable angina or an acute myocardial infarction. Such patients should be referred immediately to the medical team (in hospital) or an ambulance should be called.

Dyslipidaemia

Dyslipidaemia is a disorder of lipoprotein metabolism, including lipoprotein overproduction or deficiency. Dyslipidaemias may be manifested by elevation of the total cholesterol, 'bad' low-density lipoprotein (LDL) cholesterol and triglyceride concentrations, and a decrease in the 'good' high-density lipoprotein (HDL) cholesterol concentration in the blood.

PHYSIOTHERAPY PRACTICE POINTS: DYSLIPIDAEMIA

Dyslipidaemia is a common feature of patients with CAD and other patients requiring physiotherapy, for example post surgery (e.g. cardiac bypass grafting, gastric bypass surgery) or major medical events (e.g. stroke or myocardial infarction). Dyslipidaemia itself rarely requires special consideration by physiotherapists, and the pharmacological treatments tend not to cause problems during exercise.

Antiplatelet agents

Antiplatelet agents are used to reduce the likelihood of platelets clumping together and becoming the trigger for a platelet-rich thrombus. They are NOT anticoagulants. Antiplatelet agents are the mainstay of therapy in CAD as the clots that form are platelet rich. A summary of the properties and uses of the antiplatelet agents can be found in Table 2.5.

Clotting occurs following injury and is stimulated by many cytokine factors. A fibrin matrix forms that entraps erythrocytes (red blood cells) and platelets. Anticoagulants reduce fibrin formation and antiplatelet agents reduce the ability of the platelets to adhere to each other and the fibrin.

Beta-blockers

Beta-blockers act as competitive antagonists at beta-adrenergic receptors. There are beta-1 and beta-2 receptors in various tissues throughout the body. Stimulating beta receptors has a relaxing effect on the tissue where they are found, except the heart, where they stimulate. Some beta-blockers also antagonise alpha-1 adrenoceptors.

TABLE 2.5 Antiplatelet agents and their properties[a]

Indication	Glycoprotein IIb/IIIa inhibitors[b]			Thienopyridines			Other antiplatelet drugs		
	Abciximab	Eptifibatide	Tirofiban	Clopidogrel	Prasugrel	Ticlopidine	Aspirin	Dipyridamole	Ticagrelor
Ischaemic heart disease (angina, MI, after CABG and PCI)				X			X		
Before PCI				X	X				
Heart failure (occasional)							X		
Acute myocardial infarction (STEMI)				X	X		X		X
Acute myocardial infarction (non-STEMI)	X	X	X	X	X		X		X
Primary and secondary prevention of stroke and TIA				X		X (2°)	X	X (2°)	
Unstable angina	X	X	X				X		

[a]For further information see Table 2.9 at the end of the chapter.
[b]Injection only – used in hospitals.
CABG = coronary artery bypass grafting; MI = myocardial infarction; PCI = percutaneous coronary intervention; STEMI = ST-elevation myocardial infarction; TIA = transient ischaemic attack.
Adapted from: Australian Medicines Handbook Pty Ltd, 2015. Australian Medicines Handbook (online). Adelaide: Australian Medicines Handbook Pty Ltd <http:amhonline.amh.net.au/>.

PHYSIOTHERAPY PRACTICE POINTS: BETA-BLOCKERS

Beta-blockers are mainly used for treating myocardial ischaemia and dysrhythmias. These drugs primarily reduce the contractility of the myocardium and heart rate to reduce blood pressure and, to a lesser extent, have an effect on the renin–angiotensin–aldosterone system through neurohormonal mechanisms. Beta-blockers may limit the normal increase in heart rate seen during exercise, and therefore physiotherapists need to bear this in mind if using heart rate as a target for training intensity (e.g. 'perceived exertion' scores may prove to be more consistent when heart rate is unreliable). Patients taking beta-blockers may also struggle with basic daily activities such as stair climbing, due to the rapid increase in heart rate that usually accompanies this exertion but which is slowed or absent with beta-blockade. Due to the presence of beta-2 receptors in the smooth muscle of the airway, bronchospasm is also a possible side effect of beta-blocker therapy, so wheezes may appear in a patient in the absence of a diagnosis of asthma (particularly with non-selective beta-blockers). Beta-blocker selectivity and indications are covered in Table 2.6. Due to ongoing relative bradycardia, fatigue or lethargy may also be an issue for patients taking beta-blockers, but this may be partly improved through a program of regular exercise that maintains muscle efficiency as much as possible.

TABLE 2.6 Selectivity and indications for beta-blockers

	Receptor(s)			Indications									
	Beta-1	Beta-2	Alpha-1	Hypertension	Angina	Tachyarrhythmias	Myocardial infarction	Heart failure (stable)	Hyperthyroidism symptoms	Migraine prevention	Essential tremor	Phaeochromocytoma	Glaucoma (topical)
Atenolol	X			X	X	X	X						
Bisoprolol	X							X					
Carvedilol	X	X	X	X				X					
Labetalol	X	X	X	X									
Metoprolol	X			X	X	X	X			X			
Metoprolol XL	X							X					
Nebivolol	X			X				X					
Oxprenolol	X	X		X	X	X							
Pindolol	X	X		X	X	X							
Propranolol	X	X		X	X	X	X			X	X	X	
Timolol	X	X											X

For further information see Table 2.9 at the end of the chapter.
Adapted from: Australian Medicines Handbook Pty Ltd, 2015. *Australian Medicines Handbook* (online). Adelaide: Australian Medicines Handbook Pty Ltd <http:amhonline.amh.net.au/>.

Dysrhythmias

Physiotherapists working with cardiovascular patients should be familiar with cardiac dysrhythmias, which are common in clinical practice (atrial fibrillation, atrial flutter) or life threatening (ventricular tachycardia and ventricular fibrillation).

PHYSIOTHERAPY PRACTICE POINTS: DYSRHYTHMIAS

Where continuous ECG monitoring is available (e.g. intensive care, coronary care, cardiac surgery unit), physiotherapists need to be able to identify life-threatening arrhythmias, which may require urgent defibrillation and prevent physiotherapy treatment from progressing. Furthermore, physiotherapists should recognise dysrhythmias that are amenable to pharmacological treatment (e.g. atrial flutter) and wait until therapeutic drug levels are achieved before stressing the patient's cardiac output further with mobilisation and exercise. This will require discussion with medical staff to establish when physiotherapy treatment can proceed.

The physiotherapist and the patient should be careful with long-lasting arrhythmias that might induce serious symptoms such as fatigue, dizziness, light-headedness, fainting (syncope) or near-fainting spells, rapid heartbeat or pounding, shortness of breath, chest pain and in extreme cases, collapse and sudden cardiac arrest.

Treatment goals are:

1 to prevent blood clots that may produce emboli and lead to stroke

2 to improve the heart function to reduce the possibility of heart failure and insufficiency

3 to prevent cardiac arrest – collapse and death.

Effort activity (exercise) might trigger arrhythmia as well as several manoeuvres (activities) such as deep breathing or neck movements.

The physiotherapist should be aware when the arrhythmia is life threatening, as with severe bradycardia.

Ventricular ectopic beats

Occasional ventricular ectopic beats (where the ventricle contracts from an ectopic focus, generating a wide QRS complex) are relatively common even in healthy people and drug treatment is rarely indicated (Holt 2003). Ventricular ectopic beats do not preclude exercise, unless they become more frequent, trigger runs of sustained ventricular tachycardia and/or result in cardiac symptoms.

Atrial fibrillation

Patients with chronic, well-managed atrial fibrillation (AF) may be relatively symptom-free, as their body has adapted to the rhythm over time. However, they may be unable to undertake additional exercise such as cardiac rehabilitation, which will require an increase in their cardiac output. Alternatively, new onset of atrial fibrillation for a patient previously in sinus rhythm may manifest as symptoms of severe hypotension and distress as the body adapts to a compromised cardiac output. In this setting, pharmacological interventions target control of ventricular rate or rhythm correction in acute AF. Both methods have similar outcomes and can be limited by unacceptable medication side effects (Roy et al. 2000). Therefore, physiotherapists must balance the benefits of exercise with the risk of further destabilising the patient's cardiac output. Monitoring the patient's blood pressure, pallor and symptoms is critical and treatment should be abandoned if the patient's signs and symptoms deteriorate. Manual palpation of the patient's pulse may be useful in detecting atrial fibrillation, but this is a skill that requires significant clinical experience and practice that is not normally associated with new graduate entry-level physiotherapy competency.

Atrial flutter

Physiotherapists may most commonly observe atrial flutter in cardiac patients postoperatively, where the heart is still adapting to change. Pharmacological management is likely to be attempted in the postoperative period (e.g. digoxin, amiodarone), and usually it is advisable to postpone mobilisation until the atrial flutter has reverted to sinus rhythm, due to the compromised cardiac output. Occasionally, atrial flutter will not respond to pharmacological intervention and will require cardioversion.[2]

Ventricular tachycardia/ventricular flutter

Due to compromised cardiac output generated by these rhythms, physiotherapists involved in the care of this patient group are advised to immediately cease treatment and seek urgent medical review (Collins 2002). These patients are likely to undergo cardioversion with ongoing pharmacological management, including anticoagulation that may have implications for physiotherapy treatment. Following establishment of a stable rhythm, physiotherapy can be resumed dependent upon the adequacy of cardiac output and medical advice.

---

[2]Cardioversion is a medical procedure performed to restore a normal heart rhythm for people who have certain types of abnormal heartbeats (arrhythmias).

■ Heart failure

Heart failure affects approximately 2% of Australians (National Heart Foundation of Australia and Cardiac Society of Australia and New Zealand 2011), and the symptoms are caused by an inability of the ventricles to fill or eject sufficient blood to meet the body's demands. Heart failure can be acute or chronic, manifesting as symptoms of dyspnoea and fatigue. These symptoms can be classified based on their severity and whether they occur during physical activity or only at rest (The Criteria Committee of the New York Heart Association 1994).

Physiotherapists need to be aware of the signs and symptoms of heart failure:

◆ dyspnoea – shortness of breath can occur during activity (the physiotherapist must apply caution), at rest or while sleeping, and may come on suddenly and cause the patient to awaken

◆ persistent coughing or wheezing; development of oedema

◆ tiredness, fatigue

◆ lack of appetite, nausea

◆ confusion; impaired thinking and increased heart rate.

PHYSIOTHERAPY PRACTICE POINTS: HEART FAILURE

Exercise is a key treatment strategy for patients with chronic heart failure and has been shown to improve quality of life and reduce heart failure-related hospital admissions (Davies et al. 2010). It is imperative that physiotherapists understand the relationship between the pharmacological management of the disease process and the potential impact on exercise training.

Patients being managed with beta-blockers may fail to show a normal heart rate increase in response to exercise, which is required to increase the cardiac output in order to tolerate exercise. This failure to increase cardiac output may require an adjustment of the exercise parameters (e.g. lower heart rate targets as a percentage of maximum heart rate). Over time, these patients tend to become more tolerant to the effects of beta-blockers, and so ongoing exercise prescription adjustment will be required.

Patients with heart failure are likely to be taking a combination of medications with different mechanisms of action and side effects. The majority of medications used for heart failure will lower the blood pressure to some extent via different mechanisms of action: vasodilatation (angiotensin-converting enzyme [ACE] inhibitors and angiotensin II receptor antagonists [A2RA]), bradycardia (beta-blockers) and volume depletion and vasodilatation (loop diuretics). Consequently, physiotherapists should be aware that rapid changes in posture for these patients may precipitate symptoms of hypotension. Additional time or rest stops during exercise may facilitate mobilisation and exercise. Seated exercise (e.g. stationary cycling or seated strength training) may be advantageous in patients particularly prone to episodes of postural hypotension (for further information see Table 2.9 at the end of the chapter).

Loop diuretics are used in heart failure to reduce the intravascular blood volume and hence the amount returning to the heart (pre-load), which reduces the likelihood of the heart failing. Diuretic drugs may affect blood pressure (e.g. hypotension if diuretics have been increased), which could limit exercise performance. Acutely, even simple mobilisation of a patient out of bed should take into account whether diuretics, and other medications, may affect blood pressure, manifesting as postural hypotension until the patient's body adapts to changes in overall fluid balance. Conversely, inadequate diuresis in patients with heart failure may result in acute pulmonary oedema (APO), peripheral oedema or ascites. Physiotherapists should be suspicious of APO in a patient with heart failure who presents acutely with widespread fine crackles on auscultation and a moist sounding cough that does not clear with coughing and expectoration. Deep breathing exercises and sputum clearance techniques have no effect on APO; however, continuous positive airway pressure (CPAP) can reverse APO by physically pushing the excess fluid back into the vascular space and assisting cardiac function. Physiotherapists may assist in the set-up and titration of comfortable CPAP (with medical consultation) to improve oxygenation and work of breathing until better fluid balance can be achieved.

Patients with heart failure should be encouraged to weigh themselves daily at the same time each day: first thing in the morning upon getting out of bed, but post-micturition is recommended. This provides the most stable weight over time. As each litre of fluid weighs approximately 1 kg, it is a crude, but simple and non-invasive method for patients to monitor their fluid balance at home. Any daily gain of 2 kg or more should be immediately reported to the patient's treating doctor.

Exercise is an essential element of management of heart failure, both acutely and chronically. Physiotherapists should work closely with medical staff and patients to ensure that exercise is achievable in combination with drug treatments to optimise quality of life and potentially slow the progression of heart failure. In the intensive setting, active physiotherapy, including early mobilisation, is feasible for patients even with severe acute heart failure (e.g. for an intubated and ventilated patient on inotropes), so long as cardiovascular and respiratory parameters are being monitored closely and remain within pre-agreed limits. These limits (e.g. acceptable blood pressure and respiratory rate) will need to be negotiated between medical and physiotherapy staff on an individual basis although guidelines are available (Hodgson et al. 2014). At the other end of the spectrum, patients with stable chronic heart failure should be encouraged to attend cardiac rehabilitation classes (O'Connor et al. 2009) and may also benefit from inspiratory muscle training (Dall'Ago et al. 2006) to reduce shortness of breath and enhance quality of life. Both of these approaches require the physiotherapist to appreciate the relationship between pharmacological management of heart failure and both cardiac and respiratory signs and symptoms (e.g. breathlessness).

Abnormal blood pressure

Hypertension

Hypertension (high blood pressure), defined as blood pressure >140/90 mmHg (National Heart Foundation of Australia 2010), affects 32% of adult Australians and is the most common cardiovascular disease (Australian Bureau of Statistics 2012). More than 52% of patients diagnosed with hypertension take medication to control their blood pressure (National Heart Foundation of Australia 2012), and it is therefore essential for physiotherapists to be familiar with the possible effects and side effects of these commonly prescribed drugs. Most patients will receive an angiotensin-converting enzyme (ACE) inhibitor, dihydropyridine calcium channel blocker (or potentially a combination of both) and, particularly in older patients, thiazide diuretics (National Heart Foundation of Australia 2010). For further information see Table 2.9 at the end of the chapter.

PHYSIOTHERAPY PRACTICE POINTS: HYPERTENSION

Whenever treating a patient with hypertension, the physiotherapist must be aware of the prescribed goal blood pressure, or any strict limits, as these may deviate from the generally accepted 'normal' blood pressure. Exercise prescription is based upon these adjusted goals, but may need to account for the multiple effects and side effects of the medications taken by each patient. Where exercise is not possible in a patient with hypertension, for example due to extreme headaches or hypotension, the physiotherapist is advised to discuss this with the treating doctor as a matter of priority. Given the potential of exercise to contribute to lowering blood pressure in the long term, it is optimal to coordinate the pharmacological and physiotherapeutic management of these patients.

ACE inhibitors
ACE inhibitors lower blood pressure through relaxation of the blood vessels and reducing sodium and water retention. Due to the possibility of postural hypotension, in the context of recent bed rest (e.g. following surgery), physiotherapists should take extra care when mobilising patients taking ACE inhibitors. These patients may feel dizzy and unsteady during this period and extra caution should be taken to prevent falls (e.g. gait aids, additional support, frequent rest stops).

A persistent dry cough is a side effect to be aware of in this patient-group (Paz & West 2002) although this is not amenable to physiotherapy and requires medical review.

Beta-blockers
Beta-blockers are not used in isolation in the management of uncomplicated hypertension (see section above).

Calcium channel blockers
Calcium channel blockers reduce blood pressure by reducing myocardial contractility (verapamil and diltiazem only) or causing peripheral vasodilation (dihydropyridine drugs) by slowing transport of calcium across cell membranes. Vasodilation can cause headache and dizziness, which may be challenging when physiotherapists are encouraging mobilisation and exercise. Furthermore, calcium channel blockers may worsen postural hypotension, so in initial therapy extra care should be taken to avoid postural hypotension (pacing of position changes, additional gait aids as required and frequent rests). Constipation is also often associated with calcium channel blockers, and has been shown to be worsened by inactivity (Simren 2002). Physiotherapists play a beneficial role in offsetting this adverse effect by facilitating early mobilisation for inpatients, and ongoing regular exercise for patients living in the community.

There are two classes of calcium channel blockers (Leon et al. 2005): dihydropyridines and non-dihydropyridines. This distinction is made on the basis of chemical structure, but also indicates the site of action. Dihydropyridines are easily identified as all of their generic names end in '-ipine' (see Table 2.7).

Pulmonary hypertension

Pulmonary hypertension is defined as wedge pressure in excess of 25 mmHg at rest in the pulmonary artery (Hammon & Dean 2006b). It may occur secondary to other pathologies (e.g. congenital heart disease, advanced lung disease, connective tissue disease) or in the absence of another cause (i.e. idiopathic pulmonary hypertension). Symptoms of pulmonary hypertension can vary widely but may include exertional dyspnoea, dizziness, palpitations, angina and fatigue. Prognosis is highly variable, but pulmonary hypertension is associated

TABLE 2.7 Calcium channel blockers[a]

Drug	Dihydropyridine or non-dihydropyridines	Site of action	Long or short acting	SR dose form[b]	IR dose form[c]
Amlodipine	Y	Peripheral vasculature	L		✓
Diltiazem	N	Peripheral and cardiac vasculature	S	✓	✓
Felodipine	Y	Peripheral vasculature	S	✓	
Lercanidipine	Y	Peripheral vasculature	L		✓
Nifedipine	Y	Peripheral vasculature	S	✓	✓
Nimodipine	Y	Peripheral vasculature	L		✓
Verapamil	N	Cardiac muscle	S	✓	✓

[a]For additional information see Table 2.9 at the end of the chapter.
[b]SR = sustained release dose form. Such dose forms cannot usually be crushed, chewed or split.
[c]IR = immediate release dose form. These can be crushed, chewed or split.
L = long acting; N = no; S = short acting; Y = yes.
Adapted from: Australian Medicines Handbook Pty Ltd, 2015. *Australian Medicines Handbook* (online). Adelaide: Australian Medicines Handbook Pty Ltd <http:amhonline.amh.net.au/>.

with a worse prognosis in patients with advanced lung disease (Presberg & Dincer 2003).

In pulmonary arterial hypertension, the blood vessels that carry blood between the heart and lungs are constricted, making it difficult for the heart to pump blood through the lungs.

Prostacyclin, a prostanoid metabolised from endogenous arachidonic acid through the cyclooxygenase (COX) pathway, is a powerful vasodilator that has been recognised as one of the most effective drugs for the treatment of pulmonary arterial hypertension. Currently, prostacyclin or its equivalents are extensively used in the clinical management of pulmonary arterial hypertension patients. Since the death rate associated with pulmonary arterial hypertension has not been significantly reduced within the past 5 years, it has been suggested that more powerful therapeutic approaches are needed, including prostacyclin synthase gene therapy and cell-based therapy using native stem cells and engineered stem cells with enhanced prostacyclin production capacity (Presberg & Dincer 2003; Ruan et al. 2010; Waxman 2013). For further information see Table 2.9 at the end of the chapter.

Exercise is known to improve ventricular function and reduce inflammatory activity, and thus should be advocated for patients with pulmonary hypertension (Gondim et al. 2015). However, to minimise increases in pulmonary pressure, physiotherapists need to be aware of the necessity to titrate exercise to a moderate intensity (modified Borg score of 3 to 4 out of 10) and avoid isometric or Valsalva manoeuvres (Heart Online 2016). In patients with severe pulmonary hypertension, prostacyclins may be prescribed so physiotherapists should be aware of potential bleeding issues (i.e. avoid invasive techniques, tissue trauma and falls).

Hypotension

Acute low blood pressure can induce symptoms of dizziness, particularly when changing position from supine to sitting or sitting to standing. Severe chronic low blood pressure can be due to dehydration, heart failure, diabetes or hypothyroidism. It also might be caused by medications and, if this is the case, changes to these medications should be made. Increasing the amount of dietary salt as well as more water input might raise blood pressure, but excess sodium can worsen heart failure. Fludrocortisone can increase blood pressure, and may be used to treat orthostatic hypotension, and compression stockings might also increase blood pressure. The following medications (Table 2.8) are used in patients with acute hypotension with a potentially reversible cause such as septic shock, and are only used as a temporary measure and require close (and often invasive) monitoring.

PHYSIOTHERAPY PRACTICE POINTS: HYPOTENSION

While transient blood pressure changes often do not require pharmacological management, there may be times when vasopressor therapy is useful in facilitating physiotherapy treatment (e.g. early mobilisation in an intensive care patient). The risks and benefits of titrating vasopressors to facilitate mobilisation should be discussed with the medical team. If utilising vasopressors to support physical therapy, the physiotherapist should monitor blood pressure closely throughout treatment (e.g. constant monitoring through an arterial line, or at least frequent non-invasive measures) and collaborate closely with the bedside nurse to maintain blood pressure within the agreed pre-specified parameters negotiated with the team.

TABLE 2.8 Acute hypotension medications[a]

Medication	Mechanism of action	Administration	Infusion or bolus
Noradrenaline	Alpha agonist (and weak beta agonist)	Central line	Infusion only
Vasporessin	Acts on vascular smooth muscle and oxytocin receptors	Central line	Infusion only
Phenylephrine	Alpha-1a agonist	Peripheral or central line	Infusion or bolus
Metaraminol	Direct and indirect (alpha agonist and increased noradrenaline)	Peripheral or central line	Infusion or bolus
Ephedrine	Direct and indirect agonist (alpha and mild beta agonist)	Peripheral or central line	Infusion or bolus

[a]For further information see Table 2.9 at the end of the chapter.
Adapted from: *Australian Medicines Handbook Pty Ltd, 2015.* Australian Medicines Handbook *(online).* Adelaide: Australian Medicines Handbook Pty Ltd <http:amhonline.amh.net.au/>.

TABLE 2.9 Overview of all cardiovascular medications

Medication class/name	Mechanism of action	Indications	Common side effects	Practice points
CLASS: **Nitrates** (Table 2.4) Glyceryl trinitrate Isosorbide dinitrate Isosorbide mononitrate	Potent vasodilators that act as nitric oxide donors	Predominantly used to treat angina, although can be used as adjunct therapy in heart failure	Headache Hypotension Flushing Palpitations	Short-acting agents should be used for acute management of angina and if pain remains medical review is required Patients require 10–12 hours/day free from any nitrate therapy to avoid developing a tolerance
CLASS: **Antiplatelet agents** (Table 2.5) *Glycoprotein IIb/IIIa inhibitors:* Abciximab Eptifibatide Tirofiban *Thienopyridines:* Clopidogrel Prasugrel Ticlopidine *Others:* Aspirin Dipyridamole Ticagrelor	Reduce platelet aggregation (the ability of platelets to stick to one another) The specific mechanisms of actions are unique to the specific class (glycoprotein IIb/IIIa inhibitors, thienopyridines and others)	Ischaemic heart disease (IHD), percutaneous coronary interventions (PCI), acute coronary syndromes (STEMI and NSTEMI), stroke and transient ischaemic attack (TIA)	Bleeding, bruising, GI upset	Some indications require dual antiplatelet therapy (DAPT) for a discrete period of time; during this time the patient will have an increased risk of bleeding

Continued

TABLE 2.9 Overview of all cardiovascular medications—cont'd

Medication class/name	Mechanism of action	Indications	Common side effects	Practice points
CLASS: **Beta-blockers** (Table 2.6) Atenolol Bisoprolol Carvedilol Labetalol Metoprolol Nebivolol Oxprenolol Pindolol Propranolol Timolol	Competitive antagonists at beta-adrenergic receptors	Hypertension, angina, tachyarrhythmias, myocardial infarction, heart failure, migraine prevention, essential tremor, phaeochromocytoma, glaucoma (topical)	Hypotension, bradycardia, bronchospasm, GI upset, fatigue and lethargy	Beta-blockers should not be discontinued abruptly as the patient may experience a rebound of cardiac symptoms (including angina, tachycardia and hypertension) May exacerbate bronchospasm in severe or poorly controlled asthma so care should be used in these patients
CLASS: **ACE inhibitors** Captopril Enalapril Fosinopril Lisinopril Perindopril Quinapril Ramipril Trandolapril	Relaxation of the blood vessels and reducing sodium and water retention by inhibiting angiotensin-converting enzyme (ACE) from converting angiotensin I to angiotensin II	Hypertension, heart failure, diabetic nephropathy, persistent proteinuria, post myocardial infarction (MI)	Hypotension, dizziness, headache, persistent dry cough	A persistent dry cough can occur at any stage during therapy and will not respond to treatment; these patients will often need to stop the ACE inhibitor The cough usually resolves within 4 weeks of cessation ACE inhibitors can cause a rise in serum creatinine and potassium; patients starting on ACE inhibitors should be monitored within 1–2 weeks

CLASS:				
Calcium channel blockers (Table 2.7) *Dihydropyridines:* Amlodipine Felodipine Lercanidipine Nifedipine Nimodipine *Non-dihydropyridines:* Verapamil Diltiazem	Reduce blood pressure by reducing calcium flow into the cells in vascular smooth muscle and heart	Hypertension, angina	Headache and dizziness, postural hypotension, constipation, peripheral oedema	Dihydropyridines cause peripheral oedema that does not respond to diuretics
Prostacyclin Epoprostenol Iloprost	Potent vasodilators of the pulmonary arteries	Pulmonary hypertension and acute respiratory distress syndrome (ARDS)	Hypotension, flushing, dizziness, headache, platelet dysfunction	Can be delivered via nebulisation or intravenously, in a setting where the staff are experienced and appropriate support is available
CLASS: **Vasoconstrictors** (Table 2.8) Vasopressin Noradrenaline Phenylephrine Metaraminol Ephedrine	Potent vasoconstrictors, varied mechanisms depending on the agent	Hypotension	Excessive vasoconstriction (peripheral ischaemia), hyptertension, headache	Most need to be administered via a central access device; however, depending on the agent some may be given for a short duration via a large peripheral line Should only be administered in an acute care setting where appropriate monitoring is available

GI = gastrointestinal; STEMI = ST-elevation myocardial infarction.
Adapted from: Australian Medicines Handbook Pty Ltd, 2015. *Australian Medicines Handbook* (online). Adelaide: Australian Medicines Handbook Pty Ltd <http:amhonline.amh.net.au/>.

■ References

Australian Bureau of Statistics, 2012. Australian Health Survey: First Results, 2011/12. Cat. No. 4364.0. Australian Bureau of Statistics, Canberra.

Australian Medicines Handbook Pty Ltd, 2015. Australian Medicines Handbook (online). Australian Medicines Handbook Pty Ltd, Adelaide. <http:amhonline.amh.net.au/>.

Collins, S.M., 2002. Cardiac system. In: Paz, J.C., West, M.P. (Eds.), Acute Care Handbook for Physiotherapists, 2nd ed. Butterworth-Heinemann, Boston, pp. 76–77.

Dall'Ago, P., Chiappa, G.S., Guths, H., et al., 2006. Inspiratory muscle training in patients with heart failure and inspiratory muscle weakness: a randomized trial. Journal of the American College of Cardiology 47 (4), 757–763. doi:10.1016/j.jacc.2005.09.052.

Davies, E.J., Moxham, T., Rees, K., et al., 2010. Exercise based rehabilitation for heart failure. The Cochrane Database of Systematic Reviews (4), CD003331. doi:10.1002/14651858; CD003331. pub3.

Gondim, O.S., de Camargo, V.T., Gutierrez, F.A., et al., 2015. Benefits of regular exercise on inflammatory and cardiovascular risk markers in normal weight, overweight and obese adults. PLoS ONE 10 (10), e0140596.

Hammon, W.E., Dean, E.W., 2006a. Cardiopulmonary pathophysiology. In: Frownfelter, D.L., Dean, E.W. (Eds.), Cardiovascular and Pulmonary Physical Therapy: Evidence and practice, 4th ed. Mosby/Elsevier, St Louis, p. 102.

Hammon, W.E., Dean, E.W., 2006b. Cardiopulmonary pathophysiology. In: Frownfelter, D.L., Dean, E.W. (Eds.), Cardiovascular and Pulmonary Physical Therapy: Evidence and practice, 4th ed. Mosby/Elsevier, St Louis, p. 107.

Heart Online, 2016. *Exercise for pulmonary artery hypertension* [Internet]. <http://www.heartonline.org.au/articles/exercise/exercise-for-specific-conditions#pulmonary-artery-hypertension> (accessed 29.06.16.).

Hodgson, C.L., Stiller, K., Needham, D.M., et al., 2014. Expert consensus and recommendations on safety criteria for active mobilization of mechanically ventilated critically ill adults. Critical Care : The Official Journal of the Critical Care Forum 18 (6), 658. doi:10.1186/s13054-014-0658-y.

Holt, A., 2003. Management of specific arrhythmias. In: Bersten, A.D., Soni, N.Oh, T.E. (Eds.), Oh's Intensive Care Manual, 5th ed. Butterworth-Heinemann, London, p. 165.

Leon, A.S., Franklin, B.A., Costa, F., et al., 2005. Cardiac rehabilitation and secondary prevention of coronary heart disease: an American Heart Association scientific statement from the Council on Clinical Cardiology. Circulation 111, 369–376.

National Heart Foundation of Australia, 2012. *High blood pressure statistics (based on Heart Watch Survey 2011)* [Internet]. <http://heartfoundation.org.au/about-us/what-we-do/heart-disease-in-australia/high-blood-pressure-statistics> (accessed 29.06.16.).

National Heart Foundation of Australia and Cardiac Society of Australia and New Zealand, October 2011. *Quick reference guide. Diagnosis and management of chronic heart failure* [Internet]. <https://heartfoundation.org.au/images/uploads/publications/CHF-QRG-updated-2014.pdf> (accessed 18.06.16.).

National Heart Foundation of Australia (National Blood Pressure and Vascular Disease Advisory Committee), 2010. *Guide to management of hypertension 2008*, p. 3 [Internet]. <https://heartfoundation.org.au/images/uploads/publications/HypertensionGuidelines2008to2010Update.pdf> (accessed 18.06.16.).

Niebauer, J., Hambrecht, R., Schlierf, G., et al., 1996. Five years of physical exercise and low fat diet: effects on progression of coronary artery disease. Journal of Cardiopulmonary Rehabilitation 15, 47–64.

O'Connor, C., Whellan, D., Lee, K., et al., 2009. Efficacy and safety of exercise training in patients with chronic heart failure: HF-ACTION randomised controlled trial. Journal of the American Medical Association 301, 1439–1450.

Paz, J.C., West, M.P., 2002. Appendix IV Pharmacologic agents. In: Acute Care Handbook for Physiotherapists, 2nd ed. Butterworth-Heinemann, Boston, p. 842.

Presberg, K.W., Dincer, H.E., 2003. Pathophysiology of pulmonary hypertension due to lung disease. Current Opinion in Pulmonary Medicine 9 (2), 131–138.

Roy, D., Talajic, M., Dorian, P., et al., 2000. Amiodarone to prevent recurrence of atrial fibrillation. New England Journal of Medicine 342, 913–920.

Ruan, C.H., Dixon, R.A.F., Willerson, J.T., et al., 2010. Prostacyclin therapy for pulmonary arterial hypertension. Texas Heart Institute Journal 37 (4), 391–399.

Simren, M., 2002. Physical activity and the gastrointestinal tract. European Journal of Gastroenterology & Hepatology 14:1053–1056.

The Criteria Committee of the New York Heart Association, 1994. Nomenclature and Criteria for Diagnosis of Diseases of the Heart and Great Vessels, 9th ed. Little, Brown & Co., Boston, pp. 253–256.

Waxman, A.B., 2013. Oral prostacyclin therapy for pulmonary arterial hypertension: another step forward. Circulation 127 (5), 563–565.

World Health Organization, 2016. 'Cardiovascular diseases' fact sheet. WHO, Geneva [Internet]. <http://www.who.int/mediacentre/factsheets/fs317/en/> (accessed 18.06.16.).

Respiratory system

Bernie Bissett, Imogen Mitchell, Karlee Johnston, Richard Talbot

This chapter will discuss the roles of medications in the supplementary management of the most common respiratory conditions encountered by physiotherapists. By the end of this chapter (including cross-referencing with other relevant chapters) the reader should have an understanding of:

- pharmacotherapy options for the major respiratory disorders and respiratory symptoms
- usual dosages, routes of administration and major contraindications and precautions of these medications
- any potential impact of these medications on physiotherapeutic management.

Chronic respiratory disorders
Asthma
Chronic obstructive pulmonary disease
Conditions associated with pulmonary secretions
Cough
Mucus production in cystic fibrosis and bronchiectasis

Severe respiratory decompensation and end-of-life respiratory symptoms
Severe acute respiratory illness
End-of-life respiratory symptoms

■ Introduction

Physiotherapists are extremely likely to be directly involved in the care of patients with respiratory pathologies in an inpatient setting, in the community and in private practice. Effective exercise prescription for these patients requires not only a clear understanding of the underlying pathophysiology, but also knowledge of the likely impact of drug therapy and side effects of the medications on exercise tolerance and other physiotherapy treatments.

Although oxygen may be considered a drug, oxygen prescription and titration is beyond the scope of this chapter and is comprehensively addressed in physiotherapy textbooks elsewhere.

Overview of general factors affecting choice of medication

This chapter follows the Australian approved indications as specified on the MIMS registry. Emphasis will be placed on those signs and symptoms and conditions most frequently treated by physiotherapists, and where the physiotherapist's input is vital in monitoring the effects of the prescribed medications in both acute and chronic clinical presentations. The focus of this chapter will be on the major drugs prescribed for specific respiratory disorders and their relevance for the physiotherapist (Table 3.1).

Each category and the specific subgroup of drugs will be reviewed in terms of mechanism of action, route of administration, effects and adverse effects. Examples will be provided for the different clinical situations in which particular drugs would be used. It is important that physiotherapists have an understanding of the mechanism of action of respiratory medications, particularly as it relates to the timing of medications and physiotherapy intervention.

Table 3.2 describes the structure, location and signs and symptoms of respiratory disorders in terms of the sites of action for associated medication.

TABLE 3.1 Drugs used in respiratory disorders

General category	Specific group	Relevance for physiotherapist	Where addressed
Drugs used for airways disease	Chronic obstructive pulmonary disease (COPD)	+++	This chapter
	Asthma	+++	This chapter
Drugs used for pulmonary secretions	Sputum clearance	+++	This chapter
	Cough	++	This chapter
Drugs used for fluid overload	Pulmonary oedema	+	Chapter 2
Acute decompensation and end of life	Acute respiratory conditions	+++	This chapter
	End-of-life secretions	++	This chapter

TABLE 3.2 Structure, location, signs and symptoms in respiratory disorders

Structure	Location	Signs and symptoms[a]
Bronchial smooth muscle	Bronchi and bronchioles	Bronchoconstriction, shortness of breath
Sensory nerve fibres (Gibson et al. 2010)	Brain stem	Cough
Mucous membrane	Bronchioles, bronchi, trachea	Sputum production: moist and/or productive cough, crackles on auscultation, palpable fremitus

[a]See Table 3.3 for descriptions of the various signs and symptoms.

Disease specific information and detailed clinical characteristics are described in Table 3.3.

Table 3.3 provides information on the clinical characteristics of the respiratory conditions most commonly encountered by physiotherapists where medication also plays a role. They have been divided into the different characteristics that a patient may be provided medication for.

TABLE 3.3 Definitions, clinical features and likely causes of major signs and symptoms seen in respiratory disorders

Condition	Signs/symptoms	Clinical characteristics and pathophysiology
Chronic obstructive pulmonary disease (COPD) (Abramson et al. 2015)	Shortness of breath	Airflow limitation due to airway narrowing (e.g. from inflammation, bronchoconstriction, sputum plugging or loss of airway elasticity secondary to airway damage)
	Cough	Can be productive or non-productive
	Sputum production	Related to infective process or chronic bronchitis resulting in excessive sputum production
	Chest tightness and wheeze	Airway narrowing (bronchoconstriction, sputum plugging, dynamic airway compression)
Asthma (National Asthma Council Australia 2014)	Shortness of breath	Bronchoconstriction and inflammation
	Wheeze	Bronchoconstriction
	Chest tightness and cough	Bronchoconstriction and inflammation (less commonly due to sputum)
Acute and chronic cough	Cough	Cough reflex (protective mechanism) – both peripheral and central nerve input
End-of-life care	Increased secretions	Accumulation of secretions due to general decline in patient condition including weakness and reduced gag reflex
	Dyspnoea	Multifactorial including physiological and psychological mechanisms
	Cough	Multifactorial related to disease progression

TABLE 3.3 Definitions, clinical features and likely causes of major signs and symptoms seen in respiratory disorders—cont'd

Condition	Signs/symptoms	Clinical characteristics and pathophysiology
Acute respiratory decompensation	Moist cough	Due to increased sputum production in airways
	Crackles on auscultation	
	Palpable fremitus	
	Dyspnoea	Multifactorial including physiological and psychological mechanisms (worsened due to respiratory muscle weakness in prolonged mechanical ventilation)
	Increased sputum production	Related to infective process, possibly secondary due to ventilator-associated pneumonia (if invasively ventilated)
	Impaired oxygenation	Due to respiratory failure (multifactorial)

Chronic respiratory disorders

Asthma

Asthma is a chronic inflammatory respiratory disease, characterised by bronchoconstriction as a result of bronchospasm, mucus hypersecretion, oedema and/or smooth muscle damage (Kaufman 2011). Approximately 8% of the Australian population suffer from asthma (Harrison et al. 2013), and therefore many patients seeking physiotherapy will be managing this disease process, through either their general practitioner or a respiratory specialist. Given this prevalence, physiotherapists should be familiar with the pharmacological management of asthma, whether they are treating the asthma as the primary problem or simply as a co-morbidity. In particular, physiotherapists should be aware of the side effects of asthma drugs that may be relevant during physiotherapy treatment.

Pharmacological management for asthma

Pharmacological management for asthma is a stepwise approach (Therapeutic Guidelines Limited 2014a):

1 Short-acting beta-2 agonist (SABA) prn for symptom relief
2 Inhaled corticosteroid (ICS) + SABA prn[1]
3 ICS (low dose) + long-acting beta agonist (LABA) + SABA prn
4 ICS (medium to high dose) + LABA + SABA prn (consider leukotriene receptor antagonist).

For additional information see the overview in Table 3.11 at the end of the chapter.

---

[1]Note that prn means when necessary.

TABLE 3.4 Characteristics of SABAs

Drug	Onset of action	Duration of action	Administration
Salbutamol	5–15 minutes	3–6 hours	Inhalation: • MDI (optimally delivered with a spacer) • Nebulised (no more effective than MDI and spacer) Intravenous
Terbutaline	5–15 minutes	3–6 hours	Inhalation: • DPI Subcutaneous

DPI = dry powder inhaler; MDI = metered dose inhaler.
Adapted from: Australian Medicines Handbook Pty Ltd, 2015. *Australian Medicines Handbook* (online). Adelaide: Australian Medicines Handbook Pty Ltd <http://amhonline.amh.net.au/>.

Symptom relievers

Short-acting beta agonists (SABAs): salbutamol and terbutaline: Beta agonists relax bronchial smooth muscle by stimulating the beta-2 adrenoreceptors. There are both short-acting beta-2 agonists (SABAs), which are discussed here (see also Tables 3.4 and 3.11), and long-acting beta-2 agonists (LABAs), which are discussed later.

SABAs are used for symptomatic control of bronchoconstriction in asthma and COPD and are the first-line agents for management of acute decompensation of airways disease.

The side effect profile of these agents is dose-dependent and includes tachycardia, tremor, palpitations, headache, agitation, hypokalaemia and, rarely, lactic acidosis.

Medications that block beta adrenoreceptors (see beta-blockers in Chapter 2) should be used with extreme caution in patients with asthma as they can worsen bronchoconstriction and compete with the beta agonists (SABAs and LAMAs) decreasing their efficacy.

For acute management of bronchoconstriction salbutamol may be administered via inhalation continuously (either using a metered dose inhaler [MDI] and spacer, or nebulisation) until improvement or, in serious life-threatening situations, it can also be administered intravenously by infusion.

Short-acting muscarinic antagonist (SAMA): ipratropium: There is only one medication in this class, ipratropium. Ipratropium is used primarily in acute severe asthma attacks where SABA therapy is inadequate. It is also used in mild COPD as an alternative to SABAs. Long-acting muscarinic antagonists (LAMAs) are used in COPD and will be discussed below. If using a SAMA for acute decompensations, the LAMA should be withheld for that period of time (Therapeutic Guidelines Limited 2014a).

LAMAs and SAMAs exert their bronchodilatory effects by antagonising the bronchoconstriction that results from activation of bronchial muscarinic receptors by acetylcholine. Their side effect profile is dose-dependent and related to the anticholinergic nature of the agents and includes dry mouth and throat, blurred vision, urinary retention, constipation and dizziness (Australian Medicines Handbook Pty Ltd 2015).

Ipratropium is available as an MDI and as nebulisation solution (for additional information see Table 3.11 at the end of the chapter).

Symptom controllers
Long-acting beta agonists (LABAs): eformeterol, salmeterol, indacaterol, vilanterol: These agents must **NOT** be used in asthma unless they are combined with an inhaled corticosteroid (ICS), due to increased risk of serious asthma attacks and also potentially increased mortality risk.

See the COPD section for further information.

Long-acting muscarinic antagonists (LAMAs): aclidinium, glycopyrronium, tiotropium, umeclidinium: These agents are only indicated in COPD **NOT** asthma.

See the COPD section for further information.

Preventers
Inhaled corticosteroids (ICS): beclomethasone, budesonide, ciclesonide, fluticasone: ICS can be used in both asthma and COPD and reduce airway inflammation and bronchial hyper-reactivity (see Tables 3.5 and 3.11). They are available both alone and in fixed combination inhalers with LABAs. There is no evidence to suggest superiority of one ICS over another. ICS should be started at a low dose and the dose titrated upwards. There are some situations where a higher dose may be required initially, which is then titrated downwards over a period of time (Therapeutic Guidelines Limited 2014a).

ICS have a flat dose–response curve meaning that the upper limit of the dosing range is unlikely to provide additional clinical benefit, but the risk of side effects is much higher (Australian Medicines Handbook Pty Ltd 2015).

Adverse effects can be divided into local and systemic effects and are dependent on the degree of systemic absorption, which is influenced by dose,

TABLE 3.5 Inhaled corticosteroids

Drug	Device	Available alone	Available with LABA
Beclomethasone	MDI	Yes	No
Budesonide	DPI Nebulised solution	Yes	Eformeterol
Ciclesonide	MDI	Yes	No
Fluticasone propionate	MDI DPI (accuhaler) Nebulised solution	Yes	Salmeterol Eformeterol
Fluticasone furoate	DPI	No	Vilanterol

DPI = dry powder inhaler; MDI = metered dose inhaler.
Adapted from: Therapeutic Guidelines Limited, 2014a. 'Respiratory'. In: eTG complete [Internet]. Melbourne: Therapeutic Guidelines Limited.

duration and device (these effects may be minimised by MDI and spacer as well as by rinsing the mouth with water and spitting after each dose). Major local side effects include dysphonia (hoarse voice) and oral candidiasis (thrush). The systemic side effects are considered more serious and include adrenal suppression, decrease in bone mineral density, glaucoma and skin thinning and bruising (Australian Medicines Handbook Pty Ltd 2015).

Patients should be informed that these medications should not be used for immediate symptom relief (with the exception of budesonide/eformeterol in some patients), and should be taken regularly every day, even if feeling well, to reduce the incidence of attacks. Due to the risk of adrenal suppression these medications should not be abruptly ceased without directive from a doctor (Australian Medicines Handbook Pty Ltd 2015). For additional information see Table 3.11 at the end of the chapter.

The addition of a LABA to an ICS in asthma is indicated in patients who have a suboptimal response to ICS alone. This can be done by the addition of a LABA inhaler or swapping the patient to a fixed-dose combination inhaler, which may aid in compliance. The fixed-dose combinations also ensure that the LABA is never used without an ICS in asthma as LABA monotherapy has been associated with worse outcomes, including death, in asthma patients (Therapeutic Guidelines Limited 2014a). For additional information see Tables 3.6 and 3.11.

Non-corticosteroid preventers: montelukast, cromones and omalizumab: (For additional information see also Table 3.11 at the end of the chapter.)

TABLE 3.6 Fixed-dose inhalers

Medications	Device available	Doses available
Budesonide/eformeterol	Pressurised MDI	50/3 mcg 100/3 mcg 200/6 mcg
	DPI (turbuhaler)	100/6 mcg 200/6 mcg 400/12 mcg
Fluticasone propionate/ salmeterol	DPI (accuhaler)	100/50 mcg 250/50 mcg 500/50 mcg
	MDI	50/25 mcg 125/25 mcg 250/25 mcg
Fluticasone proprionate/ eformeterol	MDI	50/5 mcg 125/5 mcg 250/10 mcg
Fluticasone furoate/ vilanterol	DPI (device with dry powder capsules)	100/25 mcg 200/25 mcg

DPI = dry powder inhaler; MDI = metered dose inhaler.
Adapted from: Australian Medicines Handbook Pty Ltd, 2015. *Australian Medicines Handbook* (online). Adelaide: Australian Medicines Handbook Pty Ltd <http://amhonline.amh.net.au/>.

Montelukast: Montelukast, a leukotriene receptor antagonist, is an oral agent that inhibits bronchoconstriction induced by inflammation and smooth muscle contraction caused by leukotrienes. It is used most commonly in exercise-induced bronchoconstriction, and also as an additional agent for patients with severe asthma. Common side effects include headache, gastrointestinal discomfort and diarrhoea, and less commonly may include psychiatric symptoms such as nightmares, mood and behavioural changes. Tablets are taken regularly once a day and an effect is likely to be seen within days (Australian Medicines Handbook Pty Ltd 2015).

Cromones: cromoglycate, nedocromil: These mast cell stabilisers are most often used to manage exercise-induced bronchoconstriction but may not be effective for all patients. They have a good safety profile with limited side effects that are usually limited to local effects such as cough and a bitter taste (Australian Medicines Handbook Pty Ltd 2015).

Omalizumab: Omalizumab is a monoclonal antibody against immunoglobulin E (IgE) and is indicated in severe asthma with a proven allergic component (elevated IgE level). Omalizumab is administered by subcutaneous injection every 2 to 4 weeks. It is expensive and tightly restricted by the Pharmaceutical Benefits Scheme. It may be associated with injection site reactions, decrease in platelet count and increased bleeding, such as nose bleeds and bruising, as well as headache and muscle pain (Australian Medicines Handbook Pty Ltd 2015).

PHYSIOTHERAPY PRACTICE POINTS: ASTHMA

In the acute setting, where physiotherapists work closely with patients who have been admitted with an exacerbation of asthma, it is prudent for physiotherapy treatments to be scheduled with respect to bronchodilator therapy. For example, where bronchoconstriction, and its associated increased work of breathing, is a major limitation for the patient, physiotherapists should aim for exercise to occur approximately 15 minutes following administration of SABA drugs. This allows for peak bronchodilation to maximise airflow and thereby maximise exercise capacity.

Physiotherapists should also be aware of the potential side effects of SABAs in asthmatic patients, which are likely to be exaggerated during an acute exacerbation where dosage is higher than baseline. In particular, patients may demonstrate clinically relevant tachycardia at rest that is directly related to the SABA rather than an underlying cardiovascular or oxygen-delivery problem. Patients may also struggle with tremor and palpitations secondary to the SABA, and physiotherapists should provide reassurance that these transient side effects will resolve when the SABA dosage is reduced again.

Whether in the hospital setting or the community, physiotherapists are well-placed to review metered dose inhaler (MDI) techniques for patients with asthma and provide guidance as necessary[2]. While larger hospitals may employ specific asthma educators who focus on MDI technique correction, physiotherapists in other settings should not presume that the patient's MDI technique is optimal. Physiotherapists should also reinforce the benefits of spacers with MDIs in patients who struggle with MDI technique. As many exercise and physiotherapy treatments are best timed around bronchodilator administration, physiotherapy-driven correction of MDI technique may be a worthwhile investment in the management of this chronic disease.

Continued

---

[2]A useful reference for teaching MDI techniques may be found on the National Asthma Council website (http://www.nationalasthma.org.au/how-to-videos/using-your-inhaler).

Regarding other asthma medications, a major side effect of chronic administration of inhaled corticosteroids is the propensity for bruising. The risk of bruising is even higher if patients are also taking oral steroids. In our experience, these patients also appear to have a higher likelihood of developing 'tissue paper'-like skin, which is much more prone to skin tears. For both these reasons, physiotherapists should be cognisant of the risk of trauma during mobilisation and exercise, and additional precautions (e.g. extra layers of padding on equipment or bony prominences) may be warranted. Should skin tears or bruises occur as a result of physiotherapy treatment, these should be discussed with the medical and nursing teams for further management.

Over many years the prolonged use of inhaled corticosteroids is likely to reduce bone mineral density and increase the risk of spontaneous crush fractures. This risk is particularly relevant if the patient is presenting with a seemingly unrelated complaint; for example, a patient with a long history of asthma presenting to a private practice complaining of back pain. In this example, a comprehensive subjective assessment, which includes a complete medication inventory, would be very helpful as the physiotherapist should be concerned about the links between chronic steroid use and pathological fractures and refer to medical staff for further investigation. Furthermore, chronic use of steroids may result in weight gain and, at least anecdotally, asthma patients may complain that 'my steroids make me fat'. As steroids are known to stimulate appetite, this should be taken into consideration if the physiotherapist is targeting weight loss as part of a holistic patient management plan. Collaboration with a dietician may be useful in this case.

While ipratropium can be associated with blurred vision and dizziness, in our experience these side effects are rare and do not usually impact on physiotherapy treatments. Finally, although it is much less commonly used, omalizumab can result in low platelets and bleeding and, for patients taking this drug, physiotherapists should carefully consider the risks of more invasive procedures such as nasopharyngeal suction. If the physiotherapist is in doubt about the safety of any treatments that may cause bleeding, he or she should discuss their concerns with the treating medical team.

For additional medication information see Table 3.11 at the end of the chapter.

Chronic obstructive pulmonary disease

Chronic obstructive pulmonary disease (COPD) is an umbrella term for a group of pathologies that manifest as chronic airflow limitation, including emphysema, chronic bronchitis and chronic asthma. The main symptom of COPD is breathlessness, while excessive sputum production is also present for many (either acutely during an exacerbation, or chronically). In Australia, 14% of people over 40 have COPD, rising to 29% in people over 75 (Lung Foundation Australia 2016). Physiotherapists are highly likely to encounter patients with COPD in the hospital context; that is, during an acute exacerbation of COPD or as a co-morbidity for another presentation, or in the community setting (e.g. in a private practice or pulmonary rehabilitation program). Thus physiotherapists should be familiar with the pharmacological management of COPD as both the drug effects and side effects should be considered alongside exercise prescription and other non-pharmacological interventions in this group (see Table 3.7).

Pharmacological management of COPD

Symptom relievers
Short-acting beta agonists (SABA): salbutamol and terbutaline and short-acting muscarinic antagonist (SAMA): ipratropium: The features of SABAs and LAMAs are discussed in detail in the section on asthma. They are indicated in COPD for

TABLE 3.7 **Pharmacological management for COPD (like asthma) is a stepwise approach**

Stage	Pharmacological interventions	Non-pharmacological interventions
1 (mild disease)	SABA or SAMA	Smoking cessation, vaccination, exercise, general health optimisation
2 (moderate disease)	LAMA and/or LABA	Smoking cessation Pulmonary rehab and action plan
3 (severe disease)	LAMA + LABA/ICS (consider theophylline)	Smoking cessation, oxygen therapy, palliative care plans and advanced care directives

Note: for additional information see Table 3.11 at the end of the chapter.
Adapted from: Therapeutic Guidelines Limited, 2014a. Respiratory. In: eTG complete [Internet]. Melbourne: Therapeutic Guidelines Limited.

TABLE 3.8 **LABAs**

Drug	Device	Available alone	Available with LAMA
Eformeterol	DPI	Yes	No
Indacaterol	DPI (device + capsule)	Yes	Yes (glycopyrronium)
Salmeterol	DPI	Yes	No
Vilanterol	DPI (device + capsule)	No	Yes (umeclidinium)

DPI = dry powder inhaler.
Adapted from: Australian Medicines Handbook Pty Ltd, 2015. Australian Medicines Handbook (online). Adelaide: Australian Medicines Handbook Pty Ltd <http://amhonline.amh.net.au/>.

symptom relief and, although the LAMAs may be slightly more effective, the quick onset of action and better side effect profile of the SABAs means they are usually used as a first-line treatment. However, for patients who do not have an optimal response from SABAs, a SAMA should be trialled (and a combination of the two classes may offer additional benefits) (Australian Medicines Handbook Pty Ltd 2015).

Symptom controllers
Long-acting beta agonists (LABAs): eformeterol, salmeterol, indacaterol, vilanterol: These agents (see Table 3.8) are indicated when a symptom reliever is not offering optimal symptom relief. The LAMAs are added as a reliever therapy when necessary. These agents relieve symptoms, reduce exacerbations and improve quality of life.

Their mechanism of action, which is the same as the SABAs, is relaxation of bronchial smooth muscle by stimulating beta-2 adrenoreceptors. The side effect profile of these agents is dose-dependent and includes tachycardia, tremor, palpitations, headache, agitation, hypokalaemia and, rarely, lactic acidosis.

Medications that block beta adrenoreceptors (see beta-blockers in Chapter 2) should be used in extreme caution in patients with asthma as they can worsen bronchoconstriction and compete with the beta agonists (SABA and LAMAs) decreasing their efficacy.

A combination of LABA and LAMA has also been shown to provide additional benefit in lung function and quality of life.

For additional information see Table 3.11 at the end of the chapter.

Long-acting muscarinic antagonists (LAMAs): aclidinium, glycopyrronium, tiotropium, umeclidinium: Like the LABAs, the LAMAs (see Table 3.9) are indicated when a symptom reliever is not offering optimal symptom relief. They are also added as a reliever therapy when necessary. These agents relieve symptoms, reduce exacerbations and improve quality of life.

LAMAs achieve their bronchodilatory effects by antagonising the bronchoconstriction that results from activation of bronchial muscarinic receptors by acetylcholine. The side effect profile is dose-dependent and related to the anticholinergic nature of the agents and includes dry mouth and throat, blurred vision, urinary retention, constipation and dizziness (Australian Medicines Handbook Pty Ltd 2015).

The choice of agent is based on patient preference, adverse effects and response as there is no good evidence of superiority of one agent over another. These agents may be used in addition to a LABA, either by using in separate inhalers or by using a fixed-dose combination inhaler. This option should be considered for patients who do not get optimal symptom control with either a LAMA or LABA alone.

For additional information see Table 3.11 at the end of the chapter.

Inhaled corticosteroids (ICS): beclomethasone, budesonide, ciclesonide, fluticasone: ICS in COPD reduce exacerbations and slow the rate of general decline (Therapeutic Guidelines Limited 2014a). They are indicated as an additional therapy to LAMAs or LABAs for patients who are experiencing increasing exacerbations and declining lung function as measured by forced expiratory volume in 1 second (FEV_1), and also in patients who have documented responsiveness to ICS,

TABLE 3.9 **LAMAs**			
Drug	Device	Available alone	Available with LABA
Aclidinium	DPI (device + capsule)	Yes	No
Glycopyrronium	DPI (device + capsule)	Yes	Yes (indacaterol)
Tiotropium	DPI (device + capsule)	Yes	No
Umeclidinium	DPI (device + capsule)	Yes	Yes (vilanterol)

DPI = dry powder inhaler.
Adapted from: Australian Medicines Handbook Pty Ltd, 2015. *Australian Medicines Handbook* (online). Adelaide: Australian Medicines Handbook Pty Ltd <http://amhonline.amh.net.au/>.

particularly if the patient has an overlapping asthma diagnosis. Currently, there are no fixed-dose ICS + LAMA inhalers available so, if this combination is required, separate inhalers may be used; however, there are LABA + ICS fixed-dose inhalers available (Table 3.5).

For additional information see Table 3.11 at the end of the chapter.

Theophylline: Theophylline is an older medication that has been used, in lower doses, as one of the last-line pharmacological agents for COPD. The exact mechanisms of action for the benefits seen in COPD are not known but are thought to be anti-inflammatory, bronchodilatory and increased diaphragm contractility. Theophylline has a narrow therapeutic window, meaning that there is a narrow window in which doses are used for efficacy and outside of which doses result in toxicity and, as such, it is an agent that requires therapeutic drug monitoring. The side effects of theophylline include gastrointestinal upset, headache, tachycardia and palpitations and insomnia (Australian Medicines Handbook Pty Ltd 2015).

Theophylline has the potential for many drug interactions, including with common medications such as the macrolide antibiotics (e.g. clarithromycin) and phenytoin. Therefore, care should be taken when altering medication regimens of patients taking theophylline.

For additional information see Table 3.11 at the end of the chapter.

PHYSIOTHERAPY PRACTICE POINTS: CHRONIC OBSTRUCTIVE PULMONARY DISEASE

As with asthma drugs, it is helpful for the physiotherapist to be aware of the potential side effects of drugs used to manage COPD. Similar to SABAs, LABA drugs have been associated with tachycardia, tremor and palpitations; however, in our experience these appear to occur less frequently for COPD patients. In contrast, patients taking LAMA drugs frequently report frustration with dry mouth and throat, which is often irritating and sometimes painful. Ensuring water is available before, during and after exercise can be helpful in these cases.

Another important potential side effect of inhaled corticosteroids is oral thrush, which patients often report if they have not closely followed instructions regarding mouth rinsing. Unfortunately, the unpleasant experience of oral thrush may deter patients from taking their inhaled corticosteroids reliably. If patients with COPD report oral thrush, physiotherapists should reiterate the importance of mouth rinsing following inhalation and encourage compliance with the prescribed regimen.

As patients with COPD take a combination of mostly long-acting drugs, there is typically less practical pressure to time physiotherapy interventions around drug administration. However, during an exacerbation of COPD, if patients have a significant reversible component to their airflow limitation that is responsive to SABA, then ideally physiotherapy intervention should be timed at 15 minutes following administration to optimise airway patency and minimise breathlessness during therapy. If sputum is present and likely to be trapped due to reversible bronchoconstriction, clearly SABA administration should precede specific sputum clearance techniques (e.g. positive expiratory pressure therapy).

In the setting of pulmonary rehabilitation, physiotherapists collaborate with pharmacists to provide specific education about the pharmacological management of COPD. In our experience, many patients benefit from clarification of both how the drugs work and how they should be administered (e.g. some patients have been erroneously swallowing tablets instead of crushing and inhaling them). For patients with COPD who do not attend pulmonary rehabilitation programs (e.g. due to transport issues),

Continued

community-based physiotherapists have the potential to provide this education and reinforcement at an individual level. Optimisation of pharmacological management in conjunction with physical exercise is the cornerstone of the COPD-X guideline that informs COPD management practices in Australia.[3] Every interaction with physiotherapy should be seen as an opportunity to optimise management of COPD. Where physiotherapists have concerns that a patient's pharmacological management is not optimised, they should refer the patient back to the respiratory specialist or general practitioner for review.

◼ Conditions associated with pulmonary secretions

Cough

Cough is a common transient ailment but, if reported as a chronic ongoing symptom, it requires an accurate diagnosis. Coughing is a reflex action with some degree of voluntary control. A diagnosis should initially be performed to rule out any serious medical diseases such as malignancy and to identify a likely cause. Many respiratory conditions will result in an increase in cough frequency. Examples include a lower respiratory tract infection, acute asthma and pulmonary oedema. In response to an increase in sputum load, increased cough frequency is an appropriate physiological response. Other possible causes of cough should be considered in patients with normal spirometry and chest X-ray, such as gastro-oesophageal reflux disease, smoking and as a side effect of some medications. For example, angiotensin converting enzyme inhibitors (ACEIs) are known to cause a persistent dry cough in some patients and should be considered when differentiating a patient's intractable cough (see Chapter 2).

Pharmacological management for cough

Medications are unlikely to benefit patients with cough, particularly acute cough (Gibson et al. 2010); however cough therapies are available. For dry coughs the aim of treatment is to reduce the urge to cough, whereas for productive cough the aim is to facilitate sputum clearance.

Opioid cough suppressants: codeine, dextromethorphan, dihydrocodeine

These agents have limited evidence for efficacy over placebo (Gibson et al. 2010) and could be used for a short duration in adult patients with acute dry cough (not for children). They work on the medullary cough centre to depress the reflex to cough. Like all opioid medications these agents should be used with caution in patients with respiratory disease as they may cause respiratory depression and drowsiness.

Expectorants: guaifenesin, ammonia salts, senega, sodium citrate

These expectorant agents are marketed to facilitate sputum expectoration for a productive cough. These agents also do not have evidence for efficacy (Australian Medicines Handbook Pty Ltd 2015).

---

[3]Refer to the COPD-X plan on the Lung Foundation website (http://copdx.org.au/copd-x -plan/).

Mucolytics: bromhexine, acetylcysteine

Bromhexine is used to decrease the viscosity of secretions and increase ease of expectoration. Like all the other medications used for managing a cough there is inadequate evidence for their use to facilitate expectoration (Australian Medicines Handbook Pty Ltd 2015). Its role in chronic lung conditions will be discussed below. Acetylcysteine is administered by nebulisation to decrease the viscosity of secretions; however, it is also used as an oral agent in idiopathic pulmonary fibrosis.

PHYSIOTHERAPY PRACTICE POINTS: COUGH

Patients may seek physiotherapy advice regarding cough suppression, and physiotherapists should remember that a persistent dry cough can be a side effect of some drugs (as listed above, and see also Chapter 2 regarding ACEIs), or could be a sign of a sinister pathology. As a general rule, cough suppression is not ideal as it will impair sputum clearance, and drugs used to achieve this (e.g. codeine) have a host of other side effects that must be considered. However, cough suppression may be appropriate in end-of-life care if the goal is patient comfort (see the section on end-of-life respiratory symptoms). To our knowledge there is no evidence that physiotherapy intervention of any kind is effective in reducing a persistent dry cough; therefore this problem should be referred to medical staff for further management.

Conversely, physiotherapists play a direct role in improving cough and sputum clearance through a variety of techniques. Patients may ask for advice regarding the use of expectorants, many of which do not require prescription (e.g. senega). As described above, physiotherapists can confidently advise that there is a lack of evidence to support over-the-counter expectorants in sputum clearance and instead should focus on non-pharmacological techniques to improve cough efficacy as required; for example, the active cycle of breathing technique, wound support to improve a pain-inhibited cough following surgery or trauma, or exercise to enhance airflow.

Mucus production in cystic fibrosis and bronchiectasis

Many respiratory conditions result in increased mucus production. Two chronic conditions are particularly worth mentioning in the physiotherapy context due their suppurative nature, namely cystic fibrosis (CF) and bronchiectasis. CF is a progressive chronic lung disease featuring mucus plugging, airway inflammation and infection, caused by genetic mutation of a transmembrane conductance regulator (Mall & Boucher 2014). A common feature of CF is bronchiectatic change with associated decreased lung function.

Bronchiectasis is a permanent abnormal dilation of the bronchi, with chronic airway inflammation and infection leading to the main clinical manifestation of a productive cough (King 2009). Bronchiectasis can also be non-genetic in origin, and considered a separate disease. While the pathophysiology of these conditions will not be discussed in further detail in this chapter, particular symptoms will be addressed in terms of physiotherapy and pharmacology management.

Pharmacological management for mucus production in CF

One of the treatment aims for patients with CF is airway clearance with specific mucolytic agents.

Mucolytics

(For additional information see Table 3.11 at the end of the chapter.)

Dornase alpha: Dornase alpha is used exclusively for cystic fibrosis. It is a recombinant human DNAse that cleaves extracellular DNA reducing the viscosity of sputum and facilitating clearance and consequently maximising lung function. It is generally well tolerated; however, alterations in voice, laryngitis and pharyngitis have been reported. Patients nebulise dornase alpha with a high flow nebuliser (8 L/min) once or twice a day (Therapeutic Guidelines Limited 2014a).

Hypertonic saline: Nebulised hypertonic saline (3–7% sodium chloride solution) improves lung function and reduces exacerbations of cystic fibrosis (Therapeutic Guidelines Limited 2014a). A single randomised trial demonstrated that, during hospital admission for exacerbation of CF, inhalation of 7% hypertonic saline improved CF symptoms more than inhalation of non-therapeutic saline (0.12%) (Dentice et al. 2016). The only common side effect of hypertonic saline is potential bronchoconstriction or airway irritation (Therapeutic Guidelines Limited 2014a).

Mannitol: Mannitol draws fluid into the airway via osmosis and increases the water content in mucus to decrease its viscosity. Dry powder mannitol is administered from capsules by an inhalation device and has been shown to increase mucus clearance and lung function in CF patients (Therapeutic Guidelines Limited 2014a). Mannitol has been associated with bronchospasm, and therefore patients must have a test dose and undergo pulmonary function tests with increasing doses of mannitol before regular dosing can be prescribed. Other side effects that may be experienced include cough, haemoptysis, vomiting, headache and dizziness. Any patients who experience haemoptysis (>240 mL/24 hours or >100 mL/daily over several days) should seek urgent medical attention about ceasing mannitol (Australian Medicines Handbook Pty Ltd 2015).

Anti-inflammatory agents

Medications to reduce airway inflammation in CF and bronchiectasis can also be used to manage mucus production and reduce lung injury. There are a few medication classes that are used for this indication; for example, macrolide antibiotics (azithromycin, clarithromycin and erythromycin), as well as oral corticosteroids and ICS (see COPD section). Macrolide antibiotics, particularly azithromycin, have been shown to effectively reduce exacerbations (Therapeutic Guidelines Limited 2014a), resulting in reduced decline in lung function and better quality of life in CF patients when administered 3 times a week. Other macrolides have also been shown to provide pulmonary anti-inflammatory action (Suresh Babu, Kastelik & Morjaria 2013).

PHYSIOTHERAPY PRACTICE POINTS: CYSTIC FIBROSIS AND BRONCHIECTASIS

When treating a patient during an acute exacerbation of CF, timing physiotherapy treatment around pharmacological treatment is essential. As a general rule, bronchodilators and/or hypertonic saline should be taken prior to airway clearance techniques (e.g. positive expiratory pressure therapy, percussion, exercise etc) to maximise the patency of the airway and the hydration of the mucus, thereby facilitating sputum expectoration. In our experience, a time frame of 15–30 minutes between bronchodilators/saline and physiotherapy intervention works well. In contrast, mucolytics should be given after sputum clearance techniques (rather than before) as these will be more effective the longer they remain in the airways. For this reason, many patients with CF take mucolytics at night after their final airway clearance session for the day, so that the mucolytic can be maximally effective overnight.

Physiotherapists may recommend hypertonic saline as an adjunct to airway clearance during an exacerbation of CF, as this is well supported by the available evidence (Dentice et al. 2016). While saline itself does not appear to have any particular side effects, some patients have been known to experience bronchoconstriction, so administration of SABA prior to hypertonic saline may be useful in these cases. Physiotherapists should monitor for signs of bronchoconstriction during hypertonic saline therapy, and also encourage the patient to drink water before and afterwards to minimise the discomfort of the salty taste and/or thirst.

The effective management of CF presents patients with a significant time burden in terms of both pharmacological and physiotherapy treatments, and compliance with either regimen may suffer at times. In our experience, some patients can be intermittently resistant to more time-consuming therapies and refuse to participate, perhaps re-establishing some feeling of control (particularly in the teenage years). Physiotherapists should be aware of this challenge, and reinforce the importance of medication compliance, particularly with respect to the timing of airway clearance techniques. Sensitivity to the psychological dimension of treatment refusal is required and, in the case of persistent non-compliance, referral to a psychologist may be warranted.

■ Severe respiratory decompensation and end-of-life respiratory symptoms

Severe acute respiratory illness

There are many respiratory conditions that may result in severe life-threatening illnesses such as acute asthma, exacerbation of COPD, pneumonia and acute respiratory distress syndrome (ARDS). The varied nature of these conditions and their treatments make it difficult to discuss them in detail here. This section will describe general therapies that are utilised in many acute respiratory conditions, but this description is by no means exhaustive. A more detailed description of these conditions is beyond the scope of this handbook.

Pharmacological management for severe acute respiratory illness

Systemic corticosteroids
Systemic corticosteroids (see Table 3.10), either oral or intravenous, may be used in the acute management of airway inflammation that might occur in any acute respiratory decompensation such as asthma, COPD, ARDS and interstitial lung disease. Corticosteroids are required for many inflammatory diseases for their anti-inflammatory and immunosuppressant effects and also for when

TABLE 3.10 **Available corticosteroids for systemic therapy in severe acute respiratory illness**

Corticosteroid	Routes(s)	Dosing frequency	Anti-inflammatory potency (relative to hydrocortisone)	Indications for acute treatment/ comments
Dexamethasone	Oral/IV	Variable (1–4 doses per day)	25	Use IV for acute airway swelling associated with croup, tonsillitis etc
Hydrocortisone	Oral/IV/IM	Variable (1–4 doses per day)	1	Use IV for acute inflammation associated with asthma, COPD, airways disease
Methylprednisolone	IV/IM	Variable (1–4 doses per day)	5	Use high dose (IV) for severe inflammatory conditions such as multiple sclerosis or other autoimmune disorders
Prednisolone/prednisone	Oral	Daily (rarely, bd)	4	Acute inflammatory respiratory conditions no longer requiring IV therapy

bd = twice daily; IM = intramuscular; IV = intravenous.
Note: for additional information see Table 3.11 at the end of the chapter.
Adapted from: Australian Medicines Handbook Pty Ltd, 2015. *Australian Medicines Handbook* (online). Adelaide: Australian Medicines Handbook Pty Ltd <http://amhonline.amh.net.au/>.

corticosteroid replacement is required, such as adrenal insufficiency (Australian Medicines Handbook Pty Ltd 2015).

There are many potential side effects of corticosteroids that physiotherapists need to be aware of, including muscle weakness and wasting, osteoporosis and fractures, weight gain, hyperglycaemia, skin atrophy and bruising. Corticosteroids can also increase sodium and water retention leading to oedema and hypertension, as well as psychiatric effects such as mood disturbances, sleep and behavioural disturbances, mania and depression. Side effects are less likely with short courses of high-dose therapy than with longer courses of lower doses. While these agents are preferably limited to short-term use in the acute setting, there are conditions that may require long-term therapy with corticosteroids. Depending on the indication, dose and duration of therapy, a gradual dose reduction may be required to avoid adrenal crisis (Australian Medicines Handbook Pty Ltd 2015).

Intravenous bronchodilators

Intravenous salbutamol and aminophylline have been largely superseded in the acute management of asthma; however, they are still used in some severe cases. Details of these agents can be found in the asthma section. Other intravenous agents that have been used for bronchodilation include magnesium and ketamine (Goyal & Agrawal 2013; Therapeutic Guidelines Limited 2014a).

Nebulised prostacyclins
Nebulised prostacyclins such as epoprostenol and iloprost cause pulmonary artery vasodilation and are used in severe cases of ARDS in mechanically ventilated patients with significant hypoxaemia. They are nebulised via the inspiratory limb of the ventilator in an ICU setting and would usually be used as an adjunct to optimised medical therapy with corticosteroids and bronchodilators. They are also used for pulmonary hypertension both in the acute hospital setting and in the more chronic phases of the condition (iloprost is indicated for pulmonary hypertension via nebulisation at home; see Chapter 2). Side effects of these agents are related to the vasodilatory effects and include hypotension, flushing and dizziness (Australian Medicines Handbook Pty Ltd 2015).

Antibiotic therapy
Antibiotic therapy is a broad and complex subject and an in-depth description of respiratory antibiotics is beyond the scope of this chapter. In acute respiratory conditions there is often the possibility of a bacterial or viral trigger that can contribute to the decompensation of a chronic respiratory illness. There are many respiratory infections that should be considered:

- community-acquired pneumonia (CAP)
- hospital-acquired pneumonia (HAP)
- aspiration pneumonia
- influenza (and other respiratory viruses)
- exacerbation of bronchiectasis
- exacerbations of COPD.

Each of these conditions is often caused by a specific organism, and empirical therapy is based on the likely pathogens. Consideration should be given to the patient's condition, allergies, organ function and general environment (in terms of likely pathogens) before deciding on appropriate therapy. The usual approach to treatment is to treat the patient empirically with antibiotics that will cover the likely or presumed pathogens, and then to de-escalate therapy to direct antimicrobial cover to the isolated organism where possible (Therapeutic Guidelines Limited 2014b).

The most common antibiotic classes used for respiratory conditions are described below (Therapeutic Guidelines Limited 2014b).

1 Penicillins

  a Narrow spectrum: benzylpenicillin

    Intravenous therapy used as first-line agent for CAP and aspiration pneumonia that has activity against Gram-positive organisms such as streptococcus

  b Moderate spectrum: amoxicillin, ampicillin

    Used as IV or oral treatment for COPD exacerbations and CAP and to cover the Gram-positive organisms similar to the narrow spectrum penicillins

2 Cephalosporins

   a Moderate spectrum: cefuroxime, cefaclor

   Oral therapy for respiratory infections as it covers Gram-positive organisms and also has activity against *Haemophilus influenza*

   b Broad spectrum: ceftriaxone

   IV agent of choice in respiratory infections that are severe or where patients cannot have a penicillin. Ceftriaxone has a much broader spectrum of activity and should be used with consideration for the risk of general antimicrobial resistance

3 Doxycycline

   a Broad spectrum of activity that covers many likely respiratory pathogens such as Gram-positive and some atypical organisms (*Chlamydia, Mycoplasma*); used often as a single agent, but also in combination with a penicillin or cephalosporin

4 Macrolides: erythromycin, clarithromycin, roxithromycin, azithromycin

   a These agents are active against atypical organisms that are commonly seen in respiratory infections, and are often used in combination with a penicillin or cephalosporin; erythromycin is rarely used as an antibiotic as its side effect profile prohibits optimal compliance

This section offers a small introduction to a very select number of antibiotics. For more information about the role of antibiotics in certain conditions please refer to 'Therapeutic Guidelines: Antibiotic' (Therapeutic Guidelines Limited 2014b).

PHYSIOTHERAPY PRACTICE POINTS: SEVERE ACUTE RESPIRATORY ILLNESS

Physiotherapists are most likely to treat patients with severe respiratory failure in an intensive care unit (ICU) setting. In this highly monitored environment, the side effects of some respiratory medications may be even more apparent (e.g. with continuous electrocardiogram monitoring, extreme tachycardia may be observed in response to high-dose SABA administration). A working knowledge of the effects of respiratory medications is even more important in this context, as the ICU physiotherapist carefully titrates exercise and mobilisation intensity based on many inter-related factors.

Physiotherapists play a direct role in sputum clearance in many patients in ICU, particularly those who are invasively ventilated as they are at increased risk of ventilator-associated pneumonia. The physiotherapist should be aware of whether the patient is susceptible to reversible bronchoconstriction and, if so, should time sputum clearance and exercise treatments with respect to the timing of bronchodilator drugs (in our experience, approximately 15 minutes following administration is ideal). In an invasively ventilated patient, drugs usually delivered via MDI can often be delivered directly through a port in the inspiratory limb of the ventilator, while nebulised drugs can also be delivered through the inspiratory limb of the ventilator via an attachment.

Another important difference with invasively ventilated patients is that, due to frequent suction, physiotherapists are readily able to assess sputum amount, colour and viscosity and are sensitive to changes in these parameters. In our experience, physiotherapists are often the first to be aware of sputum changes (e.g. from white and mucoid to pale green and purulent) and should alert the medical team regarding these changes to inform antibiotic prescription and/or humidification requirements as soon as possible.

The diagnosis of pneumonia does not automatically mean that physiotherapy treatment for sputum clearance is indicated. There is often a 'consolidation' phase in an acute respiratory infective process where the patient has impaired oxygenation and chest X-ray signs of consolidation, but does not have any objective signs of excessive sputum production or sputum retention (i.e. moist cough, coarse crackles on auscultation and/or palpable fremitus). There may be several days between commencement of antibiotic therapy and the 'resolution' phase of pneumonia, where antibiotics have taken effect and the patient's sputum load increases, manifesting as a more productive cough (or difficulty clearing sputum). Physiotherapists should be mindful of the timing of these processes and avoid unnecessary sputum clearance interventions during the consolidation phase.

However, while antibiotics are taking effect during the consolidation phase, there is still a role for physiotherapy input to maximise mobilisation and functional independence (Stiller 2013). There is clear evidence that early mobilisation of patients with respiratory failure in ICU is safe (Leditschke et al. 2012; Needham et al. 2010) and is associated with improved outcomes (Needham et al. 2010; Schweickert et al. 2009), including mortality (Morris et al. 2011). When mobilising patients with severe acute respiratory illness, physiotherapists should be aware of any respiratory medications that are likely to increase the risk of bleeding (e.g. omalizumab), and take additional precautions with manual handling and protection of fragile skin and bony prominences. Further guidelines for the mobilisation of invasively ventilated patients in ICU are available elsewhere (Green et al. 2016) and should be interpreted with a working understanding of the medications affecting each individual patient. Although physiotherapists cannot directly affect the underlying process of respiratory infection, they can work in tandem with the antibiotic therapy to minimise adverse sequelae through optimal airway clearance and early proactive rehabilitation.

End-of-life respiratory symptoms

There are medications that can provide respiratory symptom relief to patients at the end of their lives. The two medications that are commonly used in this setting are glycopyrrolate for respiratory secretions and morphine for dyspnoea (Therapeutic Guidelines Limited 2014c).

For additional information see Table 3.11 at the end of the chapter.

Glycopyrrolate

Glycopyrrolate is an anticholinergic agent that works to dry up respiratory secretions. It is administered subcutaneously as required or via continuous subcutaneous infusion. Other anticholinergic agents include hyoscine butylbromide, hyoscine hydrobromide and atropine. Both hyoscine hydrobromide and atropine cross the blood–brain barrier and can cause confusion and delirium and are therefore not used in conscious patients. Due to the anticholinergic effects if these agents their side effect profile includes constipation, bradycardia, urinary retention, glaucoma etc. The use of these agents is for symptom control only as they do not treat the underlying cause of excessive respiratory secretions, and treatment should be ceased if the patient does not benefit from the treatment (Therapeutic Guidelines Limited 2014c).

TABLE 3.11 Overview of respiratory drugs

Medication class/name	Mechanism of action	Indications	Common side effects	Practice points
CLASS: Short-acting beta agonists (SABAs) – Table 3.4 Salbutamol Terbutaline	Stimulate beta-2 adrenoreceptors leading to bronchodilation	Symptomatic control of bronchoconstriction	Tachycardia, tremor, palpitations, headache, agitation, hypokalaemia	Caution in patients on beta-blockers (see Chapter 2) Fast onset of action and short duration of action
CLASS: Short-acting muscarinic antagonist (SAMA) Ipratropium	Antagonist of bronchoconstricting muscarinic receptors resulting in bronchodilation	Symptomatic control of bronchoconstriction most commonly in COPD Used with SABA for acute management of asthma	Dry mouth and throat, blurred vision, urinary retention	Metered dose inhaler or nebules available
CLASS: Long-acting beta agonists (LABAs) Eformeterol Salmeterol Indacaterol Vilanterol	Stimulate beta-2 adrenoreceptors leading to bronchodilation	Symptom control in COPD and asthma (in combination with an inhaled corticosteroid)	Tachycardia, tremor, palpitations, headache, agitation, hypokalaemia Less common than with the SABAs	Not for use in asthma unless combined with an inhaled corticosteroid
CLASS: Long-acting muscarinic antagonists (LAMAs) Tiotropium Aclidinium Glycopyrronium Umeclidinium	Antagonist of bronchoconstricting muscarinic receptors resulting in bronchodilation	Symptom control in COPD	Dry mouth and throat, blurred vision, urinary retention	Available as monotherapy or in combination with LABA (see below)
LABA + LAMA Glycopyrronium/indacaterol Umeclidinium/vilanterol	See individual mechanisms of action for LABA and LAMA (above)	Symptom control in COPD for patients who get inadequate relief from either agent alone	See side effects from LABA and LAMA (above)	Increased compliance with fixed-dose combinations, compared with using two separate inhalers

CLASS: **Inhaled corticosteroids** **(ICS)** – Table 3.5 Fluticasone (propionate/furoate) Budesonide Betamethasone Ciclesonide	Relieve airway inflammation and bronchial hyper-responsiveness	Preventative agents in asthma and severe COPD	Dysphonia, oral candidiasis, adrenal suppression, decreased bone mineral density, glaucoma, skin thinning and bruising	Available as monotherapy and in fixed-dose combination (see below)
ICS + LABA Fluticasone/salmeterol Budesonide/eformeterol Fluticasone/vilanterol	See individual mechanisms of action for ICS and LABA (above)	Preventative agent in asthma and COPD	See side effects from ICS and LABA (above)	Increased compliance with fixed-dose combinations, compared with using two separate inhalers
CLASS: **Leukotriene receptor** **antagonist** Monteleukast	Inhibits bronchoconstriction induced by inflammation and leukotrienes	Asthma (especially exercise-induced)	Headache, GI discomfort, diarrhoea and nightmares	Oral tablet that is taken daily
CLASS: **Cromones** Cromoglycate Nedocromil	Mast cell stabilisers	Exercise-induced bronchoconstriction	Cough and bitter taste	Not to be used for symptoms of an asthma attack
CLASS: **Monoclonal antibody** Omalizumab	Antibody against immunoglobulin E (IgE)	Severe asthma with allergic component	Injection site reactions, bruising, bleeding, headache and muscle pain	Subcutaneous injection every 2–4 weeks Expensive and highly restricted by the Pharmaceutical Benefits Scheme (PBS)

Continued

TABLE 3.11 Overview of respiratory drugs—cont'd

Medication class/name	Mechanism of action	Indications	Common side effects	Practice points
CLASS: Methylxanthines Theophylline Aminophylline	Anti-inflammatory, bronchodilatory and increased diaphragmatic contractility	Low-dose theophylline is used as an adjunct in severe COPD Intravenous aminophylline is used as a last-line agent in an acute asthma attack	Tachycardia, palpitations, GI upset and headache as well as insomnia	Therapeutic drug monitoring can be performed if required to assess for side effects (and efficacy in the acute setting when using IV aminophylline) Many medications interact with these agents
CLASS: Opioid cough suppressants Codeine Dextromethorphan Dihydrocodeine	Depress cough reflex in the medulla	Dry cough	Constipation, drowsiness, respiratory depression	Limited evidence for efficacy Not indicated for children Can increase risk of respiratory depression
CLASS: Cough expectorants Guaifenesin Ammonia salts Senega Sodium citrate	Facilitate sputum expectoration in a productive cough	Productive cough	GI upset, nausea	No evidence for efficacy
CLASS: Mucolytics for cough Bromhexine Acetylcysteine	Decrease viscosity of sputum and increase ease of expectoration	Productive cough	GI upset	Acetylcysteine has many different indications but is nebulised for this indication
Dornase alpha	Recombinant human DNAse that reduces viscosity of sputum and facilitates sputum clearance	Sputum clearance in cystic fibrosis	Voice alterations, laryngitis and pharyngitis	Only indicated for cystic fibrosis Nebulised therapy that is administered daily

Drug	Mechanism	Indication	Side effects	Notes
Hypertonic saline	Increases expectoration of sputum	Chronic lung disease such as CF and bronchiectasis for sputum expectoration	Airway irritation, bronchoconstriction	Nebulised (as 3–7%) solution
Mannitol	Osmosis draws fluid into the airway and decreases mucous viscosity	Chronic lung disease such as CF and bronchiectasis for sputum expectoration	Bronchospasm, cough, haemoptysis, headache, GI upset	Inhaled capsule contents via an inhalation device
CLASS: **Systemic corticosteroids** Dexamethasone Hydrocortisone Methylprednisolone Prednisolone/prednisone	Anti-inflammatory and immunomodulatory effects via regulation of gene expression	Acute management of airway inflammation (many other indications that are not discussed here)	Muscle weakness, osteoporosis, weight gain, hyperglycaemia, skin atrophy, bruising	Choice of agent depends on the condition being treated. Where possible shorter courses should be used
CLASS: **Nebulised prostacyclines** Epoprostenol Iloprost	Direct vasodilation of pulmonary arteries	May be used in severe acute respiratory distress syndrome (ARDS) in ventilated patients	Hypotension, flushing, dizziness	These agents are also used for pulmonary hypertension (see Chapter 2)
CLASS: **Anticholinergic agents** Glycopyrrolate Hyoscine butylbromide Hyoscine hydrobromide Atropine	Blocks muscarinic effects including excessive salivation and bronchial secretions	Dry up secretions in palliative care patients	Bradycardia, urinary retention, constipation, glaucoma, delirium and confusion	These agents are for symptom control only as they do not treat the underlying condition. Glycopyrrolate is the agent of choice as it does not cross the blood–brain barrier and therefore is less likely to cause delirium and confusion
CLASS: **Opioids** Morphine	Activates opioid receptors resulting in analgesia, sedation and respiratory depression	Relieves dyspnoea and reduces the feeling of breathlessness and anxiety	Nausea, constipation, drowsiness and dizziness	Can be administered orally, parenterally and nebulised

Morphine

Morphine can be administered via different routes, including parenteral, oral and nebulised, for the relief of dyspnoea. Morphine is used in this setting to reduce the sensation of breathlessness without causing respiratory depression, and also to provide some relief from anxiety. Most often patients are treated with oral morphine (up to every 30 minutes), and if that is ineffective the subcutaneous route is used. Once the dose required for symptom control is achieved, a slow release morphine can be given twice a day (and additional doses of immediate release as required) (Therapeutic Guidelines Limited 2014c). Although the evidence suggests that nebulised opioids are less effective than oral or parenteral opioids, and in fact are probably no more effective than nebulised saline, nebulised morphine is occasionally used for patients who 'feel' that it benefits them. The side effects associated with morphine include nausea, constipation, dizziness and drowsiness, and are far less in nebulised therapy compared with oral or parenteral therapy (Jennings et al. 2002).

**PHYSIOTHERAPY PRACTICE POINTS:
END-OF-LIFE RESPIRATORY SYMPTOMS**

In end-of-life care, physiotherapists should be involved with a focus on patient-centred goals, which often means maximising patient comfort. Understanding the pharmacological approach is essential, as many end-of-life respiratory drugs also affect cognitive function (e.g. morphine, hyoscine). Furthermore, physiotherapists should use their assessment skills to differentiate between pulmonary oedema and excessive mucus production, as these require different pharmacological and physiotherapy approaches; that is, frusemide and continuous positive airway pressure for pulmonary oedema (refer to Chapter 2) as opposed to saline and sputum clearance techniques for excessive mucus. Errors in this differentiation can lead to uncomfortable and futile treatments (e.g. invasive suction of pulmonary oedema), which should be avoided at all times but particularly when the focus is comfort care.

A well-informed physiotherapist can advocate for the patient who is dying, whether to suggest to the treating team that drying of secretions would make the patient more comfortable (e.g. hyoscine) or to suggest humidification to facilitate sputum clearance. In some instances, optimising pharmacological management is much more comfortable for the patient than invasive physiotherapy techniques (e.g. nasopharyngeal suction), and therefore collaboration between the physiotherapist, pharmacist and medical team is ideal in end-of-life care.

■ References

Abramson, M., Crockett, A.J., Dabscheck, E., et al.; on behalf of Lung Foundation Australia and the Thoracic Society of Australia and New Zealand. 2015. *The COPD-X Plan. Australian and New Zealand Guidelines for the management of Chronic Obstructive Pulmonary Disease,* V2.45, March. <http://copdx.org.au/copd-x-plan/> (accessed 13.06.16.).

Australian Medicines Handbook Pty Ltd, 2015. Australian Medicines Handbook (online). Adelaide: Australian Medicines Handbook Pty Ltd [Internet]. <http://amhonline.amh.net.au/>.

Dentice, R.L., Elkins, M.R., Middleton, P.G., et al., 2016. A randomised trial of hypertonic saline during hospitalisation for exacerbation of cystic fibrosis. Thorax 71 (2), 141–147.

Gibson, P.G., Chang, A.B., Glasgow, N.J., et al., 2010. CICADA: Cough in Children and Adults: Diagnosis and Assessment. Australian cough guidelines summary statement. Medical Journal of Australia 192 (5), 265–271.

Goyal, S., Agrawal, A., 2013. Ketamine in status asthmaticus: a review. Indian Journal of Critical Care Medicine : Peer-Reviewed. Official Publication of Indian Society of Critical Care Medicine 17 (3), 154–161.

Green, M., Marzano, V., Leditschke, I.A., et al., 2016. Mobilization of intensive care patients: a multidisciplinary practical guide for clinicians. Journal of Multidisciplinary Healthcare 9, 247–256.

Harrison, C., Britt, H., Miller, G., et al., 2013. Prevalence of chronic conditions in Australia. PLoS ONE 8 (7), e67494. doi:10.1371/journal.pone.0067494.

Jennings, A.L., Davies, A.N., Higgins, J.P., et al., 2002. A systematic review of the use of opioids in the management of dyspnoea. Thorax 57 (11), 939–944.

Kaufman, G., 2011. Asthma: pathophysiology, diagnosis and management. Nursing Standard 26 (5), 48–56, quiz 58.

King, P.T., 2009. The pathophysiology of bronchiectasis. International Journal of Chronic Obstructive Pulmonary Disease 4, 411–419.

Leditschke, I.A., Green, M., Irvine, J., et al., 2012. What are the barriers to mobilizing intensive care patients? Cardiopulmonary Physical Therapy Journal 23 (1), 26–29.

Lung Foundation Australia, 2016. COPD: the statistics. Milton, Qld: Lung Foundation Australia [Internet]. <http://lungfoundation.com.au/health-professionals/clinical-resources/copd/copd-the-statistics/>.

Mall, M.A., Boucher, R.C., 2014. Pathophysiology of cystic fibrosis lung disease. In: Mall, M.A., Elborn, J.A. (Eds.), Cystic Fibrosis. European Respiratory Society, Lausanne, pp. 1–13.

Morris, P.E., Griffin, L., Berry, M., et al., 2011. Receiving early mobility during an intensive care unit admission is a predictor of improved outcomes in acute respiratory failure. American Journal of the Medical Sciences 341 (5), 373–377.

National Asthma Council Australia, 2014. Australian Asthma Handbook. South Melbourne: National Asthma Council Australia [Internet]. <http://www.asthmahandbook.org.au>.

Needham, D.M., Korupolu, R., Zanni, J.M., et al., 2010. Early physical medicine and rehabilitation for patients with acute respiratory failure: a quality improvement project. Archives of Physical Medicine and Rehabilitation 91 (4), 536–542.

Schweickert, W.D., Pohlman, M.C., Pohlman, A.S., et al., 2009. Early physical and occupational therapy in mechanically ventilated, critically ill patients: a randomised controlled trial. Lancet 373 (9678), 1874–1882.

Stiller, K., 2013. Physiotherapy in intensive care: an updated systematic review. Chest 144 (3), 825–847.

Suresh Babu, K., Kastelik, J., Morjaria, J.B., 2013. Role of long term antibiotics in chronic respiratory diseases. Respiratory Medicine 107 (6), 800–815.

Therapeutic Guidelines Limited, 2014a. Respiratory. In: eTG complete [Internet]. Melbourne: Therapeutic Guidelines Limited.

Therapeutic Guidelines Limited, 2014b. Antibiotic. In: eTG complete [Internet]. Melbourne: Therapeutic Guidelines Limited.

Therapeutic Guidelines Limited, 2014c. Palliative care. In: eTG complete [Internet]. Melbourne: Therapeutic Guidelines Limited.

Women's and men's health

Kathryn Vine, Miriam Lawrence, Roberto Orefice

OBJECTIVES

This chapter will discuss the role that medications have in the supplementary management of the common gynaecological, obstetric and urological conditions treated by physiotherapists that affect women and men throughout their adult lifespan. By the end of this chapter (including cross-referencing with other relevant chapters) the reader should have an understanding of:

+ the major common gynaecological, obstetric and urological disorders according to structure, location, signs and symptoms
+ pharmacotherapy options for common gynaecological, obstetric and urological disorders
+ usual dosages, routes of administration and major contraindications and precautions of these medications
+ any potential impact of these medications on physiotherapeutic management.

■ Introduction

This chapter outlines specific conditions affecting women, men or both during their adult life in four sections.

1 *Conditions of the child-bearing year*[1]: these include the musculoskeletal sequelae of the 40 weeks of the gestation pregnancy and include conditions such as pelvic girdle pain and carpal tunnel syndrome as well as difficulties experienced in the 12-week postnatal period (e.g. perineal trauma, mastitis and caesarean section recovery).

2 *Incontinence*: in Australia, up to 13% of men and up to 37% of women are incontinent of urine (Australian Institute of Health and Welfare [AIHW] 2013) and up to 20% of men and up to 12.9% of women are faecally incontinent (AIHW 2013). It is widely recognised that both forms of incontinence go underreported. In 2008–09, $1.6 billion were spent on incontinence via hospital and residential care, and continence aids.

3 *Gynaecological conditions*: many women suffering from incontinence will have concomitant pelvic organ prolapse (International Continence Society 2015), which affects up to half of parous women (Hagen & Stark 2011) and one-third of all women (Brækken et al. 2010). Pelvic viscera can be one of a myriad of potential sources of chronic pelvic pain, which affects 20% of adult, pre-menopausal Australian women (Pitts et al. 2008) and can be particularly debilitating for sufferers.

4 *Specific men's health problems*: albeit at a lower incidence, men can experience incontinence, prolapse and pelvic pain similar to female counterparts. However, they alone face the sequelae of prostate surgery, which increases their risk of urinary incontinence and erectile dysfunction.

Where applicable, the chapter follows the International Continence Society diagnostic nomenclature and guidelines and the Australian approved indications. Emphasis will be placed on those signs and symptoms and conditions most frequently treated by physiotherapists, and where the input of the physiotherapist is vital in monitoring the effects of the prescribed medications. The focus of this chapter will be on the major drugs prescribed for specific gynaecological, obstetric and urological disorders and their relevance for the treating physiotherapist (Table 4.1). As indicated in Table 4.1 many of the drugs prescribed for gynaecological, obstetric and urological conditions are discussed in other chapters of this handbook. The reader is directed to the relevant chapter.

Each category and the specific subgroup of drugs will be reviewed in terms of mechanism of action, route of administration, effects and side effects (adverse effects). Examples will be provided for the different clinical situations in which particular drugs would be used. Ranges of medication options are available for the treatment and/or management of gynaecological, obstetric and urological disorders and physiotherapists must be aware of the impact of drug intervention on their own treatment.

Table 4.2 describes the diverse group of structures, their locations and the signs and symptoms that arise from their dysfunction in the gynaecological, obstetric and urological context.

---

[1]This section specifically refers to the time of the pregnancy and the 12-week period immediately post birth.

TABLE 4.1 Drugs used in gynaecological, obstetric and urological disorders

General category	Specific group	Relevance for physiotherapist	Where addressed
Drugs used for specific gynaecological, obstetric and urological disorders – system oriented	Neuro-urological	++	This chapter
	Hormonal	+	This chapter
	Gastroenterological	+	This chapter
	Gynaecological	++	This chapter
	Reproductive	+	This chapter
Drugs used for specific gynaecological, obstetric and urological disorders – condition oriented	Drugs used in urge incontinence	+++	This chapter
	Drugs used in overactive bladder	+++	This chapter
	Drugs used in anal incontinence	+	This chapter (Table only)
	Drugs used in neurogenic incontinence	+	This chapter Chapter 6
	Drugs used in pelvic organ prolapse	++	This chapter
	Drugs used in erectile dysfunction	++	This chapter
	Drugs used in mastitis	++	This chapter
Adjuvant drugs that are used to treat gynaecological, obstetric and urological disorders	Pain Anti-inflammatory	+++ +++	See Chapter 7 See Chapters 5, 7

TABLE 4.2 Structure, location, signs and symptoms

Structure	Location	Signs and symptoms[a]
Viscera	Bladder	Incontinence, pain
	Bowel	Incontinence, constipation, pain
CNS	Ventral horn Dorsal horn	Incontinence, pain
PNS	Peripheral nerves (parasympathetic, sympathetic and somatic)	Incontinence, paraesthesia, weakness, erectile dysfunction (post prostatectomy)
Tissue level	Muscle, fascia, breast	Pain, inflammation, muscle spasm, pelvic organ prolapse, infection (mastitis)

[a]See Table 4.3 for descriptions of the various signs and symptoms.
CNS, central nervous system; PNS, peripheral nervous system.

Table 4.3 provides an outline of the conditions encountered within the four sections of this chapter (see 'Overview'). It defines each condition and the affected anatomy. Table 4.4 lists the mechanisms by which gynaecological, obstetric and urological disorders may produce the conditions described above. It is these mechanisms that are commonly targeted with pharmaceutical intervention.

Conditions of the child-bearing year

Common antenatal problems

Pelvic girdle pain

Definition
Pelvic girdle pain (PGP) 'between the posterior iliac crest and the gluteal fold, particularly in the vicinity of the sacroiliac joints (SIJs)' (Vleeming et al. 2008) is commonly attributed to a proposed laxity of the SIJs and pubic symphysis (PS) due to the production of the hormone relaxin.

Clinical features
Women with PGP in pregnancy will report pain at the buttocks with or without pain at the PS. Pain may refer down the posterior thigh, but distribution can be variable throughout the pregnancy (Kanakaris, Roberts & Giannoudis 2011). Women will often report difficulties with walking, standing and sitting (Vleeming et al. 2008). Feasibly, any activities that load the pelvis asymmetrically can aggravate the symptoms.

Clinical significance
The incidence of PGP in pregnant women is 20% (Vleeming et al. 2008).

Pharmacological management
Analgesia with paracetamol is first-line treatment[2] (Therapeutic Guidelines Limited 2010).

Carpal tunnel syndrome

Carpal tunnel syndrome (CTS) is a peripheral entrapment of the medial nerve at the wrist and results in paraesthesia or numbness of the median nerve distribution, mainly in the mornings, pain at the wrist and weakness or clumsiness of grip. Its incidence in pregnancy may be as high as 60%. Half of women with CTS in pregnancy report sleep disruption (Osterman, Ilyas & Matzon 2012). Unlike the incidence in other populations, CTS in pregnancy is related to the physiological consequences of pregnancy including fluid retention, hormonal changes and neural sensitivity (Osterman, Ilyas & Matzon 2012). Hence, non-steroidal anti-inflammatories (NSAIDS), which have potential for miscarriage and harm to the foetus, and corticosteroid injections are not routinely indicated (Therapeutic Guidelines Limited 2010). Conservative treatment by the use of nocturnal splinting for CTS is the mainstay of treatment; rarely is surgical intervention indicated (Osterman, Ilyas & Matzon 2012).

---

[2]See Chapter 7 for further information.

TABLE 4.3 Definitions and clinical features of the major signs and symptoms seen in gynaecological, obstetric and urological disorders

	Condition	Clinical characteristics	Anatomical location
Child-bearing year (ante- and postnatal)	Pelvic girdle pain (PGP)	Pain in the region of the buttocks and groin, attributable to hormonal and postural changes in pregnancy	Sacroiliac joints, pubic symphysis, buttocks, groin and thigh
	Carpal tunnel syndrome (CTS)	Pain and paraesthesia	Median nerve distribution of the hand
	Perineal trauma	Pain and inflammation due to varying degrees of tissue damage of the muscle, nerves and vessels of the perineum during child birth	Perineum
	Caesarean section	Incision wound pain	Lower abdomen
	Mastitis	Inflammation, pain, erythema, possible fevers, muscle soreness	Breast tissue, ducts, nipples, systemic
Incontinence	Stress urinary incontinence (SUI)	Incontinence during exertion	Pelvic floor, urethral neck, urethra
	Urge urinary incontinence (UUI)	Incontinence in the presence of urinary urge	Bladder, PNS, CNS, pelvic floor
	Mixed urinary incontinence (MUI)	Combined condition of stress and urge	Bladder, urethral neck, urethra, PNS, CNS, pelvic floor
	Urgency/overactive bladder (OAB)	A syndrome characterised by symptoms of urgency (overwhelming sense of bladder fullness), urge urinary incontinence and associated increased urinary frequency (International Continence Society 2015)	Bladder, PNS, CNS, pelvic floor
	Neurogenic incontinence	Incontinence as a sequela of neurological conditions (e.g. spinal cord injury, Parkinson's disease and stroke)	CNS, PNS, bladder, bowel, pelvic floor, internal and external anal sphincters
	Anal incontinence (AI)	Involuntary loss of faeces (solid or liquid) or flatus	Colon, rectum, internal and external anal sphincters, pelvic floor
	Male incontinence	Aside from UI or AI listed above, which can affect both sexes, men can suffer from incontinence secondary to prostate surgery	Urethra, bladder neck, rhabdosphincter, pelvic floor, PNS
Gynaecological	Pelvic organ prolapse	Loss of support for the uterus, bladder, colon or rectum leading to the affected organ's descent	Uterus, vaginal walls, cervix, bladder, urethra, rectum
	Pelvic pain	Pain in the lower abdomen or pelvis of at least 6 months' duration	Lower abdomen, pelvic cavity, pelvic floor, perineum
Erectile dysfunction		Inability to develop and maintain an erection	PNS, pelvic floor

CNS, central nervous system; PNS, peripheral nervous system.

TABLE 4.4	**Disease mechanisms in gynaecological, obstetric and urological disorders**
Mechanism(s)	**Disorder(s)**
Weakness	SUI, PGP, UUI
Cognitive	Urgency, UUI, frequency
Inflammatory/autoimmune	Inflammatory mastitis, PGP, CTS
Infection	Infective mastitis, UTI
Degenerative/genetic	Incontinence
Neurogenic	CTS, OAB, UUI, erectile dysfunction, neurogenic incontinence
Endocrinological	CTS, UI in women (deoestrogenisation), PGP (relaxin)
Trauma	Perineal trauma, postnatal SUI, wound pain post caesarean section, UI in men post prostatectomy, erectile dysfunction

CTS, carpal tunnel syndrome; OAB, overactive bladder; PGP, pelvic girdle pain; SUI, stress urinary incontinence; UI, urinary incontinence; UTI, urinary tract infection; UUI, urge urinary incontinence.

Medication use in pregnant women

Care must be taken when using medications in pregnant women, or those of child-bearing age (see Table 4.5). Harm can occur at any time during pregnancy. In the first trimester, teratogenic medications can cause congenital malformations; in the second and third trimesters, drugs can affect foetal growth and functional development. Medications can affect the foetus or can have adverse effects on labour or the baby once born (Australian Medicines Handbook Pty Ltd 2015a; Therapeutic Goods Administration 2011).

PHYSIOTHERAPY PRACTICE POINTS: MEDICINES USE IN PREGNANCY

- Balance the risks and benefits of prescribing medicines in pregnancy. Some medicines may have the potential to harm the unborn baby; not treating an illness or medical condition during pregnancy may also have negative consequences.

- Few drugs have been shown conclusively to be teratogenic in humans, but no drug is safe beyond all doubt in early pregnancy.

- Some medications have been used extensively in pregnant patients and appear to be safe. In general, these should be prescribed rather than new or untested medications.

- Take care when discussing risk with pregnant patients. Overly cautious advice may have negative consequences including suboptimal treatment or the cessation of necessary medicines.

- Information sources may not always provide the right context for an individual's situation. Always refer patients to specialist advice available via the state-based obstetric drug information services (see http://www.tga.gov.au/obstetric-drug-information-services#.UztO07T2Msg).

- Follow rational prescribing guidelines in pregnancy such as those from *Therapeutic Guidelines* or the *Australian Medicines Handbook*. Always consider non-pharmacological management where available.

Adapted from: NPS Medicinewise, 2014. Medicines in pregnancy – safe? Health News and Evidence [Internet]. <*http://www.nps.org.au/publications/health-professional/health-news-evidence/2014/pregnancy-medicine-safety*>.

TABLE 4.5 Australian categories for use of medicines in pregnancy

Category	Description
A	Drugs that have been taken by a large number of pregnant women and women of child-bearing age, without any proven increase in the frequency of malformations or other direct or indirect harmful effects on the foetus having been observed
C	Drugs that, owing to their pharmacological effects, have caused or may be suspected of causing, harmful effects on the human foetus or neonate without causing malformations. These effects may be reversible. Specialised texts should be consulted for further details
B1	Drugs that have been taken by only a limited number of pregnant women and women of child-bearing age, without an increase in the frequency of malformation or other direct or indirect harmful effects on the human foetus having been observed. Studies in animals have not shown evidence of an increased occurrence of foetal damage
B2	Drugs that have been taken by only a limited number of pregnant women and women of child-bearing age, without an increase in the frequency of malformation or other direct or indirect harmful effects on the human foetus having been observed. Studies in animals are inadequate or may be lacking, but available data show no evidence of an increased occurrence of foetal damage
B3	Drugs that have been taken by only a limited number of pregnant women and women of child-bearing age, without an increase in the frequency of malformation or other direct or indirect harmful effects on the human foetus having been observed. Studies in animals have shown evidence of an increased occurrence of foetal damage, the significance of which is considered uncertain in humans
D	Drugs that have caused, are suspected to have caused or may be expected to cause, an increased incidence of human foetal malformations or irreversible damage. These drugs may also have adverse pharmacological effects. Specialised texts should be consulted for further details
X	Drugs that have such a high risk of causing permanent damage to the foetus that they should not be used in pregnancy or when there is a possibility of pregnancy

Reproduced with permission from: Prescribing medicines in pregnancy database, 2016, Therapeutic Goods Administration, used by permission of the Australian Government <https://www.tga.gov.au/prescribing-medicines-pregnancy-database>. © Commonwealth of Australia This work is copyright. You may download, display, print and reproduce the whole or part of this work in unaltered form for your own personal use or, if you are part of an organisation, for internal use within your organisation, but only if you or your organisation do not use the reproduction for any commercial purpose and retain this copyright notice and all disclaimer notices as part of that reproduction. Apart from rights to use as permitted under the Copyright Act 1968 or allowed by this copyright notice, all other rights are reserved and you are not allowed to reproduce the whole or any part of this work in any way (electronic or otherwise) without first being given specific written permission from the Commonwealth to do so. Requests and inquiries concerning reproduction and rights are to be sent to the TGA Copyright Officer, Therapeutic Goods Administration, PO Box 100, Woden ACT 2606 or emailed to tga.copyright@tga.gov.au Disclaimer: The Australian categorisation system and database for prescribing medicines in pregnancy have been developed by medical and scientific experts based on available evidence of risks associated with taking particular medicines while pregnant. This information is presented for the use of health professionals prescribing medicines to pregnant women, rather than for the general public to use. It is general in nature and is not presented as medical advice to health professionals or the public. It is not intended to be used as a substitute for a health professional's advice.

These pregnancy classifications are used by the Therapeutic Goods Administration for categorising medications on registration for use in Australia; however, their relevance in clinical practice is limited due to (Australian Medicines Handbook Pty Ltd 2015a; NPS Medicinewise 2014):

◆ categories not indicating which stage of foetal development the medication may affect

◆ categories not being updated, even if new information or evidence becomes available

◆ incorrect assumption that the alphabetical code indicates a scale of safety

◆ categories not indicating any balance between risks and benefits.

Both Australian and American medication references are moving towards providing clinically relevant information on medication use in pregnancy based on human data and clinical experience and away from these categories (Australian Medicines Handbook Pty Ltd 2015a).

Medicines use in breastfeeding mothers

Care must also be taken with medicines use in breastfeeding mothers (Australian Medicines Handbook Pty Ltd 2015f). If a medication passes into breast milk in pharmacologically significant quantities, this may have toxic effects on the infant. Additionally some medications may suppress lactation or impact the infant's sucking reflex.

PHYSIOTHERAPY PRACTICE POINTS:
MEDICINES USE IN BREASTFEEDING

• Only use medicines clearly documented as safe for breastfeeding women, as many medications have insufficient information available to appropriately determine risk.

• Some medications have been well investigated and/or used widely during breastfeeding and appear to be safe; in general, these should be prescribed rather than new or untried drugs.

• For some medication (with a shorter half-life), taking the medication dose immediately after a feed decreases the amount of the drug in breast milk; this may reduce effects on the infant and reassure the mother.

• Seek expert advice from state-based obstetric drug information services (see http://www.tga.gov.au/obstetric-drug-information-services#.UztOO7T2Msg).

Common postnatal problems

Perineal tears and episiotomies

Perineal trauma is common after vaginal births, particularly in primiparous women. It is classified against the anatomical consequence, with third and fourth degree tears termed obstetric anal sphincter injuries (OASIS) (see Table 4.6 and Figure 4.1).

TABLE 4.6 Classification of perineal trauma

Classification	Definition
First degree	Injury to perineal skin only
Second degree	Injury to perineum involving perineal muscles, but not involving the anal sphincter
Third degree	Partial or complete disruption of the EAS +/− IAS: • < 50% of the EAS • > 50% of the EAS • both EAS and IAS
Fourth degree	Complete tear of both EAS and IAS as well as the rectal mucosa (Therapeutic Guidelines Limited 2010)
Episiotomy	Surgical incision of the perineum This may 'extend' to involve more perineal tissue, including OASIS (Thiagamoorthy et al. 2014)

EAS, external anal sphincter; IAS, internal anal sphincter; OASIS, obstetric anal sphincter injuries.

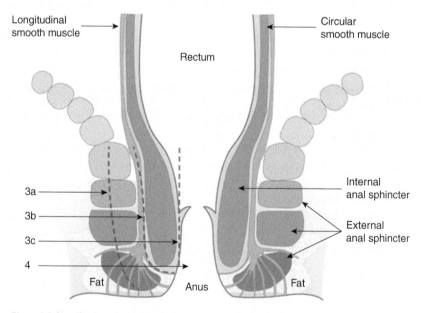

Figure 4.1 Classification of perineal trauma.
Reproduced with permission from: Lone, F., Sultan, A. & Thakar, R., 2012. Obstetric pelvic floor and anal sphincter injuries. The Obstetrician & Gynaecologist 14 (4), 257–266.

Clinical features

Symptoms of perineal trauma include pain (rated as moderate to severe by one-third of women) (East et al. 2012), urinary and/or anal incontinence, defecation dysfunction, dyspareunia, pelvic organ prolapse (POP) and psychological distress (Lone, Sultan & Thakar 2012; Skinner & Dietz 2015; Tan, Ruane & Sherburn 2013).

Clinical significance

Perineal trauma occurs in 85% of vaginal births (Lone, Sultan & Thakar 2012). OASIS incidence is cited as around 3% (Thiagamoorthy et al. 2014), but can be as high as 6.4% (Tan, Ruane & Sherburn 2013). Such injuries may have significant physical and psychological consequences, including diminished quality of life, sexual dysfunction, chronic pain, POP obstetric fistula and urinary and anal incontinence that may persist for decades (Lone, Sultan & Thakar 2012; Skinner & Dietz 2014; Tan, Ruane & Sherburn 2013). Over half of women report having to change their lifestyle as a result of sustaining an OASIS (Kumar 2012).

Pharmacological management

Analgesia: Simple analgesia with paracetamol and NSAIDs is recommended.[3]

Antibiotics: Before the repair of a third or fourth degree tear, a single preoperative dose of cephazolin is recommended. Routine use of postoperative antibiotics is not recommended; however, in the case of obstetric anal sphincter repair, a broad-spectrum antibiotic such as amoxycillin/clavulanate therapy is recommended to reduce the incidence of postoperative infections and wound dehiscence. Metronidazole is often included to cover possible anaerobic contamination from faecal matter (Royal College of Obstetricians and Gynaecologists 2007; Therapeutic Guidelines Limited 2014a).

Aperients: The use of postoperative laxatives is recommended to reduce the incidence of postoperative wound dehiscence (Royal College of Obstetricians and Gynaecologists 2007). A stool softener (e.g. docusate) and sometimes an osmotic laxative (e.g. polyethylene glycol laxatives) can be used for up to 10 days postpartum (see Table 4.7). Some recommendations suggest using fibre supplements to produce voluminous but soft stools, while others suggest avoiding fibre supplements as they can be associated with more frequent incontinence episodes (Toglia 2011).

Text continued on p. 86

---

[3]For further details see Chapter 7.

TABLE 4.7 Medications used in postnatal conditions

Drug name	Mechanism of action	Indications	Common side effects	Practice points	Common dosage range
			CLASS: Stool softeners		
Docusate	Softens stool by increasing the amount of water drawn into the faeces	Constipation and to prevent straining	Adverse effects are rare (<0.1%), but include abdominal cramps, diarrhoea, nausea, rash	Takes 1–3 days to work	• 50–500 mg daily in one or two doses • Comes in combined tablets with senna, given 1–4 tablets per day
Liquid paraffin	Acts as a lubricant to assist faecal material to move through the bowel	Constipation	Adverse effects are Infrequent (0.1–1%), but can include: anal leakage and with high doses or long-term use rectal irritation. With regular or long-term use, reduction in fat soluble vitamins (A, D, E, K) can occur	• Emulsions are given orally and therefore more acceptable • Onset of effect after oral administration is 2–3 days	*Oral*, 40 mL daily (emulsion 50%) *Rectal*, 120 mL daily (unemulsified liquid) Doses can be adjusted by 5 mL (up or down to achieve regular bowel motions)
			CLASS: Stimulant laxatives		
Bisacodyl **Senna** **(also comes in combined products with docusate)** **Sodium picosulfate**	Directly stimulates colonic mucosal nerve endings to increase intestinal motility Can additionally cause a build-up of water and electrolytes in the bowel May also cause accumulation of water and electrolytes in the colonic lumen	Constipation	Adverse effects are Infrequent, but can include diarrhoea, abdominal pain, cramps, nausea and with excessive or long-term use fluid and electrolyte imbalance	• Used long term for constipation in patients with spinal injuries, chronic neuromuscular disease and for patients taking opioids • No evidence that chronic use is harmful to the colon • Laxative class most often associated with misuse	**Bisacodyl** *Oral*, 5–15 mg at night *Rectal*, 10 mg once daily when required Onset of action: • 6–12 hours (oral) • 15–60 minutes (suppository) • 5–15 minutes (enema) **Senna** ***(also comes in combined products with docusate)*** 7.5–30 mg at bedtime Onset of action: • 6–12 hours **Sodium picosulfate** 10–20 drops (5–10 mg) at night Onset of action: • 6–12 hours

CLASS: Osmotic laxatives

Glycerol	Draws water into the stool and lubricates bowel. It also has local irritant effects which may act as a stimulant	Constipation	Infrequently causes rectal discomfort	Onset of action: 5–60 minutes	1 adult suppository once daily when required
Lactulose	Draws water into the colon and causes an increase in intraluminal pressure which stimulates peristalsis	Constipation Hepatic encephalopathy	Flatulence, abdominal discomfort, cramps Less common are nausea and vomiting	Onset of action: 1–3 days	15–45 mL daily in 1 or 2 doses
Macrogol	Macrogols or polyethylene glycols (PEGs) are large polymers with osmotic activity which minimises electrolyte and water loss. Some products also contain sodium sulfate, a saline laxative that stimulates peristalsis	Constipation Faecal impaction Bowel preparation before surgery and diagnostic procedures	Nausea, vomiting, diarrhoea, anal irritation, abdominal distension, cramps or pain Fluid and electrolyte disturbances are less of a risk with macrogol laxatives than with other osmotic laxatives (e.g. saline laxatives)	Macrogol is not significantly absorbed from the GIT	Doses will vary depending on the product, dosed between once and three times per day

Continued

TABLE 4.7 Medications used in postnatal conditions—cont'd

Drug name	Mechanism of action	Indications	Common side effects	Practice points	Common dosage range
Saline laxatives	Contain magnesium, sulfate, phosphate and citrate which are poorly absorbed and cause the colon to retain fluid due to their osmotic effect; and also stimulate peristalsis	Constipation Bowel preparation, for GI diagnostic or surgical procedures	Nausea, bloating, fluid and electrolyte disturbance, rectal irritation Sodium phosphate laxatives can cause serious fluid and electrolyte disturbance. Acute renal failure, cardiac arrest and deaths have been reported	Onset of action: • 0.5–3 hours post oral administration • 2–30 minutes post rectal administration • Patients must be well hydrated to reduce the risk of electrolyte disturbance • Picolax®, PicoPrep® and Picosalax® also contain sodium picosulfate, which is a stimulant laxative	Wide range of products available – see directions on label
Sorbitol	Non-absorbable sugar which produces osmotic action in the colon	Constipation	Flatulence, abdominal distension and cramping	Ineffective in treating hepatic encephalopathy	20 mL once to three times a day as required

CLASS: Bulk-forming laxatives

| **Psyllium, Ispaghula, Sterculia** | Draws water into the colon to increase faecal bulk which also stimulates peristalsis | Constipation when dietary modification is inadequate

To improve or regulate stool consistency in diarrhoea, faecal incontinence, colostomy and ileostomy | Flatulence, bloating, abdominal discomfort | • Give with extra fluid to ensure laxative effect, or with minimal fluid to harden stool
• Full effect may take several days
• Some products contain frangula (buckthorn) bark, which is one of the stimulant laxatives | Wide range of products available – see directions on label
Should not be taken immediately before going to bed |

GIT, gastrointestinal tract; NSAIDs, non-steroidal anti-inflammatories.
Adapted from: Australian Medicines Handbook Pty Ltd, 2015e. Gastrointestinal drugs. Australian Medicines Handbook [Online]. <https://amhonline-amh-net-au/chapters/chap-12/gastrointestinaldrugs.t>.

PHYSIOTHERAPY PRACTICE POINTS: PERINEAL TEARS AND EPISIOTOMIES

It is recommended the OASIS are followed up in a dedicated multidisciplinary (MDT) perineal clinic (Lone, Sultan & Thakar 2012; Tan, Ruane & Sherburn 2013). Physiotherapy treatment should be undertaken in conjunction with the above-mentioned pharmacological management and includes advice regarding rest, ice, compression, elevation (RICE) and supervised pelvic floor muscle (PFM) re-training rehabilitation (Tan, Ruane & Sherburn 2013). The treating physiotherapist needs to be aware of the half-life of the pain medication to maximise treatment outcomes. If conservative management fails and symptoms continue, secondary repair or salvage colorectal surgery may be indicated (Lone, Sultan & Thakar 2012; Roos, Thakar & Sultan 2010).

Mastitis

Definition

Lactational mastitis is an often painful inflammation or infection of the breast during breastfeeding (Betzold 2007). The condition is considered a continuum of ailments including engorgement, blocked ducks, inflammation, infection and abscess (Betzold 2007). Engorgement is congestion of the breast due to insufficient drainage. If milk backs up behind an area of congestion, localised milk stasis occurs and presents as a blocked duct (Betzold 2007). Inflammatory mastitis is caused by cytokines released in response to milk stasis caused by ineffective and/ or obstructed drainage of milk from the breast. Infectious mastitis can result from untreated milk stasis and/or colonisation with pathogenic bacteria, most commonly *Staphylococcus aureus*. A breast abscess is a collection of pus within the breast tissue, resulting from untreated or inadequately treated mastitis (Cusack & Brennan 2011).

Clinical features

Both inflammatory and infectious mastitis typically present as a locally warm, tender, reddened wedge-shaped area of breast tissue, usually affecting only one breast, which may or may not be accompanied by systemic flu-like symptoms such as fever, chills and muscle aches (Betzold 2007; Cusack & Brennan 2011). Symptoms that persist for more than 24 hours are more indicative of infection (Betzold 2007).

Engorgement is characterised by bilateral, hard, enlarged, shiny, flushed and painful breasts. Venous and lymphatic drainage is obstructed resulting in vascular congestion and oedema, which prevents normal milk ejection reflex (Betzold 2007).

Symptoms of abscess are similar to mastitis, but include a discrete, erythematous, tender lump. This can be tense or fluctuant and the overlying skin may be necrotic (Cusack & Brennan 2011). Rarely, the lump may be non-tender and colourless (Cusack & Brennan 2011).

Clinical significance

Mastitis is a painful and distressing condition, associated with depression, distress, anxiety, feelings of helplessness and concerns about milk supply (Lumley & Amir 2006).

Pharmacological management

Acute bacterial mastitis is usually caused by *Staphylococcus aureus* and associated with breastfeeding. If no systemic symptoms are present, increased feeding and gentle expression on the affected side can prevent progression. However, early treatment with oral antibiotics covering *S. aureus* (dicloxacillin/flucloxacillin, cephalexin, cephalexin or clindamycin) is required to prevent the formation of an abscess if systemic symptoms develop (Therapeutic Guidelines Limited 2014b).

PHYSIOTHERAPY PRACTICE POINTS: MASTITIS

Physiotherapeutic management targets the early inflammatory phase of mastitis. Inspect the breast for colour and temperature changes, nipple condition (as a tract for infection). Palpate for engorgement, blocked ducts or abscess. If possible, feeding can be observed to gain information regarding infant and maternal behaviour, feeding positioning and ease of attachment (Cusack & Brennan 2011).

Therapeutic, continuous ultrasound performed at 1 MHz, 0.5–2 W/cm² daily for 1 minute/1 cm² over 2–3 days may be useful. Lymphatic massage, performed toward the axilla and avoiding firm pressure, is also endorsed (Callinan-Moore 2012). Kinesiotape may assist lymphatic drainage by lifting the superficial skin and opening initial lymphatics, directing fluid to the axillary lymph nodes (Kase et al. 2003). If symptoms of infective mastitis are present, or if conservative treatments fail, the woman should be referred for consideration of antibiotic management. If abscess is suspected, the mother should be referred for diagnostic ultrasound (Cusack & Brennan 2011) – see pharmacological management highlighted above.

Caesarean section

Definition

Caesarean section is the surgical delivery of a baby via an abdominal incision. It may be medically indicated prior to labour or performed as an emergency procedure. Maternally elected caesareans may represent 17% of births in Australia (Robson et al. 2009).

Clinical features

Women who have undergone a caesarean section will have incisional pain that may affect their mobility, slower postnatal recovery times, including slower return to physical activity (Royal Australian and New Zealand College of Obstetricians and Gynaecologists 2013), and higher complication rates (Allen, O'Connell & Baskett 2006).

Clinical significance

Women who deliver their babies via caesarean section have many of the same postnatal sequelae as those who birth vaginally. Caesareans may be associated with slower return to physical conditioning and may be a predictor of poor mental quality of life in the postpartum period (Torkan et al. 2009).

Pharmacological management

Pain: Pain management post caesarean section may include simple analgesia (paracetamol and NSAIDs) together with opioids (both oral and intravenous).

Approximately 6% of mothers have persistent postoperative pain, and 1% have severe postoperative pain (Therapeutic Guidelines Limited 2012).[4]

Antibiotics: A single dose of an antibiotic (cephazolin or clindamycin) is usually given as prophylaxis within 60 minutes of the surgical incision. This reduces the rate of postoperative infection, including endometritis, after elective and non-elective caesarean section (Therapeutic Guidelines Limited 2014c).

If postoperative infection does develop, surgical drainage and irrigation with sodium chloride 0.9% is adequate to treat minor infection. If moderate infection develops with associated cellulitis, oral antibiotic therapy is warranted (dicloxacillan/flucloxacillin, cephazolin or clindamycin). If this progresses to severe infection with systemic symptoms intravenous antibiotics are required. The use of topical antibiotics is not recommended for treatment or prophylaxis of surgical site infections, and they are associated with increased resistance and hypersensitivity reactions (Therapeutic Guidelines Limited 2014d).

PHYSIOTHERAPY PRACTICE POINTS: CAESAREAN SECTION

In addition to routine postpartum care outlined above, physiotherapy management following caesarean section should include screening for risk factors for respiratory complications and treatment should ensue only if necessary, but is not routinely indicated. Early mobilisation is recommended, but should not rely on physiotherapy input; however, postsurgical pain can limit mobilisation and analgesia should be considered. Education should be provided about specific incisional protection and return to physical activity and sport. The treating physiotherapist should monitor symptoms of postoperative infection and refer on for assessment and pharmacological intervention where indicated. PFM training is provided as caesarean sections are not protective of pelvic floor function in the long term (MacArthur et al. 2011).

Incontinence

Stress urinary incontinence

Definition

Stress urinary incontinence (SUI) is defined as any involuntary loss of urine during physical exertion, coughing or sneezing (International Continence Society 2015).

Clinical significance

There are numerous secondary complications following the development of SUI including urinary tract infections (UTIs), skin excoriation and infection, constipation, social isolation and avoidance of physical activity with its myriad of health sequelae. Following appropriate assessment, physiotherapy interventions should be the first-line treatment and are usually highly successful with cure rates (defined as less than 2 g leakage on a pad test) cited as high as 80% (Bø 2012).

---

[4]For further details on pain management see Chapter 7.

Pharmacological management

There are no identified pharmaceutical interventions for SUI (Therapeutic Guidelines Limited 2014c).

PHYSIOTHERAPY PRACTICE POINTS: STRESS URINARY INCONTINENCE

Since there are no pharmacological interventions for SUI, pelvic floor physiotherapy, primarily focused on pelvic floor muscle (PFM) strengthening, should be first-line treatment (International Continence Society 2015). A regimen established by Bø and colleagues (1990) of 6–8-second contractions, 8–12 repetitions, 3 times a day, progressing from supine to erect is commonly adopted (Brækken et al. 2010; Frawley et al. 2010). Adjunct techniques including e-stimulation, vaginal cones and biofeedback (International Continence Society 2015) may be helpful (MacArthur et al. 2011; Bø et al. 2007; Bø 2007). Failing physiotherapeutic interventions, urethral slings or injectable urethral bulking agents may be indicated (International Continence Society 2015).

Overactive bladder syndrome

Definition

Overactive bladder syndrome (OAB) is characterised by symptoms of urgency, urge urinary incontinence (UUI) and associated increased urinary frequency (International Continence Society 2015). Urgency is the sensation of an abrupt, compelling need to urinate (International Continence Society 2015). When associated with involuntary urine loss, UUI is diagnosed (International Continence Society 2015). If involuntary detrusor contractions are observed during bladder filling upon urodynamic testing, a diagnosis of detrusor overactivity (DO) also can be made (International Continence Society 2015). DO may be present in the absence of the clinical diagnosis of OAB (International Continence Society 2015).

Clinical features

Patients with OAB syndrome will describe an overwhelming need to void, with a decreased ability to delay the urge (urgency). UI of variable volumes may result due to premature contraction of the detrusor (UUI). Both urgency and UUI are associated with increased day and night time frequency (International Continence Society 2015). Increasing frequency may be adopted in an attempt to reduce bladder volumes and episodes of urgency or UUI (International Continence Society 2015) and may be associated with decreased functional bladder capacity and a worsening of symptoms.

Clinical significance

It is estimated that one in five women across the world is affected by OAB (Irwin et al. 2011). It has a substantial negative effect on the quality of life of sufferers. It is associated with lower SP-36 scores for quality of life, higher depression and poorer quality of sleep (Stewart et al. 2003). Due to the risk of embarrassing urinary loss, sufferers often avoid social outings (International Continence Society 2015). It is associated with a modest increase in falls (Chiarelli, Mackenzie

& Osmotherly 2009) and increased morbidity and mortality in the elderly (International Continence Society 2015).

Pharmacological management

Always consider other medications as a potential cause for incontinence, such as selective alpha-blockers (e.g. prazosin), diuretics, anticholinesterases (e.g. donepezil) and sedatives. Medications with anticholinergic effects (see Box 4.1) and opioids can cause urinary retention and subsequent overflow incontinence (Australian Medicines Handbook Pty Ltd 2015c).

Anticholinergics are the mainstay of treatment for urge incontinence. They reduce bladder contractility and increase bladder capacity. They include darifenacin, oxybutynin, propantheline, solifenacin and tolterodine (Australian Medicines Handbook Pty Ltd 2015c).

Mirabegron is a beta-3-adrenoceptor agonist; it relaxes bladder muscle during the storage phase of micturition, increasing bladder capacity, and is also used for urge incontinence (Australian Medicines Handbook Pty Ltd 2015c).

PHYSIOTHERAPY PRACTICE POINTS: OVERACTIVE BLADDER SYNDROME

Physiotherapists can provide valuable insight into the efficacy of drugs used for OAB through their assessment and observing symptom severity as well as monitoring women for side effects such as urinary retention, blurred vision, dry mouth, constipation and confusion (Australian Medicines Handbook Pty Ltd 2015b). Changes can be qualified by use of a bladder diary, which reflects fluid intake, urinary frequency and volume (International Continence Society 2015) but may also include parameters such as degree of urgency at void, episodes of incontinence, triggers and emotions (Marti, Valentini & Robain 2014).

Neurogenic bladder

Definition

Many neurological conditions can have detrimental effects on bladder and urinary tract function. The nature and severity of symptoms is dependent on the site and extent of neurological lesion and disease (see Table 4.8). Most commonly implicated disorders include spinal cord injury, multiple sclerosis, stroke, Parkinson's disease, dementia, spina bifida and neuropathy (International Continence Society 2013a, 2013b).

Clinical features

Central nervous system insults and spinal cord lesions above the sacral level result in detrusor overactivity and symptoms akin to OAB, while sacral spinal cord lesions will cause hypocontractability of the bladder and subsequent overflow incontinence (see Table 4.9). Peripheral neuropathy will result in weakness of the pelvic floor, the results of which are also described above (International Continence Society 2013b).

Clinical significance

Incontinence can be a devastating sequela of neurological disease and injury. For example, up to half of all stroke victims, 90% of people with multiple sclerosis

BOX 4.1 Drugs with anticholinergic effects

Aclidinium, amantadine, amitriptyline, atropine

Belladonna alkaloids, benzhexol, benztropine, biperiden, brompheniramine

Chlorpheniramine, chlorpromazine, clomipramine, clozapine, cyclizine, cyclopentolate, cyproheptadine

Darifenacin, dexchlorpheniramine, dimenhydrinate, diphenhydramine, disopyramide, dothiepin, doxepin

Glycopyrronium

Homatropine, hyoscine (butylbromide or hydrobromide)

Imipramine, ipratropium (nebulised)

Levomepromazine

Mianserin

Nortriptyline

Olanzapine, orphenadrine, oxybutynin

Pericyazine, pheniramine, pizotifen, prochlorperazine, promethazine, propantheline

Solifenacin

Tiotropium, tolterodine, trimeprazine, triprolidine, tropicamide

Umeclidinium

Adapted from: Australian Medicines Handbook Pty Ltd, 2015b. Anticholinergics (genitourinary). Australian Medicines Handbook [Online]. <https://amhonline-amh-net-au./chapters/chap-13/urinary-incontinence/anticholinergics-02>.

TABLE 4.8 Overview of neurological supply affecting continence

	Sympathetic T10–L1	Parasympathetic S2–4	Somatic S3–5
Bladder	Inhibitory	Facilitatory	–
Bladder neck	Facilitatory	Inhibitory	Facilitatory
External urethral sphincter	Proposed*	Proposed*	–
Bowel	–	Facilitatory	–
Internal anal sphincter	Facilitatory	Inhibitory	–
External anal sphincter	Proposed*	Proposed*	Facilitatory
Pelvic floor	–	–	Facilitatory

*As determined in animal-based studies.
Adapted from: Drake, M.J., Apostolidis, A., Emmanuel, A., et al., 2013. Neurologic urinary and faecal incontinence. In: Abrams, P., Cardozo, L., Khoury, S., et al. (Eds.), Incontinence, fifth ed. International Continence Society, Paris, France.

TABLE 4.9 Characterisation of neurological lesions affecting continence

	Congenital and perinatal	Acquired stable conditions	Acquired progressive conditions
Brain and brainstem	Cerebral palsy	Stroke Acquired brain injury	Multiple sclerosis Parkinson's disease Dementia Multiple system atrophy
Suprasacral spinal cord	Hereditary spastic paraparesis Spinal dysraphism	Trauma	Multiple sclerosis Spondylosis with myelopathy
Sacral spinal cord	Spinal dysraphism Sacral agenesis Anorectal anomaly	Conus injury	Tumour
Subsacral	Spinal dysraphism Familial dysautonomia	Cauda equina injury Pelvic nerve injury	Tumour Peripheral neuropathy

Adapted from: Drake, M.J., Apostolidis, A., Emmanuel, A., et al., 2013. Neurologic urinary and faecal incontinence. In: Abrams, P., Cardozo, L., Khoury, S., et al. (Eds.), Incontinence, fifth ed. International Continence Society, Paris, France.

and two-thirds of cerebral palsy sufferers will have urological dysfunction, with the majority of these having some degree of subsequent incontinence (Drake et al. 2013).

Pharmacological management

The pharmaceutical management of neurogenic incontinence targets the same mechanism as that of other causes:

* anticholinergics as per Table 4.10
* selective alpha blockers as per Table 4.13 (later)
* Botox®; refer to Chapter 6.

PHYSIOTHERAPY PRACTICE POINTS: NEUROGENIC BLADDER

Assessment of neurogenic bladder relies on the general principles of pelvic floor, urinary function and incontinence quantification as for stress and urge urinary incontinence, but is often augmented with neurological and urodynamic testing (International Continence Society 2013b).

Treatment of neurogenic incontinence will depend on the individual presentation, but many strategies described above can be applied. Similarly, physiotherapists can provide valuable input into the effectiveness or complications of pharmacological management. If conservative measures are not effective, intermittent or suprapubic catheterisation may be required (Australian Medicines Handbook Pty Ltd 2015b). Physiotherapeutic attention should also be given to the functional requirements of voiding, such as mobility and hand function (International Continence Society 2013b).

TABLE 4.10 Medications used in incontinence

Drug name	Mechanism of action	Indications	Common side-effects	Practice points	Common dosage range
Anticholinergics **Darifenacin** **Oxybutynin** **Propantheline** **Solifenacin** **Tolterodine**	Reduce bladder muscle contractility and increase bladder capacity. They can also cause hesitancy and retention in susceptible people by increasing voiding dysfunction	Urinary urge incontinence	Elderly people may be more sensitive to anticholinergic adverse effects (urinary retention, blurred vision, dry mouth, constipation and confusion) Adverse effects are usually dose related; therefore start at low dosage, particularly in the elderly, and increase cautiously to the lowest effective dose Facial flushing (more common in children)	The benefit from anticholinergics varies between individuals New agents (solifenacin, darifenacin) appear to have fewer CNS adverse effects, yet the same efficacy Patient should be reviewed by prescriber after 4 weeks to monitor for adverse effects (including changes in cognitive function) and assess for improvement in symptoms; treatment should be stopped if no overall benefit; an alternative anticholinergic could be tried Avoid use in urinary retention or significant bladder outlet obstruction	**Darifenacin** 7.5–15 mg once daily; do not exceed 7.5 mg daily in people with moderate hepatic impairment or taking potent CYP3A4 inhibitors (e.g. itraconazole, ritonavir) **Oxybutynin** *Oral*, 2.5–5 mg 2 or 3 times daily; maximum 20 mg daily Lower dose range in elderly *Patch*, 1 patch applied twice a week (every 3–4 days) **Propantheline** 15–30 mg 2 or 3 times daily **Solifenacin** 5–10 mg once daily **Tolterodine** 1–2 mg twice daily

Continued

TABLE 4.10 Medications used in urinary incontinence—cont'd

Drug name	Mechanism of action	Indications	Common side-effects	Practice points	Common dosage range
Mirabegron	Relaxes bladder muscle via beta$_3$-adrenoceptor agonist activity	Urinary urge incontinence	Hypertension, nasopharyngitis, UTI	• Can take up to 8 weeks for full effect of 25 mg dose • Monitor BP at baseline and periodically, especially in pre-existing hypertension • Improved absorption if taken on an empty stomach (1 hour before or 2 hours after eating) • Mirabegron has demonstrated a reduction in incontinence episodes by about 0.8 in 48 hours compared to placebo in clinical trails • Long-term safety and efficacy data are lacking	25–50 mg once daily. Maximum 25 mg daily in people with renal or hepatic impairment

BP, blood pressure; CNS, central nervous system; UTI, urinary tract infection.
Adapted from: Australian Medicines Handbook Pty Ltd, 2015c. Drugs for urinary incontinence. Australian Medicines Handbook [Online]. <https://amhonline-amh-net-au./chapters/chap-13/urinary-incontinence/urinary-incontinence.t>.

Anal incontinence

Definition

Anal incontinence (AI) is the inability to control both or either liquid or solid stool (faecal incontinence) and flatus (International Continence Society 2015; Rømmen et al. 2012).

Clinical features

Symptoms of AI include any involuntary loss of bowel material and are most commonly associated with urgency (International Continence Society 2015). Faecal incontinence is more likely to be associated with physical exertions. AI is also associated with diarrhoea and constipation, with higher prevalence in women who fluctuate between the two (Rømmen et al. 2012). Sufferers may also experience painful skin excoriation and urinary tract infections.

Clinical significance

Prevalence of AI may be as high as one in five adult women, but is generally regarded as underreported (Rømmen et al. 2012). It can be a socially debilitating condition and sufferers often experience a poor quality of life (Norton, Cody & Hosker 2006).

Pharmacological management

The pharmacological treatment will depend on the cause of the AI identified. Adverse effects of medication or uncontrolled underlying gastrointestinal diseases such as inflammatory bowel disease should always be considered in the differential diagnosis. If overflow incontinence due to chronic constipation is the cause, laxatives may be used (see Table 4.7). If diarrhoea is the cause, in some cases anti-diarrhoeal agents such as loperamide or codeine may be used. If stool consistency is the cause, sometimes bulk-forming laxatives can be used (see Table 4.7).

PHYSIOTHERAPY PRACTICE POINTS: ANAL INCONTINENCE

Assessment should focus on establishing the nature and causes of AI, as only some will be amenable to physiotherapy. The physiotherapist may be able to provide insight into the contribution to AI by suboptimal stool consistency, for example as a result of diet, psychological stress, irritable bowel syndrome or Crohn's disease, and refer for appropriate investigation and management. Causes such as neurological dysfunction and ongoing structural defect from OASIS may require referral to the treating doctor. Thorough assessment will allow physiotherapy management of PFM strength, defaecation dynamics and behavioural re-training (as for OAB). Similar training as for UI, electrical stimulation and/ or biofeedback can augment a PFM strengthening program (Norton, Cody & Hosker 2006).

Gynaecological conditions

Pelvic organ prolapse

Definition

Pelvic organ prolapse (POP) is the urogenital herniation of pelvic organs into or through the vagina (International Continence Society 2015). It is caused by changes to the myofascial support of the pelvic floor and is closely related to SUI (International Continence Society 2015). Although difficult to ascertain on examination (International Continence Society 2015), POP can involve the bladder, urethra, uterus and bowel, or a combination of structures. POP is closely associated with SUI, UUI and mixed UI as discussed above. However, it is notable that the presence of POP may mask symptoms of SUI (International Continence Society 2015).

Clinical features

Most women with POP will report a sensation of genital heaviness or bulging (International Continence Society 2015). Due to the anatomical deficiency, some women will have difficulty with micturition and/or defaecation and may need to digitally support the vaginal walls to empty their bladder or bowel (International Continence Society 2015).

Clinical significance

POP affects up to 50% of all parous women (Hagen & Stark 2011) and one-third of all women (Brækken et al. 2010), with a lifetime incidence of 11.1% (International Continence Society 2015). Similar to UI, POP has a negative impact on quality of life (QoL) including social, psychological and sexual domains (Bartoli, Aguzzi & Tarricone 2010).

Pharmacological management

Topical vaginal oestrogen has been shown to increase the generation of mature collagen, decreases degradative enzyme activity and increases vaginal wall thickness, which helps to oestrogenise the tissue, improve symptoms and improve surgical recovery (Rahn et al. 2014).

PHYSIOTHERAPY PRACTICE POINTS: PELVIC ORGAN PROLAPSE

A urogynaecological history should be taken, including parity, incontinence, gynaecological surgery and bowel habits. It should also gain information about the nature of POP symptoms, including 24 hour variances and aggravating activities (Bump et al. 1996). The prolapse QoL (PQoL) tool is a valid and reliable questionnaire to quantify the impact of POP (Digesu et al. 2005).

The International Continence Society (2015) endorses the POP Quantification (POP-Q) tool for objective classification of POP (Bump et al. 1996) (Table 4.11). Examination of prolapse should reproduce the woman's symptomatic activities (Bump et al. 1996).

Physical examination should include PFM strength and function, signs of de-oestrogenisation (which may be amenable to topical treatments) and any relevant test for UI as described above.

Chronic pelvic pain

Definition

'Chronic pelvic pain can be defined as intermittent or constant pain in the lower abdomen or pelvis of at least 6 months' duration' (Royal College of Obstetricians and Gynaecologists 2005). There are a multitude of potential causes, which often overlap as summarised in Table 4.12.

TABLE 4.11 POP-Q classification

Stage 0	No prolapse is demonstrated
Stage 1	The most distal portion of the prolapse is more than 1 cm above the level of the hymen
Stage 2	The most distal portion of the prolapse is 1 cm or less proximal or distal to the hymental plane
Stage 3	The most distal portion of the prolapse protrudes more than 1 cm below the hymen but no further than 2 cm less than the total vaginal length (e.g. not all of the vagina has prolapsed)
Stage 4	Vaginal eversion is essentially complete

Adapted from: Bump, R.C., Mattiasson, A., Bø, K., et al., 1996. The standardization of terminology of female pelvic organ prolapse and pelvic floor dysfunction. American Journal of Obstetrics and Gynecology 175 (1), 10–17.

TABLE 4.12 Examples of causes of chronic pelvic pain

Gynaecological	Urological	Gastrointestinal	Musculoskeletal
Endometriosis	Interstitial cystitis/painful bladder syndrome	Irritable bowel syndrome	Myofascial syndrome/ trigger points
Adenomyosis	Urethral syndrome	Chronic appendicitis	Pelvic floor myalgia
Chronic pelvic inflammatory disease	Chronic urinary tract infection	Inflammatory bowel disease	Chronic visceral pain syndrome
Adhesions	Bladder dysfunction	Diverticular disease	Nerve entrapment
Ovarian cysts	Bladder stones	Hernia	Sacroiliac disorders
Pelvic congestion	Neoplasms	Neoplasms	Disc disease

Adapted from: Stacy, J., Frawley, H., Powell, G., et al., 2012. Persistent pelvic pain: rising to the challenge. Australian and New Zealand Journal of Obstetrics and Gynaecology 52 (6), 502–507.

Clinical features

As per any chronic pain condition, pelvic pain persists beyond the original nociceptive stimulus (May 2008) (such as those outlined above) as will factors such as memory and emotions (Melzack 2001). Ongoing pain is facilitated by changes to the afferent and efferent pathways within the central and peripheral nervous systems (Melzack 2001; Royal College of Obstetricians and Gynaecologists 2005). Pain can be triggered by low intensity noxious input and, significantly, by input that previously would not have triggered a pain response (Moseley 2003).

Clinical significance

Chronic pelvic pain affects one in five Australian women between 16 and 49 years of age (Pitts et al. 2008). Like other urogynaecological problems chronic pelvic pain is associated with significant deficiencies in QoL (Brotto et al. 2015), including depression, sleep disorders, relationship difficulties and loss of employment (Royal College of Obstetricians and Gynaecologists 2005; Stacy et al. 2012).

Pharmacological management

Pharmaceutical treatment will be consistent with the management of chronic pain (see Chapter 7).

PHYSIOTHERAPY PRACTICE POINTS: CHRONIC PELVIC PAIN

As with any chronic pain condition, a biopsychosocial treatment approach proffered by a multidisciplinary team is preferred (Brotto et al. 2014). The team should ideally include gynaecology, pharmacy, physiotherapy, sex therapy and psychology input (Brotto et al. 2014). However, nociceptive triggers may be reduced by physical therapies (Moseley 2003). Soft tissue mobilisation of adhered tissue can improve pain, dyspareunia and sexual satisfaction (Wurn et al. 2011). (See Chapter 7 for medications for chronic pain.)

■ Specific men's health problems

Prostate-related incontinence and sexual dysfunction

Definition

Urinary incontinence and anal incontinence are unfortunate sequelae of the surgical management of prostate cancer (Nahon et al. 2009). They may result from any or a combination of change in urethral length, neurological damage, bladder neck or rhabdosphincter–levator ani damage and OAB (Nahon et al. 2009). Erectile function is often diminished after prostatectomy due to local neuropathy (Nahon et al. 2009).

Clinical features

Incontinence is assessed very similarly to UI in women. However, it is noteworthy that most men report UI later in the day, so a 24-hour pad test may more accurately assess symptom severity (Nahon et al. 2009).

Clinical significance

Early post-prostatectomy incontinence affects half of men in the first month post surgery. Fortunately, incidence drops markedly through the first year, but may be wildly underreported by patients (Nahon et al. 2009). Similar to women, men suffering incontinence may have significantly reduced quality of life (QoL), with embarrassment and social isolation. They may also suffer a sense of loss of manhood. It is commonly understood that men may suffer this burden alone as few will seek professional help (Nahon et al. 2009).

Pharmacological management

Prostate-related urinary incontinence
Selective alpha blockers: These agents block alpha-1 receptors causing relaxation of the smooth muscle in the bladder neck and prostate that decease the resistance to urinary flow. They include alfuzosin, prazosin, tamsulosin and terazosin.

Tamsulosin is more selective for the alpha-1 receptor subtypes found in the bladder and prostate, and therefore is the most commonly used (Australian Medicines Handbook Pty Ltd 2015d).

5-Alpha-reductase inhibitors: These agents inhibit 5-alpha reductase, an enzyme that coverts testosterone to dihydrotestosterone. This reduces prostate size and improves urinary flow. They include dutasteride and finasteride (Australian Medicines Handbook Pty Ltd 2015d).

Erectile dysfunction

Phosphodiesterase type 5 inhibitors are the first-line therapy; they include sildenafil, tatalafil, vardenafil. They are generally dosed 0.5 to 1 hour before sexual activity and do not produce an erection without sexual stimulation and activity (see Table 4.13) (Therapeutic Guidelines Limited 2014e).

TABLE 4.13 Pharmacokinetic properties and doses of phosphodiesterase type 5 inhibitors

		Sildenafil	Tadalafil	Vardenafil
Indications	Erectile dysfunction	✓	✓	✓
	Pulmonary arterial hypertension[a]	✓	✓	
	BPH-related lower urinary tract symptoms			✓
Starting dose		50 mg	10 mg	10 mg
Dose range		25–100 mg	5–20 mg	5–20 mg
Dose in kidney impairment		Initial dose 25 mg if severe impairment	10 mg maximum if severe impairment	Do not use if on dialysis
Dose in hepatic impairment		Initial dose 25 mg	10 mg maximum if mild to moderate impairment	Initial dose 5 mg if mild to moderate impairment (10 mg maximum if moderate impairment)
Peak effect		1 hour (delayed by food)	2 hours	1 hour (delayed by food)
Duration of clinical effect		4–6 hours	24–36 hours	4 hours
Half-life		3–5 hours	17.5 hours	4–5 hours
Metabolism		Hepatic	Hepatic	Hepatic
Comments		Sildenafil is most likely to cause visual changes	Headaches caused by tadalafil last for 3–8 hours	Vardenafil has prolonged the QT interval in healthy volunteers

[a]*See Chapter 2.*
BPH, benign prostatic hyperplasia.
Adapted from: Therapeutic Guidelines Limited, 2014e. Erectile dysfunction [Internet], Table 5.39. <http://online.tg.org.au:2048/ip/tablet/tgc/edg52/29323.htm?rhsearch=Erectile%20dysfunction%20>.

TABLE 4.14 Medications used in prostate related incontinence and sexual dysfunction

Drug name	Mechanism of action	Indications	Common side effects	Practice points	Common dosage range
Selective alpha-blockers Alfuzosin Prazosin Tamsulosin Terazosin	Block alpha, receptors causing smooth muscles in the bladder neck and prostate to relax, and therefore decreasing resistance to urinary flow	Used for symptom relief in BPH	Hypotension, and dizziness (less frequent with alfuzosin and tamsulosin); floppy iris syndrome in cataract surgery (especially with tamsulosin), nasal congestion, urinary urgency, headache, weakness, fatigue, drowsiness	• First-dose hypotension is most serious in the elderly and in patients with fluid depletion or who are taking diuretics • If treatment with prazosin or terazosin is interrupted for several days, restart as if starting for the first time • Monitor BP (lying and standing) • Stop if there is no improvement in symptoms of BPH after 4–6 weeks of maximal treatment	**Alfuzosin** 10 mg once daily **Prazosin** 0.5–2 mg twice daily **Tamsulosin** 400 mcg once daily **Terazosin** 1–10 mg daily Also used in hypertension
5-Alpha-reductase inhibitors Dutasteride Finasteride	Reduce prostate size and BPH symptoms and improve urinary flow rate by inhibition of 5-alpha-reductase, an enzyme which converts testosterone to dihydrotestosterone (a stimulator of prostate growth) Long-term use reduces the risk of acute urinary retention and the need for surgery; finasteride also reduces the risk of of haematuria After 6 months of dutasteride or 1 year of finasteride prostate specific antigen (PSA) concentration is reduced by an average of 50%	Symptomatic BPH with prostate >30–40 cm^3	Impotence, decreased libido, ejaculation disorders	• Men with a prostate <30 cm^3 are unlikely to benefit as efficacy depends on prostate size • Symptoms may not improve until >6 months of treatment • If PSA concentration begins to rise during treatment, assess for prostate cancer • 6 months after stopping treatment, PSA concentrations have generally returned to baseline	**Dutasteride** 500 mcg once daily Available in a fixed dose combination with Tamsulosin **Finasteride** 5 mg once daily

Drug	Mechanism	Indication	Adverse effects / cautions	Dose
Phosphodiesterase 5 inhibitors **Sildenafil** **Tadalafil** **Vardenafil**	During sexual stimulation, cyclic guanosine monophosphate (cGMP) levels increase, causing smooth muscle relaxation, and an inflow of blood to the corpus cavernosum and penile erection. Phosphodiesterase 5 inhibitors stop the breakdown of cGMP, therefore increasing blood flow to the penis during sexual stimulation. Without sexual stimulation they are ineffective	Erectile dysfunction	Headache (>10%), dizziness, flushing, dyspepsia, nasal congestion/rhinitis. Significant hypotension if combined with any nitrate drug (glyceryl trinitrate in any form, isosorbide mononitrate, isosorbide dinitrate, sodium nitroprusside, amyl nitrite, nicorandil). Therefore any combination with nitrates is contraindicated	• Ideal dose should produce an erection that lasts no more than 1 hour • A smaller dose is required to maintain adequate erection at home than in the clinic See Table 4.14 above
Alprostadil (prostaglandin E1)	Relaxes smooth muscle of corpus cavernosum and spongiosum and dilates cavernosal arteries	Erectile dysfunction alone or in combination with other agents	Penile pain, erection lasting 4–6 hours, fibrotic changes (but of the injectable products, alprostadil is the least likely to cause penile fibrosis or priapism)	• Check development of fibrosis at regular follow-up visits with prescriber • Stop treatment if fibrosis develops Give by intracavernosal injection: 10–20 up to 60 mcg. Use no more than 1 injection in 24 hours; up to 3 times a week
Papaverine	Relaxation of all vascular components of the penile erectile system	Erectile dysfunction	Pain and bruising on injection, priapism, penile fibrosis	• Check possible development of fibrosis at regular follow-up visits with prescriber • Stop treatment if fibrosis develops • Tolerance may develop, requiring an increase in dosage *Intracavernosal injection,* initially 5–15 mg. Usual range 30–60 mg
Dapoxetine	A selective serotonin reuptake inhibitor (SSRI), usually used for depression, but thought to modify the ejaculatory reflex	Premature ejaculation	Vomiting (infrequently)	• In controlled trials of dapoxetine, about 62% of men treated with dapoxetine 30 mg reported improvement at week 9–12 compared with 36% of those taking placebo 30 mg taken 1–3 hours before sexual activity; limit to 1 dose in 24 hours

BP, blood pressure; BPH, benign prostatic hyperplasia; SSRI, selective serotonin reuptake inhibitors.
Adapted from: Australian Medicines Handbook Pty Ltd, 2015d. Drugs for benign prostatic hyperplasia and prostatitis. Australian Medicines Handbook [Online]. <https://amhonline-amh-net-au/chapters/chap-13/bph-drugs-for>.

Second-line treatment includes intracavernosal vasodilator injections of prostaglandin E_1 (alprostadil) (Therapeutic Guidelines Limited 2014e).

PHYSIOTHERAPY PRACTICE POINTS: PROSTATE-RELATED INCONTINENCE AND SEXUAL DYSFUNCTION

Post prostatectomy treatment aims at retraining the PFM to assume the function of the defunct intrinsic sphincter (Nahon et al. 2009). PFM training is also effective in restoring erectile function (Nahon et al. 2009). A side effect of 5-alpha-reductase inhibitors can be impotence (Australian Medicines Handbook Pty Ltd 2015b), and the physiotherapist should consider this effect as a cause of sexual dysfunction post prostatectomy. See Table 4.14 for medications patients may be taking to address these conditions.

■ References

Allen, V.M., O'Connell, C.M., Baskett, T.F., 2006. Maternal morbidity associated with cesarean delivery without labor compared with induction of labor at term. Obstetrics & Gynecology 108 (2), 286–294.

Australian Institute of Health and Welfare (AIHW), 2013. Incontinence in Australia. AIHW, Canberra.

Australian Medicines Handbook Pty Ltd, 2015a. Prescribing for pregnant women. Australian Medicines Handbook [Online]. <https://amhonline-amh-net-au.atlantis2.anu.edu.au/guides/guide-pregnancy>.

Australian Medicines Handbook Pty Ltd, 2015b. Anticholinergics (genitourinary). Australian Medicines Handbook [Online]. <https://amhonline-amh-net-au./chapters/chap-13/urinary-incontinence/anticholinergics-02>.

Australian Medicines Handbook Pty Ltd, 2015c. Drugs for urinary incontinence. Australian Medicines Handbook [Online]. <https://amhonline-amh-net-au./chapters/chap-13/urinary-incontinence/urinary-incontinence.t>.

Australian Medicines Handbook Pty Ltd, 2015d. Drugs for benign prostatic hyperplasia and prostatitis. Australian Medicines Handbook [Online]. <https://amhonline-amh-net-au/chapters/chap-13/bph-drugs-for>.

Australian Medicines Handbook Pty Ltd, 2015e. Gastrointestinal drugs. Australian Medicines Handbook [Online]. <https://amhonline-amh-net-au/chapters/chap-12/gastrointestinaldrugs.t>.

Australian Medicines Handbook Pty Ltd, 2015f. Prescribing for breastfeeding women. Australian Medicines Handbook [Online]. <https://amhonline.amh.net.au/>.

Bartoli, S., Aguzzi, G., Tarricone, R., 2010. Impact on quality of life of urinary incontinence and overactive bladder: a systematic literature review. Urology 75 (3), 491–500.

Betzold, C.M., 2007. An update on the recognition and management of lactational breast inflammation. Journal of Midwifery & Women's Health 52 (6), 595–605.

Bø, K., 2007. Pelvic floor muscle training for stress urinary incontinence. In: Bø, K., Berghmans, B., Morkved, S. (Eds.), Evidence-based Physical Therapy for the Pelvic Floor: Bridging science and clinical practice. Elsevier Health Sciences.

Bø, K., 2012. Pelvic floor muscle training in treatment of female stress urinary incontinence, pelvic organ prolapse and sexual dysfunction. World Journal of Urology 30 (4), 437–443.

Bø, K., Hagen, R.H., Kvarstein, B., et al., 1990. Pelvic floor muscle exercise for the treatment of female stress urinary incontinence: III. Effects of two different degrees of pelvic floor muscle exercises. Neurourology and Urodynamics 9 (5), 489–502.

Bø, K., Morkved, S., 2007. Motor learning. In: Bø, K., Berghmans, B., Morkved, S. (Eds.), Evidence-based Physical Therapy for the Pelvic Floor: Bridging science and clinical practice. Elsevier Health Sciences.

Brækken, I.H., Majida, M., Engh, M.E., et al., 2010. Can pelvic floor muscle training reverse pelvic organ prolapse and reduce prolapse symptoms? An assessor-blinded, randomized, controlled trial. American Journal of Obstetrics and Gynecology 203 (2), 170.e1–170.e7.

Brotto, L.A., Yong, P., Smith, K.B., et al., 2015. Impact of a multidisciplinary vulvodynia program on sexual functioning and dyspareunia. The Journal of Sexual Medicine 12 (1), 238–247.

Bump, R.C., Mattiasson, A., Bø, K., et al., 1996. The standardization of terminology of female pelvic organ prolapse and pelvic floor dysfunction. American Journal of Obstetrics and Gynecology 175 (1), 10–17.

Callinan-Moore, K., The Lymphatic system. Course notes from The Lactating Breast for Physiotherapists Level 1, 2012.

Chiarelli, P.E., Mackenzie, L.A., Osmotherly, P.G., 2009. Urinary incontinence is associated with an increase in falls: a systematic review. The Australian Journal of Physiotherapy 55 (2), 89–95.

Cusack, L., Brennan, M., 2011. Lactational mastitis and breast abscess: diagnosis and management in general practice. Australian Family Physician 40 (12), 976.

Digesu, G.A., Khullar, V., Cardozo, L., et al., 2005. P-QOL: a validated questionnaire to assess the symptoms and quality of life of women with urogenital prolapse. International Urogynecology Journal and Pelvic Floor Dysfunction 16 (3), 176–181.

Drake, M.J., Apostolidis, A., Emmanuel, A., et al., 2013. Neurologic urinary and faecal incontinence. In: Abrams, P., Cardozo, L., Khoury, S., et al. (Eds.), Incontinence, fifth ed. International Continence Society, Paris, France.

East, C.E., Sherburn, M., Nagle, C., et al., 2012. Perineal pain following childbirth: prevalence, effects on postnatal recovery and analgesia usage. Midwifery 28 (1), 93–97.

Frawley, H.C., Phillips, B.A., Bø, K., et al., 2010. Physiotherapy as an adjunct to prolapse surgery: an assessor-blinded randomized controlled trial. Neurourology and Urodynamics 29 (5), 719–725.

Hagen, S., Stark, D., 2011. Conservative prevention and management of pelvic organ prolapse in women. The Cochrane Database of Systematic Reviews (12), CD003882, doi:10.1002/14651858.CD003882.pub4.

International Continence Society, 2013a. ICS factsheets: Faecal incontinence. The International Continence Society, 2013.

International Continence Society, 2013b. ICS factsheets: Neurogenic bladder. The International Continence Society, 2013.

International Continence Society, 2015. ICS factsheets: A background to urinary and faecal incontinence. The International Continence Society. Bristol, United Kingdom.

Irwin, D.E., Kopp, Z.S., Agatep, B., et al., 2011. Worldwide prevalence estimates of lower urinary tract symptoms, overactive bladder, urinary incontinence and bladder outlet obstruction. BJU International 108 (7), 1132–1138.

Kanakaris, N.K., Roberts, C.S., Giannoudis, P.V., 2011. Pregnancy-related pelvic girdle pain: an update. BMC Medicine 9 (1), 15.

Kase, K., Wallis, J., Kase, T., 2003. Clinical Therapeutic Applications of the Kinesio Taping Method, second ed. Ken Ikai Co Ltd, Tokyo.

Kumar, R., 2012. Anal incontinence and quality of life following obstetric anal sphincter injury. Archives of Gynecology and Obstetrics 285 (3), 591–597.

Lone, F., Sultan, A., Thakar, R., 2012. Obstetric pelvic floor and anal sphincter injuries. The Obstetrician & Gynaecologist 14 (4), 257–266.

Lumley, J., Amir, L., 2006. Women's experience of lactational mastitis: 'I have never felt worse'. Australian Family Physician 35 (9), 745.

MacArthur, C., Glazener, C., Lancashire, R., et al., 2011. Exclusive caesarean section delivery and subsequent urinary and faecal incontinence: a 12-year longitudinal study. BJOG: An International Journal of Obstetrics & Gynaecology 118 (8), 1001–1007.

Marti, B.G., Valentini, F.A., Robain, G., 2014. Contribution of behavioral and cognitive therapy to managing overactive bladder syndrome in women in the absence of contributive urodynamic diagnosis. International Urogynecology Journal 1–5.

May, A., 2008. Chronic pain may change the structure of the brain. Pain 137, 7–15.

Melzack, R., 2001. Pain and the neuromatrix in the brain. Journal of Dental Education 65 (12), 1378–1382.

Moseley, G.L., 2003. A pain neuromatrix approach to patients with chronic pain. Manual Therapy 8 (3), 130–140.

Nahon, I., Waddington, G.S., Dorey, G., et al., 2009. Assessment and conservative management of post-prostatectomy incontinence after radical prostatectomy. The Australian and New Zealand Continence Journal 15 (3), 70.

Norton, C., Cody, J.D., Hosker, G., 2006. Biofeedback and/or sphincter exercises for the treatment of faecal incontinence in adults. The Cochrane Database of Systematic Reviews (3), CD002111.

NPS Medicinewise, 2014. Medicines in pregnancy – safe? Health News and Evidence [Internet]. <http://www.nps.org.au/publications/health-professional/health-news-evidence/2014/pregnancy-medicine-safety> (accessed 19.04.16.).

Osterman, M., Ilyas, A.M., Matzon, J.L., 2012. Carpal tunnel syndrome in pregnancy. Orthopedic Clinics of North America 43 (4), 515–520.

Pitts, M.K., Ferris, J.A., Smith, A., et al., 2008. Prevalence and correlates of three types of pelvic pain in a nationally representative sample of Australian women. The Medical Journal of Australia 189 (3), 138–143.

Rahn, D.D., Good, M.M., Roshanravan, S.M., et al., 2014. Effects of preoperative local estrogen in postmenopausal women with prolapse: a randomized trial. Journal of Clinical Endocrinology and Metabolism 99 (10), 3728–3736.

Robson, S.J., Tan, W.S., Adeyemi, A., et al., 2009. Estimating the rate of cesarean section by maternal request: anonymous survey of obstetricians in Australia. Birth (Berkeley, Calif.) 36 (3), 208–212.

Roos, A.M., Thakar, R., Sultan, A., 2010. Outcome of primary repair of obstetric anal sphincter injuries (OASIS): does the grade of tear matter? Ultrasound in Obstetrics & Gynecology 36 (3), 368–374.

Royal Australian and New Zealand College of Obstetricians and Gynaecologists, Caesarean Delivery on Maternal Request (CDMR). 2013.

Royal College of Obstetricians and Gynaecologists, 2005. Greentop Guideline No. 41: The initial management of chronic pelvic pain. Royal College of Obstetricians and Gynaecologists, London.

Royal College of Obstetricians and Gynaecologists, 2007. Green-top Guideline No. 29: The management of third and fourth degree perineal tears. Royal College of Obstetricians and Gynaecologists, London.

Rømmen, K., Schei, B., Rydning, A., et al., 2012. Prevalence of anal incontinence among Norwegian women: a cross-sectional study. BMJ Open 2 (4), doi:10.1136/bmjopen-2012-001257.

Skinner, E.M., Dietz, H.P., 2015. Psychological and somatic sequelae of traumatic vaginal delivery: a literature review. Australian and New Zealand Journal of Obstetrics and Gynaecology 55 (4), 309–314.

Stacy, J., Frawley, H., Powell, G., et al., 2012. Persistent pelvic pain: rising to the challenge. Australian and New Zealand Journal of Obstetrics and Gynaecology 52 (6), 502–507.

Stewart, W., Van Rooyen, J., Cundiff, G., et al., 2003. Prevalence and burden of overactive bladder in the United States. World Journal of Urology 20 (6), 327–336.

Tan, J.-L., Ruane, T., Sherburn, M., 2013. The role of physiotherapy after obstetric anal sphincter injury: an overview of current clinical practice. The Australian and New Zealand Continence Journal 19 (1), 6–11.

Therapeutic Goods Administration, 2011. Australian Categorisation System for Prescribing Medicines in Pregnancy [Internet]. <https://www.tga.gov.au/australian-categorisation-system-prescribing-medicines-pregnancy> (accessed 19.04.16.).

Therapeutic Guidelines Limited, 2010. Musculoskeletal conditions in pregnancy: common conditions [Internet]. <http://online.tg.org.au:2048/ip/tablet/tgc/rhg/5381.htm?rhsearch=Musculoskeletal%20conditions%20in%20pregnancy%3A%20common%20conditions%20> (accessed 07.05.).

Therapeutic Guidelines Limited, 2012. The transition from acute to chronic pain: postsurgical pain syndromes [Internet]. <http://online.tg.org.au:2048/ip/tablet/tgc/agg/7858.htm?rhsearch=The%20transition%20from%20acute%20to%20chronic%20pain%3A%20postsurgical%20pain%20syndromes%20> (accessed 03.15.).

Therapeutic Guidelines Limited, 2014a. Antibacterial prophylaxis in obstetric patients [Internet]. <https://tgldcdp-tg-org-au.atlantis2.anu.edu.au/viewTopic?topicfile=infection-prevention-medical&guidelineName=Antibiotic#toc_d1e1177> (accessed 04.15.).

Therapeutic Guidelines Limited, 2014b. Mastitis [Internet]. <http://online.tg.org.au:2048/ip/tablet/tgc/abg/23386.htm?rhsearch=mastitis> (accessed 03.15.).

Therapeutic Guidelines Limited, 2014c. Prophylaxis: obstetric and gynaecological surgery [Internet]. <http://online.tg.org.au:2048/ip/tablet/tgc/abg/13264.htm?rhsearch=Prophylaxis%3A%20obstetric%20and%20gynaecological%20surgery%20> (accessed 03.15.).

Therapeutic Guidelines Limited, 2014d. Wound infections [Internet]. <http://online.tg.org.au:2048/ip/tablet/tgc/abg/25255.htm?rhsearch=Surgical%20site%20infection%20> (accessed 03.15.).

Therapeutic Guidelines Limited, 2014e. Erectile dysfunction [Internet]. <http://online.tg.org.au:2048/ip/tablet/tgc/edg52/29323.htm?rhsearch=Erectile%20dysfunction%20> (accessed 03.15.).

Thiagamoorthy, G., Johnson, A., Thakar, R., et al., 2014. National survey of perineal trauma and its subsequent management in the United Kingdom. International Urogynecology Journal 1–7.

Toglia, M.R., 2011. Repair of episiotomy and perineal lacerations associated with childbirth. UpToDate [Internet]. <http://www.uptodate.com/contents/repair-of-episiotomy-and-perineal-lacerations-associated-with-childbirth> (accessed 19.04.15.).

Torkan, B., Parsay, S., Lamyian, M., et al., 2009. Postnatal quality of life in women after normal vaginal delivery and caesarean section. BMC Pregnancy and Childbirth 9 (1), 4.

Vleeming, A., Albert, H.B., Östgaard, H.C., et al., 2008. European guidelines for the diagnosis and treatment of pelvic girdle pain. European Spine Journal 17 (6), 794–819.

Wurn, B.F., Wurn, L.J., Patterson, K., et al., 2011. Decreasing dyspareunia and dysmenorrhea in women with endometriosis via a manual physical therapy: results from two independent studies. Journal of Endometriosis 3, 188–196.

CHAPTER 5

Orthopaedic and musculoskeletal systems

Joanne Morris, Miriam Lawrence, Bryan Ashman

OBJECTIVES

This chapter will discuss the role that medications have in the supplementary management of the most common musculoskeletal conditions treated by physiotherapists. By the end of this chapter (including cross-referencing with other relevant chapters) the reader should have an understanding of:

+ the major classification of musculoskeletal disorders according to structure, location, signs and symptoms
+ pharmacotherapy options for the major musculoskeletal disorders
+ usual dosages, routes of administration and major contraindications and precautions of these medications
+ any potential impact of these medications on physiotherapeutic management.

OVERVIEW

Arthritis
Osteoarthritis
Septic arthritis
Rheumatoid arthritis and other synovial joint disorders
Psoriatic arthritis
Crystal arthropathies

Joint conditions
Adhesive capsulitis
Avascular necrosis
Osteomyelitis
Tumours

Maxillofacial disorders
Trigeminal neuralgia
Temporomandibular joint disorders
Bell's palsy

Soft tissue conditions
Soft tissue injuries – sprains, strains and contusions
Acute tendon pain
Subacute/chronic tendon pain

Nerve compression syndromes
Bursitis
Connective tissue disorders

Spinal conditions
Ankylosing spondylitis
Spondylosis/spondyloarthropathy

Trauma
Fractures/acute trauma
Dislocation

Miscellaneous

■ Introduction

Musculoskeletal conditions are conditions of the bones, muscles and their attachments (e.g. joints and ligaments) (Australian Institute of Health and Welfare [AIHW] 2015).

According to the Australian Institute of Health and Welfare (AIHW) 28% of Australians, approximately 6.1 million people, have arthritis and other musculoskeletal conditions (AIHW 2015) (see Figure 5.1).

Fourteen percent of Australians (3.0 million) are affected by back conditions, 8% with osteoarthritis (1.8 million), 3% with osteoporosis (728,000) and 2% with rheumatoid arthritis (445,000) according to 2011–12 self-reported figures (AIHW 2015).

Physiotherapists are key members of the primary and secondary care treating teams for patients with musculoskeletal disorders (MSD) and often are the primary treating clinician. Physiotherapy is a clinically- and cost-effective management strategy for patients with a musculoskeletal disorder. The most common complaints of patients with an MSD are pain, swelling and altered function. Therefore, the predominant reason a patient with an MSD takes medication is to manage pain and inflammation.

In this chapter the classification of musculoskeletal disorders proposed by the National Institute for Health and Care Excellence (NICE) will be followed (NICE 2015):

1 arthritis
2 congenital conditions (not included)
3 joint conditions
4 maxillofacial conditions
5 soft tissue conditions
6 spinal conditions
7 trauma
8 vasculitis.

Overview of general factors affecting choice of medication
This chapter follows the Australian approved indications as specified in the Therapeutic Goods Administration approved product information. Emphasis

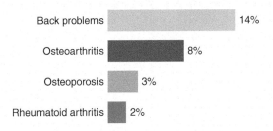

Figure 5.1 Percentage of Australians with musculoskeletal conditions.
Adapted with permission from: Australian Institute of Health and Welfare (AIHW), 2015. Arthritis, Osteoporosis and Other Musculoskeletal Conditions. <http://www.aihw.gov.au/arthritis-and-musculoskeletal-conditions/>.

will be placed on those signs and symptoms and conditions most frequently treated by physiotherapists and where the physiotherapist's input is vital in monitoring the effects of the prescribed medications. The focus of this chapter will be on the major medications prescribed for specific musculoskeletal disorders and their relevance for the physiotherapist (Table 5.1). As indicated, many of the medications prescribed for musculoskeletal disorders are discussed in detail in other chapters of this handbook.

Each category and the specific subgroup of medications will be reviewed in terms of mechanism of action, route of administration, effects and adverse effects. A range of medication options are available for the treatment and/or management of musculoskeletal disorders and physiotherapists are often involved in discussions regarding treatment options. In addition to the impact of the physiotherapy intervention on the patient, the treating physiotherapist can also monitor the impact of the medications intervention using appropriate outcome measures.

PHYSIOTHERAPY PRACTICE POINTS: MUSCULOSKELETAL DISORDERS

The main complaints of patients with an MSD are pain, swelling, stiffness and altered functional capacity. An integral component of a physiotherapist's assessment is to gain an understanding of the severity and irritability of the patient's symptoms and, through thorough assessment, the underlying disease processes. Understanding the underlying disease processes assists the clinical reasoning of the treating team in relation to the provision and monitoring of medications.

The pathophysiology of pain is addressed in Chapter 7. Figure 5.2 provides a basic understanding of the pathophysiology of inflammation at the organ and tissue level, thus providing valuable information regarding the mechanism of action of medications used to treat inflammation.

TABLE 5.1 Medications used in musculoskeletal disorders

General category	Specific group	Relevance for physiotherapist	Where addressed
Medications used for musculoskeletal disorders – symptom orientated	Pain	+++	See Chapter 7 for additional information
	Inflammation	+++	This chapter
	Muscle spasm	+++	This chapter
Medications used for musculoskeletal disorders – disease orientated	Antibiotics	+	This chapter
	Anti-inflammatories	+++	This chapter
	Autoimmune	++	This chapter
	Osteopenia/porosis	++	Chapter 8

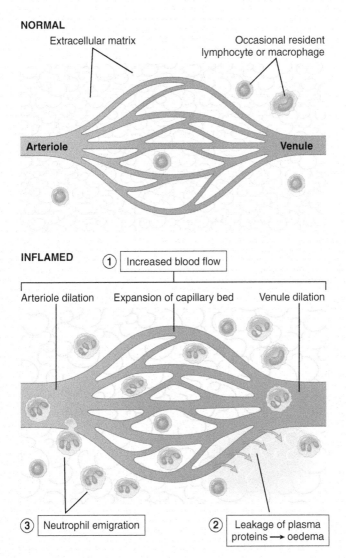

Figure 5.2 Acute inflammation.
Reproduced with permission from: Kumar, V., Abbas, A.K., Aster, J.C., 2013. Robbins Basic Pathology, ninth ed. Elsevier Sanders, Philadelphia, pp. 29–73.

Figure 5.3 highlights the mechanism of action of medications commonly used in the management of inflammation (COX-1 and COX-2 inhibitors). For further information regarding basic pharmacology and pharmacokinetic concepts please see Chapter 1.

Table 5.2 describes the structure, location and signs and symptoms of musculoskeletal disorders in terms of the sites of action for associated medication; disease-specific information and detailed medication management are described in Table 5.3.

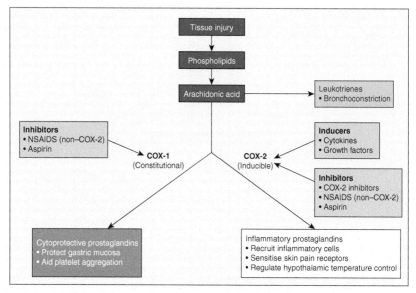

Figure 5.3 Action of non-steroidal anti-inflammatory drugs (NSAIDs).
Adapted with permission from: Stovitz, S.D., Johnson, R.J., 2003. NSAIDs and musculoskeletal treatment: what is the clinical evidence? The Physician and Sports Medicine *31*. <*http://www.chiro.org/LINKS/FULL/ NSAIDs_and_Musculoskeletal_Treatment.html*>.

TABLE 5.2 Structure, location, signs and symptoms of medication action in musculoskeletal disorders

Structure	Location	Signs and symptoms [a]
Tissue level	Local tissue trauma	Pain, swelling and muscle spasm
Central nervous system	Dorsal horn	Pain, muscle spasm

[a]See Table 5.3 for descriptions of the various signs and symptoms.

Depending on the structure(s) affected and the nature of the patient's condition (e.g. autoimmune) the clinical signs and symptoms will vary. Listed in Table 5.3 are the clinical characteristics, anatomical locations (where applicable) and signs and symptoms for which physiotherapy treatment may be applicable.

Table 5.4 outlines the disease mechanisms of some of the common MDSs treated by physiotherapists – providing further clarity regarding the mechanism of action of the medications used in the treatment of common conditions. This will be explored in greater detail under disease-specific medication regimens later in the chapter.

Conditions will be subdivided according the NICE classification of musculoskeletal disorders and common medication management will be highlighted.

Text continued on p. 115

TABLE 5.3 Definitions and clinical features of major signs and symptoms seen in musculoskeletal disorders

Musculoskeletal disorders classification	Signs/symptoms/specific diagnosis	Clinical characteristics	Anatomic location
Arthritis	Pain	Pain is the most commonly reported complaint of patients with arthritis – ranging from acute to chronic pain, which can be mild to severe in nature	Various
	Inflammation	Swelling often occurs in acute flares of arthritic complaints	Various
	Stiffness	Loss of movement in the affected joints, which may be associated with chronic synovitis	Affected joints
	Weight gain	The reasons for weight gain can be multifactorial, but include reduced activity levels (which may be secondary to pain) and co-morbidities (such as metabolic disease)	
	Muscle weakness	Muscle weakness can be driven by altered movement patterns, swelling (e.g. intraarticular swelling of the knee), reduced activity levels and co-morbidities (e.g. stroke)	
	Infection	Patients with septic arthritis are pyrexial, report acute severe pain, swelling and often erythema	Generally large joints including knee, shoulder and elbow
Joint conditions	Adhesive capsulitis	Patients with adhesive capsulitis are generally over the age of 35, with pain in the shoulder of their dominant arm that is generally worse at night There has been a global loss of range of movement; however there is often a more marked loss of external rotation range (Walmsley, Osmotherly and Rivett 2014) Risk factors include: type 1 or 2 diabetes mellitus, thyroid disease, myocardial infarction and prolonged periods of immobility (Kelley et al. 2013)	Shoulder
	Rheumatoid arthritis and other synovial joint disorders	Rheumatoid arthritis is a systemic, inflammatory, autoimmune disorder that results in joint destruction and persistent inflammation of synovial tissue (synovitis) Results in musculoskeletal pain and swelling, as a result of the destructive erosion of bone and a loss in joint integrity Reportedly affects 2% of Australians (AIHW 2015)	Various

Continued

TABLE 5.3 Definitions and clinical features of major signs and symptoms seen in musculoskeletal disorders—cont'd

Musculoskeletal disorders classification	Signs/symptoms/specific diagnosis	Clinical characteristics	Anatomic location
	Psoriatic arthritis	Psoriasis is characterised by erythematous, scaly patches of skin and nails. Patients with psoriatic arthritis (PsA) may have spondylitis, oligoarthritis [a] or polyarthritis, presenting as pain, stiffness and inflammation, but it may also affect ligaments, tendons and fascial tissue	Various
	Crystal arthropathies	Gout is often characterised by rapid onset of severe pain, swelling, warmth, erythema and decreased range of movement in the affected joint (Khanna et al. 2014). Pain is the overriding symptom	Knee, big toe, various
Maxillofacial conditions	Pain	Conditions such as trigeminal neuralgia, temporomandibular joint (TMJ) disorders (including osteoarthritis) and Bell's palsy are commonly treated by physiotherapy and are associated with pain and/or altered sensation and/or muscle weakness	TMJ, ocular pain, tingling in the cheek/mouth
	Inflammation	Acute injury and flare of arthritis may be associated with swelling to the affected area	Affected area
	Stiffness	Loss of movement in the affected joints, which may be associated with chronic synovitis	Affected area
	Infection	Dental and/or infection is a differential diagnosis for patients with maxillofacial conditions	Affected area
	Benign paroxysmal positional vertigo	Sudden onset of severe positional dizziness that can be associated with nausea and vomiting	
Soft tissue conditions – including connective tissue disorders	Pain	Sprains, strains and contusions are associated with pain to the affected area	Affected area
	Inflammation	Sprains, strains and contusions are associated with swelling and erythema to the affected area, which in some cases may result in nerve compression and therefore be associated with paraesthesia, tingling etc	Affected area. Nerve compression syndromes such as carpal tunnel syndrome

		Affected area
Stiffness	The affected area quickly becomes stiff secondary to pain, swelling and altered function	
Infection	Pain, swelling and erythema coupled with fever	Common around the olecranon bursae
Systemic lupus erythematosus	A chronic, inflammatory, multifactorial autoimmune connective tissue disorder Common features of the disease include a butterfly rash around the eyes, polyarthritis, haematological manifestations, nephritis and photosensitivity (Tarr et al. 2015; Yeun & Cunningham 2014) Characterised by unpredictable periods of exacerbation (flares) and remission (Yeun & Cunningham 2014)	Various
Scleroderma	A chronic autoimmune connective tissue disorder, of which there are two major types: localised scleroderma and systemic sclerosis Both are characterised by excess collagen in the connective tissues Localised scleroderma affects only the skin and occasionally the tissues beneath the skin, resulting in stiffness locally Systemic sclerosis also affects the skin and underlying tissues, but additionally the gastrointestinal tract, lungs, heart and kidneys can be affected (Arif et al. 2015) through widespread vascular lesions and fibrosis of the skin and internal organs	
Spinal conditions		
Pain	The symptoms of musculoskeletal spinal conditions are highly variable and have a relatively low correlation with radiographic and anatomical findings (Gibson & Waddell 2005) Presenting complaints may include spine pain, leg and/or arm symptoms (pain, paraesthesia), functional impairment and headaches	Cervical, thoracic or lumbosacral spine
Stiffness	Patients frequently report stiffness and reduced range of motion	Cervical, thoracic or lumbosacral spine
Muscle spasm	Acute or acute-on-chronic flares are often associated with muscle spasm	Cervical, thoracic or lumbosacral spine

Continued

TABLE 5.3 Definitions and clinical features of major signs and symptoms seen in musculoskeletal disorders—cont'd

Musculoskeletal disorders classification	Signs/symptoms/specific diagnosis	Clinical characteristics	Anatomic location
	Infection	Patients with septic arthritis and/or discitis are pyrexial, report acute severe pain	Cervical, thoracic or lumbosacral spine
	Ankylosing spondylitis	Patients present with pain, stiffness and reduced mobility in the lumbar spine and sacroiliac joints Commonly associated with peripheral arthritis, enthesitis and acute anterior uveitis (Dagfinrud, Kvien & Hagen 2008)	Lumbosacral spine is most commonly affected
Trauma – fractures and dislocation	Pain	Depending on the severity of the injury this is often associated with moderate to severe pain of the affected area In the case of both fracture and dislocation the possibility of neurovascular compromise is high, resulting in paraesthesia, tingling etc	Various
	Inflammation	Depending on the severity of the injury this is often associated with moderate to severe swelling of the affected area	Various
	Muscle spasm	Acute fractures and dislocations are often associated with muscle spasm	Various
	Infection (prophylactic medication)	Open fractures and dislocations require prophylactic treatment for infection	Various
Vasculitis	Pain and inflammation	The symptoms of vasculitis are highly variable and dependent on the affected area, however they may include: • fever • loss of appetite • weight loss • fatigue • general aches and pains	Various

[a]*Oligoarthritis is arthritis affecting one to four joints during the first 6 months of disease.*

TABLE 5.4 Disease mechanisms in musculoskeletal disorders and examples of disease states for each category	
Mechanism(s)	Disorder(s)
Vascular	Haematoma Avascular necrosis Deep vein thrombosis
Inflammatory/autoimmune	Rheumatoid arthritis Systemic lupus erythematosus Psoriatic arthritis Ankylosing spondylitis
Infections	Osteomyelitis Septic arthritis Infective bursitis
Degenerative/genetic	Osteoarthritis
Neoplastic	Sarcoma (Ewing's, chondrosarcoma and osteosarcoma) Soft tissue sarcoma
Trauma	Fracture, soft tissue sprain, strain and contusion
Metabolic/nutritious/toxic	Osteopenia

Arthritis

Osteoarthritis

Osteoarthritis (OA) is one of the primary causes of illness in the world, affecting 8% of the Australian population (AIHW 2015); hip and knee arthritis alone is a leading cause of global disability (Cross et al. 2014; Reid et al. 2014; Woolf & Pfleger 2003).

Pharmacological management

Oral treatment
Regular paracetamol is currently the recommended first-line treatment (see Table 5.11 later), and is combined with NSAIDs (see Table 5.12 later) if symptoms are not controlled with paracetamol alone. An anti-inflammatory dose of fish oil may also have benefit in osteoarthritis (Therapeutic Guidelines Limited 2010a).

However, a recent meta-analysis has indicated that the evidence for single therapy paracetamol is lacking, and has questioned its role as single therapy in the treatment of OA (da Costa et al. 2015).

Topical treatment
Topical NSAIDs and capsaicin treatments (see Table 5.14 later) have been shown to improve short-term (up to 10 days) pain when compared to placebo rubs (Therapeutic Guidelines Limited 2010a).

Intraarticular treatment
A single intraarticular corticosteroid injection can provide symptomatic relief for up to 4 weeks and up to 12 weeks in hip and trapeziometacarpal joint

osteoarthritis (see Table 5.15 later). The effect of repeated doses appears to be less successful, and a general guide is that an individual joint should not be injected more than 4 times per year (Therapeutic Guidelines Limited 2010a).

These injections should only be given by, or under the supervision of, experienced clinicians. Local anaesthetic may be used before, or mixed with, the corticosteroid.

Only corticosteroids specifically formulated for the purpose should be used for intraarticular injection or injection into soft tissue.

Table 5.5 gives examples of appropriate doses. The dose must be adjusted to the specific requirements of the patient according to the size of the joint or soft tissue lesion, the severity of the condition, the response obtained and the patient's tolerance of the corticosteroid. The total volume of the injection administered will vary depending on the amount of local anaesthetic (see Table 5.15).

Other treatment

Patient uptake of the use of glucosamine sulfate and chondroitin sulfate for symptomatic benefit in osteoarthritis has been widespread despite limited

TABLE 5.5 Examples of doses of local corticosteroid injections

Corticosteroid	Dose				Comments
	Small joint (e.g. hand)	Medium sized joint (e.g. wrist)	Large joint (e.g. knee)	Soft tissue (e.g. bursa)	
Betamethasone sodium phosphate + betamethasone acetate 5.7 mg/mL	0.5–1 mL	1 mL	1–2 mL	1–2 mL	Usually used for injection into smaller joints
Methylprednisolone acetate 40 mg/mL	n/a	1 mL	1–2 mL	1–2 mL	Methyprednisolone is crystalline and is formulated as a suspension It is not suitable for injection into small joints or superficial soft tissue sites, where it may cause fat atrophy and can be an irritant It could be used in a large bursa such as a trochanteric bursa
Triamcinolone acetonide 10 mg/mL	0.5–1 mL	1 mL	1–2 mL	1–2 mL	Triamcinolone acetonide is the least soluble injection and provides the longest duration of action (up to 21 weeks)
Triamcinolone acetonide 40 mg/mL	n/a	n/a	0.5 mL	n/a	

Adapted from: Therapeutic Guidelines Limited, 2010. Joint aspiration and injection, Table 12.6. In: eTG complete [Internet]. Therapeutic Guidelines Limited, Melbourne.

evidence (see Table 5.14 later). For patients with osteoarthritis of the knee who want to try alternative therapies a 3–6 month trial of glucosamine sulfate either with or without chondroitin sulfate may be indicated, although not strongly supported by evidence (Therapeutic Guidelines Limited 2010a; Towheed et al. 2005).

For patients who have uncontrolled pain and where surgery is pending or not possible, oral opioids may be tried (see Table 5.13 later). The risk of adverse effects is high and the benefit is minimal, so this approach must be made with caution (Therapeutic Guidelines Limited 2010a).

For further information see Chapter 7.

PHYSIOTHERAPY PRACTICE POINTS: OSTEOARTHRITIS

It is common practice for corticosteroid injections to be used in conjunction with physiotherapy as a means of improving functional status, strength and range of movement while the patient is experiencing lower pain levels (Hawkins & Ghazi 2012; Jowett et al. 2013; Roddy et al. 2014). Physiotherapists are therefore directly involved in the care of patients post-injection. Patients are commonly advised to undertake gentle range of movement exercises of the injected joint 0–48 hours after the injection as this will assist with the circulation of the corticosteroid around the joint. There is variability in the post-injection advice, depending on site/structure injected, however generally patients should be advised to avoid any heavy activity for 5–7 days post-injection (Brukner & Khan 2012). This is particularly important as it is possible that patients will feel significantly better post-injection and therefore are likely to increase their activity levels. Outcomes from corticosteroid injections are mixed: they are used to provide short-term relief (1–6 weeks), but no long-term benefit is evident in the majority of cases (Jüni et al. 2015).

It is widely accepted that exercise is an essential component of OA management, in which physiotherapists play a significant role (French et al. 2013). Depending on the pain medication of the patient, the physiotherapist can provide guidance regarding the best time to undertake exercise in accordance with the efficacy of the pain medication – for specific information regarding the duration of action of pain medications see Tables 5.11, 5.12, 5.13 and 5.14.

Septic arthritis

Definition

Septic arthritis is an infection of a joint that may be bacterial, fungal, mycobacterial or viral in origin (Carpenter et al. 2011).

Clinical significance

Permanent disability and increased mortality are associated with a delayed diagnosis of septic arthritis. In the presence of infection the cartilage of the joint can be destroyed in a matter of days if antibiotic management is not commenced (Carpenter et al. 2011).

Pharmacological management

Diagnostic specimens should always be taken before starting antibiotic therapy. Pus should be drained and the joint irrigated to reduce the pathogen load, protect the articular surface and improve the diffusion of the antibiotic into the joint.

Empirical therapy is the same as what would be used in long bone osteomyelitis (see 'Osteomyelitis' below). Directed therapy should then be guided by microbiology results of cultures and susceptibility testing from the aspirate.

Once directed therapy starts, antibiotic therapy must continue for the following duration (Therapeutic Guidelines Limited 2010c):

+ neonate – 3 weeks (all IV therapy)
+ child – 3 weeks (minimum of 3 days of IV therapy)
+ adult – 4 weeks (minimum of 2 weeks of IV therapy).

Rheumatoid arthritis and other synovial joint disorders

Rheumatoid arthritis

Definition

Rheumatoid arthritis (RA) is a chronic, systemic, inflammatory, progressive, autoimmune disease, with joint synovitis as its predominant clinical manifestation (Breedland et al. 2011; Iversen, Chhabriya & Shadick 2011).

Clinical significance

RA affects around 400,000 Australians and is the second most common type of arthritis, after osteoarthritis. The disease is more common among females and in older age groups (AIHW 2009). Further tests including blood tests and imaging are required to confirm a diagnosis of RA.

Pharmacological management

Rheumatoid arthritis treatment can be described in four groups as listed in Table 5.6 below.

Recommendations for treatment of early RA are described in Figure 5.4. For further pain management information see Chapter 7.

Figures 5.4 and 5.5 detail recommendations for the progression of medications in the management of early RA (under 6 months), first-line treatments and when medications should be increased or changed according to the patient's prognosis and the disease activity. Specifically, Figure 5.5 highlights the '2012 update of the 2008 American College of Rheumatology recommendations for the use of disease-modifying antirheumatic drugs and biologic agents in the treatment of rheumatoid arthritis' (Singh et al. 2012).

Psoriatic arthritis

Definition and clinical significance

Psoriatic arthritis (PsA) is a chronic, systemic inflammatory disease, classified as a seronegative spondyloarthropathy (Cinar et al. 2015). Sufferers of psoriasis include 1–3% of the population of the world, and 42% go on to develop psoriatic arthritis. It is therefore estimated that PsA has a prevalence of 0.1–1.0% in the general population (Mease & Armstrong 2014).

TABLE 5.6 Medication management of rheumatoid arthritis (RA)

Class of treatment	Examples of medications used	Place in therapy, extra information
Disease-modifying antirheumatic drugs (DMARDs)	Methotrexate (MTX) Hydroxychloroquine (HCQ) Sulfasalazine Leflunomide (LEF) Cyclosporin	Reduce or resolve synovial inflammation and therefore prevent joint damage Can be used alone or in combination and all have dose limiting side effects Choice depends on arthritis severity, patient's age, childrearing status and coexisting conditions
Corticosteroids	Prednisolone/prednisone (prednis(ol)one) Hydrocortisone Betamethoasone Ortisone Dexamethasone Methylprednisolone Triamcinolone	Used while waiting for a response from a DMARD or to achieve remission quickly, either as pulse oral, intravenous or intramuscular therapy or as intraarticular therapy Long-term significant adverse effects (e.g. cardiovascular and osteoporosis) that limit long-term use
Biological disease-modifying antirheumatic drugs (DMARDs)	Abatacept Adalimumab Certolizumab Etanercept Golimumab Infliximab Tocilizumab Anakinra	Are considered if remission is not achieved with the appropriate use of DMARDs Should only be used under the supervision of experienced specialists, and the Australian Rheumatology Association has specific recommendations for when and how they are to be used (Australian Rheumatology Association 2011) Before commencing treatment patients must be screened for tuberculosis and hepatitis B and C as the immunosuppression caused by DMARDs can cause these diseases to re-emerge
Symptom management	NSAIDs	NSAIDs improve symptoms of RA, but do not reduce joint damage and have significant adverse effects Used before DMARD therapy is started or intermittently during flare-ups
	Fish oil	Has been shown to reduce symptoms and the need for NSAIDs and may also give cardiovascular protection
	Analgesia (paracetamol and opiates)	Should be used to facilitate activity rather than to relieve pain Paracetamol should be used to reduce the NSAID load Opiates should only be added if paracetamol and NSAIDS do not adequately control pain or ability to function or exercise and should only be used for a fixed short period of time such as 3 weeks See Chapter 7 for more detail

NSAIDs, non-steroidal anti-inflammatory drugs.
Adapted from: Therapeutic Guidelines Limited, 2010. Rheumatoid arthritis: pharmacological management. In: eTG complete [Internet]. Therapeutic Guidelines Limited, Melbourne. See Table 5.19 later for further information.

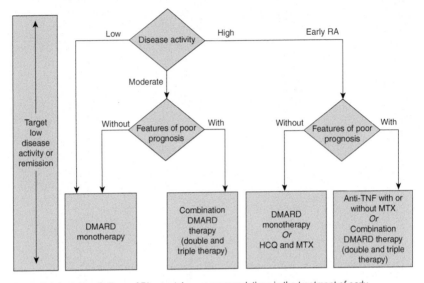

Figure 5.4 American College of Rheumatology recommendations in the treatment of early rheumatoid arthritis (disease duration less than 6 months).
Adapted with permission from: Singh, J.A., Furst, D.E., Bharat, A., et al., 2012. 2012 update of the 2008 American College of Rheumatology recommendations for the use of disease-modifying antirheumatic drugs and biologic agents in the treatment of rheumatoid arthritis (RA). Arthritis Care and Research 64 (5), 625–639. Copyright © 2012 by the American College of Rheumatology.

Pharmacological management

NSAIDs and intraarticular corticosteroid injections are usually first line, with DMARDs used in resistant cases (see Tables 5.12 and 5.15). In polyarticular cases DMARDs are always used (see Tables 5.18 and 5.19 later). Fish oil is also used as an NSAID-sparing agent, as recommended in the Australian Therapeutic Guidelines (Therapeutic Guidelines Limited 2010e).

Methotrexate is the DMARD of choice in psoriatic arthritis as it benefits both the arthritis and the skin. It is given either orally, subcutaneously or intramuscularly, but always with folic acid supplementation (see Table 5.18 later for further information). There is also evidence to support the use of sulfasalazine, leflunomide and cyclosporin for this indication.

In cases where DMARDs are poorly tolerated or not effective, good evidence supports the use of the tumour necrosis factor (TNF) inhibitors adalimumab, etanercept, golimumab and infliximab – see Table 5.19 (Therapeutic Guidelines Limited 2010f).

For further pain management information see Chapter 7.

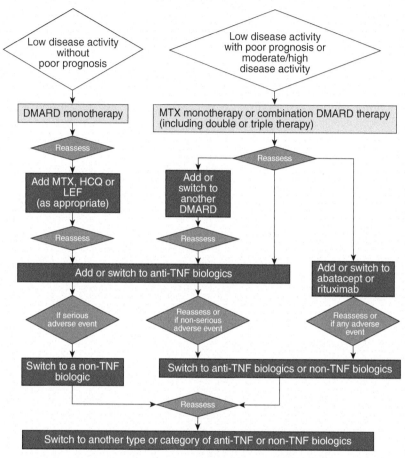

Figure 5.5 Recommendations for the use of disease-modifying anti-rheumatic medications and biologic agents in the treatment of RA. DMARD, disease-modifying anti rheumatic drugs; HCQ, hydroxychloroquine; LEF, leflunomide; MTX, methotrexate; TNF, tumour necrosis factor.
Adapted with permission from: Singh, J.A., Furst, D.E., Bharat, A., et al., 2012. 2012 update of the 2008 American College of Rheumatology recommendations for the use of disease-modifying antirheumatic drugs and biologic agents in the treatment of rheumatoid arthritis (RA). Arthritis Care and Research 64 (5), 625–639. Copyright © 2012 by the American College of Rheumatology.

Crystal arthropathies

Gout

Definition
Gout is an inflammatory disorder characterised by the deposition of monosodium urate (MSU) crystals in articular and peri-articular structures (Punzi et al. 2012). It is often associated with co-morbidities such as cardiovascular disease, chronic kidney disease, obesity and type 2 diabetes (Robinson & Horsburgh 2014).

Further tests to confirm diagnosis include blood tests to ascertain the presence of raised urate and analysis of joint aspirate.

Pharmacological management

Management involves providing rapid pain relief for acute attacks, preventing further attacks and preventing the complications of gout such as the formation of gouty tophi and destructive arthritis.

Acute gout treatment focuses on treating the inflammation only, with the following agents used:

* NSAIDs with indomethacin being the agent of choice (see Table 5.12 later)
* colchicine – use is limited by adverse effects (see Table 5.17 later)
* corticosteroids, oral or intraarticular (if more than one joint is involved or NSAIDs are contraindicated) – see Table 5.15.

Any changes to allourinol or probenecid therapy must be avoided during an attack, as sudden changes in uric acid concentrations can precipitate further acute attacks.

Urate lowering therapy with allopurinol can be commenced once the attack has settled and appropriate lifestyle factors or medication changes have been made. The aim is to reduce the plasma urate level to <0.3 mmol/L, and monthly blood test are recommended to allow appropriate dose adjustment. During the initiation and dose titration period, concurrent treatment with cholchicine or an NSAID is recommended to prevent an acute exacerbation. Oral prednis(ol)one can be used in patients in whom NSAID or colchicine is contraindicated (Therapeutic Guidelines Limited 2010g).

Some patients do develop an asymptomatic hyperuricaemia due to genetic factors, medication or concurrent medical problems. These patients should not be treated with urate lowering therapy unless they develop gout symptoms (Therapeutic Guidelines Limited 2010g).

For further pain management information see Chapter 7.

▉ Joint conditions

Adhesive capsulitis

Definition

A disorder that affects the capsule of the glenohumeral joint, it is generally accepted that adhesive capsulitis is divided into three stages: 1) the painful stage, 2) the adhesive phase and 3) the resolution stage (Walmsley, Osmotherly & Rivett 2014).

Pharmacological management

Analgesia

Simple oral analgesic such as paracetamol and NSAIDs should be used first line (see Tables 5.11 and 5.12). Limited evidence suggests that topical NSAIDs are not effective in adhesive capsulitis. If pain persists despite simple analgesia, and it is interfering with the activities of daily living, immediate release opioids (codeine, tramadol or oxycodone) can be considered for short-term use, with an active treatment plan with a defined time frame – see Table 5.13 later (Therapeutic Guidelines Limited 2010h).

Corticosteroids

Rapid pain relief can be achieved with an intraarticular corticosteroid injection (see Table 5.15); however, the effect is short-lived. Either an anterior or posterior approach to the glenohumeral joint may be used. These have been found to be most beneficial in stage 1 due to the inflammatory nature of this stage (Jain & Sharma 2014).

Oral prednis(ol)one can also alleviate pain rapidly, improve range of movement and function, and may provide a more sustained benefit (see Table 5.15). Doses such as 30 mg daily for 3 weeks, then tapered over the next 2 weeks and then ceased, have been used.

This approach provides most benefit in patients who have been symptomatic for 5–6 months, and the risk of potential side effects must be balanced against the benefits, particularly in high-risk patients (Therapeutic Guidelines Limited 2010h).

PHYSIOTHERAPY PRACTICE POINTS: ADHESIVE CAPSULITIS

There are multiple physiotherapy options that are beneficial in the management of adhesive capsulitis including stretching, manual therapy, electrotherapy and acupuncture. Use in combination with timely medication management (including injection therapy) may provide greater symptomatic relief (Jain & Sharma 2014); however, this is dependent on the stage of the disorder (Ranalletta et al. 2016).

Avascular necrosis

Definition

Avascular necrosis (AVN) is the cellular death of the bone due to a disruption in its blood supply.

There are no evidence-based pharmacological treatments for AVN; therefore the focus of this section is the implications of the patient's medications as a predisposing factor to developing AVN.

Clinical features

There are a number of factors that may predispose a patient to developing AVN. These include trauma, corticosteroid use, alcohol misuse, haemoglobinopathies, chemotherapy, radiation, collagen vascular disease, pancreatitis and pregnancy (Barile, Wu & McMahon 2014). Patients may present with a variety of symptoms and history of injury and/or pain; however, they often report a period of ongoing, non-settling pain in the affected area.

Clinical significance

Untreated AVN is frequently a progressive disorder that ultimately may lead to collapse of the affected area. Therefore, early diagnosis and appropriate management are essential (Barile, Wu & McMahon 2014).

Osteomyelitis

Definition

Osteomyelitis (OM) is an infection of the bone, almost always caused by a bacterium (Conterno & Turchi 2013). Left untreated it may lead to necrosis.

Clinical features

Osteomyelitis can occur in patients of any age. There are a number of predisposing factors including sickle cell anaemia, injury, the presence of a foreign body (such as a splinter or a surgical screw), intravenous drug use, diabetes, kidney dialysis, surgery and untreated infections of tissue near a bone. The patient may present with swelling, pain and low grade fever.

Clinical significance

Osteomyelitis is painful and can be difficult to treat. Despite advances in antibiotic and surgical treatments the recurrence rate is 20% (Conterno & Turchi 2013).

Additional tests are required to ascertain the presence of osteomyelitis; these may include: assessment of body temperature, blood tests, X-rays, MRI and bone scan.

The first-line treatment for OM is antibiotics; antibiotic treatment may be oral or intravenously.

Pharmacological management

Empirical therapy

The likely pathogen is influenced by the site of the bone infection and the presence of any of the following risk factors in the patient:

+ history of injecting drug use
+ postoperative infection
+ current or recurrent urinary tract or gastrointestinal infection
+ healthcare-acquired infection
+ high local prevalence of community-acquired methicillin-resistant *Staphylococcus aureus* (MRSA)
+ colonisation with MRSA (or history of).

Empirical and directed therapy regimens are detailed in Tables 5.7A and 5.7B, respectively (Therapeutic Guidelines Limited 2014a).

The duration of therapy depends on the type of OM and the age of the patient. This may include 3 days to 4 weeks of intravenous therapy followed by 3 weeks to many months of oral therapy (Conterno & Turchi 2013).

Tumours

Tumours are a differential diagnosis that musculoskeletal physiotherapists must be aware of as they present with symptoms commonly reported to physiotherapists such as joint and bone pain (Slipman et al. 2003). There a number of symptoms that may indicate the presence of more sinister pathology, such as:

+ night pain
+ fever

TABLE 5.7A Empirical therapy for long bone and vertebral osteomyelitis (OM)

Type of OM	Suggested empirical therapy
Long-bone osteomyelitis	First line is flucloxacillin IV Patients with penicillin hypersensitivity, use cephazolin IV Patients with immediate hypersensitivity to penicillins use vancomycin IV
Vertebral osteomyelitis	First line in adults is ceftriaxone IV AND vancomycin IV Ceftriaxone IV PLUS vancomycin IV *Staphylococcus aureus* is the most common pathogen; however, a wide variety of other pathogens may be implicated, so collection of specimens (e.g. bone or pus) to allow culture and sensitivities is critical to determine appropriate treatment

Adapted from: Therapeutic Guidelines Limited, 2014a. Osteomyelitis. In: eTG complete [Internet]. Therapeutic Guidelines Limited, Melbourne.

TABLE 5.7B Directed therapy for colonised pathogens in osteomyelitis

Colonised pathogen	Suggested directed therapy
Methicillin-susceptible *Staphylococcus aureus* (MSSA)	Flucloxacillin IV then di/flucloxacillin orally For patients with penicillin hypersensitivity: • cefalothin *or* cephazolin IV then cephalexin orally For patients with immediate hypersensitivity to penicillins: • clindamycin IV then orally *or* • vancomycin IV if the MSSA is not susceptible to macrolides (and hence lincosamides)
Methicillin-resistant *Staphylococcus aureus* (MRSA)	Vancomycin IV then oral therapy with rifampicin and fusidic acid *or*, if patient is not critically ill or bacteraemic and susceptibility is confirmed: • clindamycin IV then orally, *or* doxycycline *or* • trimethoprim/sulfamethoxazole
Gram negative infections	If infection with Enterobacteriaceae, *H. influenzae* or *K. kingae* is suspected or confirmed, use: • ceftriaxome IV or cefotaxime IV If *Pseudomonas* species are confirmed, use: • ceftazidime IV followed by oral ciprofloxacin

Adapted from: Therapeutic Guidelines Limited, 2014a. Osteomyelitis. In: eTG complete [Internet]. Therapeutic Guidelines Limited, Melbourne.

♦ unexplained weight loss
♦ previous cancer.

In the presence of potential sinister pathology the physiotherapist must refer the patient for further assessment as a matter of urgency.

Further detail in this area is beyond the scope of this handbook.

■ Maxillofacial disorders

Trigeminal neuralgia

Trigeminal neuralgia (TN) is one of the most severe and progressive forms of chronic neuropathic pain of the Vth cranial nerve. While the average age of onset for TN is usually during the fifth and sixth decades, young adults and even children may develop typical or atypical TN. There are rare occasions when TN appears to run a familial pattern (Devor, Amir & Rappaport 2002; Sarlani, Balciunas & Grace 2005).[1]

Temporomandibular joint disorders

Dysfunction of the temporomandibular joint (TMJ) is common; reported prevalence varies from 20% to 75%, and most patients are female (Ahmed et al. 2014).

Pharmacological management

If pain is the primary symptom, a simple oral analgesic such as paracetamol and NSAIDs should be used initially (see Tables 5.11 and 5.12). If pain persists despite simple analgesia, and interferes with the activities of daily living, immediate release opioids (codeine, tramadol or oxycodone) may be considered for short-term use (see Table 5.13).

There are circumstances in TMJ disorders where the use of muscle relaxants may be beneficial to relax the muscle of the jaw[2] (see Table 5.16 later).

For further pain management information see Chapter 7.

PHYSIOTHERAPY PRACTICE POINTS: TEMPOROMANDIBULAR JOINT DISORDERS

Physiotherapy is commonly used to treat temporomandibular joint disorders. Strategies include exercises, ultrasound, manual therapy, acupuncture and laser therapy. The treating therapist needs to be aware of the mechanism of action of any medications the patient may be taking, in order to maximise the benefit of the treatment (Rashid, Matthews & Cowgill 2013).

Bell's palsy

Bell's palsy is a paralysis or weakness of the muscles on one side of the face. These symptoms are caused by a lower motor neuron lesion to the VIIth cranial nerve. While stroke may cause a facial paralysis, in this case it is an upper motor neuron lesion with a slight variation of signs and symptoms.

Pharmacological management

Strong evidence exists for the early use of corticosteroids within 48 hours of onset of symptoms (Salinas et al. 2010) (see Table 5.15). However, no strong evidence supports the use of antiviral therapies for facial nerve palsy.

---

[1] Treatment of neuropathic pain is discussed in Chapter 7.
[2] See anti-spastic medication in the 'Spasticity' section in Chapter 6.

PHYSIOTHERAPY PRACTICE POINTS: BELL'S PALSY

In Bell's palsy various physiotherapy interventions, such as exercise, PNF, biofeedback, laser, electrotherapy, massage and thermotherapy, are used to speed recovery. However, the evidence for the efficacy of any of these therapies is lacking. The possibility that facial exercise reduces time to recover and adverse outcomes needs confirming with good quality controlled trials (Cardoso et al. 2008).

■ Soft tissue conditions

Soft tissue injuries – sprains, strains and contusions

Definition

Sprains, strains/tears and contusions are terms associated with many peripheral and central structures including, but not limited to, muscle, ligament, joint and nerve.

◆ Sprain is associated with injury to a ligament and ranges from mild injury to only a few fibres to a complete tear of the ligament (Brukner & Khan 2012). These are commonly graded I–III in accordance with the severity of injury: grade I involves few fibres up to grade III, which is a complete tear.

◆ Strains/tears are associated with muscle injuries and graded according to severity with the same classification as sprains (Brukner & Khan 2012).

◆ Contusion usually results from a direct blow, causing local muscle damage and bleeding (Brukner & Khan 2012).

Pharmacological management

Analgesia for mild to moderate pain including paracetamol, NSAIDs and oral opioids may be used[3] (Therapeutic Guidelines Limited 2012a) (see Tables 5.11, 5.12 and 5.13).

For muscle spasm often associated with acute back strain, muscle relaxants can be used; however, evidence for their role is conflicting and adverse effects are common. Diazepam, a benzodiazepine, is the medication of choice, given either orally or IV[4] (Australian Medicines Handbook Pty Ltd 2015b; National Institute for Health and Care Excellence 2009) (see Table 5.16).

Acute tendon pain

Definition

The pathological changes that occur with tendon pain are poorly understood (Resteghini & Yeoh 2012). Recent research suggests a continuum of three stages of tendon pathology: 1) reactive tendinopathy, 2) tendon disrepair (failed healing) and 3) degenerative tendinopathy (Cook & Purdam 2009; Fu et al. 2010; McCreesh & Lewis 2013).

---

[3]See also Chapter 7.
[4]See also Chapter 6.

Clinical features

Reactive tendinopathy (stage 1) is an acutely overloaded tendon and more common in younger people. It may also occur as a result of direct trauma to the tendon (Cook & Purdam 2009). The affected tendon may present with an erythema, swelling and acute tenderness.

Subacute/chronic tendon pain

The tendon disrepair phase (stage 2) is most commonly reported in chronically overloaded tendons in the young; however, it may present across a broad range of ages in varying loading environments. Clinically, these tendons are thickened, generally in a localised area of the tendon; however, more accurate diagnosis of this phase can be established using imaging, as commonly there are focal structural changes to the tendon (with or without increased vascularity) present. Symptoms and imaging need to be carefully mapped with loading patterns of the painful tendon (Cook & Purdam 2009).

Degenerative tendinopathy (stage 3) is predominantly seen in the older person; however, it may also be present in younger people with a chronically overloaded tendon. Generally, patients present with localised swelling and pain in the tendon. The tendon can have one or more focal nodular areas with or without general thickening. Patients usually report a history of episodic pain in the tendon that is sensitive to changes in load (Cook & Purdam 2009). Degenerative tendinopathy, if extensive enough or if the tendon is placed under high load, can result in rupture (Trobisch et al. 2010; Wiegand, Vámhidy & Lőrinczy 2010).

Pharmacological management

The use of medications is dependent on the phase of the tendon pain. In reactive tendinopathy and early disrepair phase NSAIDs have been reported to impair healing in a range of tissues and therefore, while pain may be reduced, they have a negative effect on tendon healing (Ofir et al. 2014; Su & O'Connor 2013), particularly at the enthesis[5] (Scott Backman & Speed 2015). Although other sources suggest that the inhibition of tenocyte activity may be achieved using ibuprofen and celecoxib, inhibition of aggrecan deposition with ibuprofen, naproxen or indomethacin and anti-TNFα is also beneficial in reducing pain (Cook & Purdam 2014).

Analgesia for mild to moderate pain including paracetamol and NSAIDs (in the later stages of presentation or early stages where indicated) and oral opioids may be used[6] (Therapeutic Guidelines Limited 2010i) (see Tables 5.11 and 5.12).

There is limited evidence to support the use of injection therapy in the management of tendinopathies; these are therefore not recommended at this time (Cook & Purdam 2014; Kearney et al. 2015; Scott Backman & Speed 2015).

---

[5]This is the specialist interface where tendon integrates into bone.
[6]See also Chapter 7.

> ### PHYSIOTHERAPY PRACTICE POINTS: ACUTE TENDON PAIN
>
> Depending on the stage of tendinopathy and the patient's functional requirements (employment, elite athlete), the primary treatment should involve load management/modification, a graduated loading program and manual therapy. Medication is an adjunct to these treatments, which may be beneficial in subgroups of patients with tendinopathy (Cook & Purdam 2014, Malliaras et al. 2013).

Nerve compression syndromes

Physiotherapists play a key role in the management of multiple nerve compression syndromes. This section will use carpel tunnel syndrome as an example where a combination of medication and physiotherapy management is used. These principles may be applicable to other nerve compression syndromes[7].

Carpel tunnel syndrome

Definition
Carpel tunnel syndrome (CTS) is related to increased pressure in the carpel tunnel, resulting in mechanical compression and local ischaemia, which in turn results in damage to the median nerve (Huisstede et al. 2014; Pratelli et al. 2015).

Clinical significance
The prevalence of CTS within the general population is reportedly 0.6% in men and 5.8% in women (Pratelli et al. 2015).

Pharmacological management
For management of carpel tunnel in pregnancy, please see Chapter 4.

Oral NSAIDs (see Table 5.12) may be useful and local injection of corticosteroid (see Tables 5.5 and 5.15) into the carpal tunnel can provide symptomatic relief for at least 1 month. Studies have shown that in the first 3 months corticosteroid injection was superior to surgical decompression, but after 6 months they were equally effective (Therapeutic Guidelines Limited 2010j).

Short-term relief may be obtained with oral corticosteroids (see Table 5.15), but no benefit has been demonstrated with diuretics and vitamin B6 (Therapeutic Guidelines Limited 2010j).

> ### PHYSIOTHERAPY PRACTICE POINTS: CARPAL TUNNEL SYNDROME
>
> Physiotherapists play an important role in the conservative management of CTS. The combination of the medication management highlighted above and timely physiotherapy (i.e. within 1–3 months of corticosteroid injection) such as splinting and ergonomic advice is considered an effective approach, particularly in the short term (Huisstede et al. 2014).

---

[7]For neuropathic pain see Chapter 7.

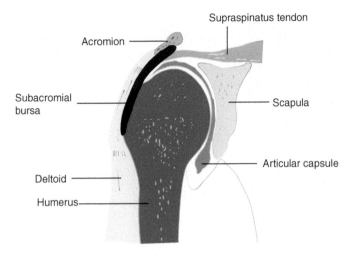

Figure 5.6 Subacromial bursa.
Adapted with permission from: Lhee, S.-H., Jo, Y.H., Kim, B.Y., et al., 2013. Novel supplier of mesenchymal stem cell: subacromial bursa. Transplantation Proceedings 45 (8), 3118–3121.

Bursitis

Definition

A bursa is defined as: 'a closed sac lined with a synovial membrane and filled with fluid, usually found in areas subject to friction, such as where a tendon passes over a bone' (The Gale Group Inc. 2008). There are more than 140 in the human body (Baumbach et al. 2014) (see Figure 5.6).

Bursitis is therefore characterised by the collection of fluid within the bursal sac, which may or may not be associated with inflammation (Baumbach et al. 2014; Sayegh & Strauch 2014). Bursitis is often triggered by repetitive trauma or mechanical overuse (Baumbach et al. 2013), and occasionally by direct, acute trauma (Buono et al. 2012).

Pharmacological management

Non-infective bursitis

Oral and topical therapies: NSAIDs can be used in conjunction with a local injection, or alone when local injection in contraindicated.

NSAIDs should be used first line in patients without any contraindications (see Table 5.12). For patients with increased risk of gastrointestinal NSAID adverse effects, a selective cyclooxygenase inhibitor NSAID may be used or prophylactic treatment with a proton-pump inhibitor may be warranted. Topical NSAID may be an option in superficial cases of bursitis where systemic NSAID treatment is contraindicated (Anderson & Todd 2015).

In cases of acute microcrystalline bursitis where NSAIDs are contraindicated, a short course of prednis(ol)one starting at 20 mg daily reducing over 10–14 days can be used (Anderson & Todd 2015) (see Table 5.15).

Intrabursal corticosteroid injections: Corticosteroid injections for superficial bursitis (olecranon, prepatellar and Achilles) are not recommended as the risk of infection, skin atrophy and development of a draining sinus tract does not outweigh the benefit. However, when inflammation is presumed in the deeper bursae, an intralesional injection of a combined local anaesthetic and corticosteroid can be beneficial from both a therapeutic and diagnostic angle (see Tables 5.5 and 5.15). If the pain is alleviated during the anaesthetic phase of injection, it is a strong indication that inflammation is in the bursa and can reduce the need for further imaging (Anderson & Todd 2015).

PHYSIOTHERAPY PRACTICE POINTS: NON-INFECTIVE BURSITIS

Post-injection treatment provides the treating physiotherapist with an opportunity to improve the biomechanics of the shoulder, through scapula-thoracic mechanics, rotator cuff strengthening and posture (Roddy et al. 2014; Jowett et al. 2013). (For specific information regarding post-injection management see earlier section on osteoarthritis.)

Infective (septic) bursitis

Septic bursitis is usually caused by *Staphylococcus aureus* following local trauma. If signs of infection are present, the bursa must be aspirated to confirm the diagnosis with microbiological cultures. If the underlying joint is involved antibiotic treatment must be commenced as per septic arthritis guidelines (Therapeutic Guidelines Limited 2014b) (see earlier section on septic arthritis and Tables 5.7a and 5.7b).

Connective tissue disorders

As primary contact clinicians physiotherapists need to be aware of the clinical features of connective tissue disorders as a differential diagnosis for patients presenting with musculoskeletal complaints and refer patients on accordingly. This section will briefly describe these conditions, their presenting features and cross-reference the medication management.

Systemic lupus erythematosus

Systemic lupus erythematosus (SLE) is a chronic autoimmune disease characterised by multi-system manifestations. It is regarded as the original connective tissue disease, where the pathology relates to a dysfunctional immune system resulting in over-production of various autoantibodies.

The prevalence of SLE varies greatly depending on race, disease definition and method of confirmation, but it is generally accepted as a rare disease, affecting less than 0.1% of the population (Apostolopoulos & Hoi 2013). In Australia, SLE is more common and more severe in Indigenous Australians and descendants from South East Asia. It is nine times more common in females. Generally speaking, SLE has a relapsing and remitting nature where patients experience episodes of symptom exacerbation interspersed with periods of relatively low disease activity (Connelly, Morand & Hoi 2013; Pons-Estel et al. 2010).

Clinical significance
SLE most commonly affects women at childbearing age; in 10–20% of cases this is before the age of 18 years (Apostolopoulos & Hoi 2013).

SLE can affect almost any organ in the body, with symptoms including rash, photosensitivity, oral ulcers, arthritis, serositis (pleuritis or pericarditis), renal impairment, seizures or psychosis, haematological and immunological symptoms.

Pharmacological management
Pharmacological treatment of SLE is determined by the severity of the inflammation and the organ involved. Severe end-organ disease of any type may result in the need for treatment with strong immunosuppressant therapy, usually under specialist care.

The following immunosuppressants may be used together with NSAIDs and corticosteroids, either oral or topical, depending on symptoms (Therapeutic Guidelines Limited 2014c):

+ azathioprine
+ cyclophosphamide
+ cyclosporin
+ hydroxychloroquine
+ immunoglobulin, normal
+ methotrexate
+ mycophenolate mofetil
+ prednis(ol)one
+ rituximab.

For pain management see Tables 5.11, 5.12 and 5.13 and also Chapter 7.

Scleroderma

Clinical significance
Scleroderma is a relatively rare condition; the Australian Rheumatology Association report a prevalence of around 20/100,000 (Australian Rheumatology Association 2015).

It is characterised by vascular abnormalities, inflammation and fibrosis usually affecting the skin but also affecting a range of other organs.

Pharmacological management
Management of scleroderma is summarised in Table 5.8.

For pain management see Tables 5.11, 5.12 and 5.13 and Chapter 7.

TABLE 5.8 Pharmacological management of scleroderma

Clinical feature	Pharmacological management
Raynaud phenomenon	Episodic, often painful blanching, cyanosis and erythema of digits Treatment includes: • amlodipine, or delodipine or nifedipine and/or • transdermal glyceryl trinitrate Alprostadil via IV infusion can be used for severe digital ischaemia See Chapter 2 for details of these medications
Skin fibrosis	Regular application of emollients (e.g. sorbolene cream) Pruritus may be helped by non-sedating antihistamines Low-dose corticosteroids and immunosuppression with cyclophosphamide, cyclosporin and mycophenolate have been beneficial in some cases
Digital ulceration	Antibiotics are required when ulcers become red and swollen: • di/flucloxacillin orally or IV or • clindamycin Together with regular analgesia
Digital calcinosis	No medications have evidence base in this setting Surgery is suggested
Oesophageal dysmotility	Proton pump inhibitors
Small bowel involvement	Delayed gastric emptying with nausea and bloating may respond to domperidone Nonspecific looseness or diarrhoea should imply lifestyle factors together with antidiarrhoeal medications such as loperamide
Large bowel involvement	Regular use of laxatives is required for constipation and rectal prolapse requires surgery
Pulmonary fibrosis	Low-dose corticosteroids are given with concurrent immunosuppression such as cyclophosphamide
Pulmonary arterial hypertension (PAH)	See Chapter 3 The following therapies are used for PAH with WHO class III and IV symptoms: • endothelian antagonists (bosentan or ambtisartan) • phosphodiesterase inhibitors (sildenafil) • inhaled prostanoids (iloprost) Warfarin is usually used to prevent pulmonary vascular thrombosis, with little evidence to support it
Hypertension and scleroderma renal crisis	Scleroderma renal crisis can develop over a few days Aggressive antihypertensive therapy with an ACE inhibitor-containing regimen must be used See Chapter 2

Adapted from: Therapeutic Guidelines Limited, 2014d. Inflammatory connective tissue diseases: scleroderma. In: eTG complete [Internet]. Therapeutic Guidelines Limited, Melbourne.

■ Spinal conditions

Non-specific low back pain is one of the leading reasons for a reduction in activity levels and absence from work. Physiotherapists are an essential member of the treating team; management may include advice, education, exercise, pacing and manual therapy (Otoo, Hendrick & Ribeiro 2015). The purpose of medication for these patients is alleviation of pain, muscle spasm and inflammation; elements of management of these symptoms are covered in other areas of this chapter. Further information on pain management is covered in detail in Chapter 7. The treating physiotherapist should be aware of the duration of action and half-life of the medications their patients are using.

Ankylosing spondylitis

Definition

Ankylosing spondylitis (AS) is a chronic inflammatory disease that predominantly affects the spine and sacroiliac joints (Stockdale, Selfe & Roddam 2014).

Clinical significance

AS is purported to affect 0.1–1.4% of Caucasian populations, with average age of onset of 24–26 years, with males being more commonly affected (Prince, McGuigan & McGirr 2014).

Further tests may be indicated to confirm the diagnosis. These may include blood tests, X-ray and MRI.

Pharmacological management

Since pain is the major complaint of these patients regular paracetamol is the recommended first-line treatment, and combined with NSAIDS if symptoms are not controlled with paracetamol alone (see Tables 5.11 and 5.12). During episodes of high disease activity corticosteroid medicines or injections may be indicated (see Table 5.15). Additionally, disease-modifying anti-rheumatic drugs (DMARDs) (see Table 5.18), biological DMARDs or anti-TNFα medication (see Table 5.19) may be required (Therapeutic Guidelines Limited 2010k).

For further pain management information see Chapter 7.

**PHYSIOTHERAPY PRACTICE POINTS:
ANKYLOSING SPONDYLITIS**

Physiotherapists play an important role in the management of patients with AS. Management strategies may include: supervised and unsupervised exercises, hydrotherapy, manual therapy, functional training, electrophysical agents and advice and information (Dagfinrud, Kvien & Hagen 2008). Timing these therapies with the peak action of medication would be most beneficial (see Table 5.5). Physiotherapists are also well-placed to monitor the need to increase a patient's medication (as above) through their compliance with exercise therapies (Stockdale, Selfe & Roddam 2014).

Spondylosis/spondyloarthropathy

Definition

Degenerative disorders of the spine are commonly grouped under the term 'spondylosis'. For the purposes of this text spondylosis includes spinal stenosis, degenerative disc disease, degeneration of the vertebrae and/or associated joints, degenerative spondylolisthesis and clinical syndromes of instability (Gibson & Waddell 2005).

Clinical significance

In 2013 a study reported the incidence of cervical spondylosis alone to be 3.3 cases per 1000 people (Wani et al. 2013), while lumbar spondylosis is considered a major cause of disability in the elderly in the majority of developed countries (Muraki et al. 2013). Physiotherapists are one of the main professional groups to provide conservative management to patients with spondylosis.

Pharmacological management

Regular paracetamol is the recommended first-line treatment, and combined with NSAIDs if symptoms are not controlled with paracetamol alone (see Tables 5.11 and 5.2).

Epidural injections of corticosteroids are not supported by the current evidence base; however, uncontrolled observational studies suggest that injections of local anaesthetics with or without corticosteroids have been associated with reduced short-term pain (Levin 2015) (see Table 5.15).

■ Trauma

Fractures/acute trauma (including simple wound management)

Definition

A fracture is a break in bone or cartilage. Although usually a result of trauma, a fracture can be the result of an acquired disease of bone, such as osteoporosis (covered in Chapter 8) or of abnormal formation of bone in a congenital disease of bone, such as osteogenesis imperfecta (Chapter 8). Fractures can be open (compound) or closed and are classified according to their character and location (e.g., spiral fracture of the fibula) (Brukner & Khan 2012).

Clinical significance

Fractures are a very common injury. In 2012 it was reported that the incidence of hip fracture alone in Australia is 150–250/100,000 per year (Kanis et al. 2012), with women being twice as likely to suffer a hip fracture as men.

Acute wound management

In some clinical settings, such as the emergency department and on the sporting field, physiotherapists are involved in the management of simple wounds. This may include the cleaning and dressing of simple wounds. Physiotherapists need to be aware of when onward referral is required for wound management.[8]

Analgesia

Simple oral analgesics such as paracetamol and NSAIDs are usually sufficient to manage pain associated with wounds; however, analgesic requirements need to be regularly reviewed and titrated as required (Therapeutic Guidelines Limited 2015) (see Tables 5.11 and 5.12).

For further information on pain and analgesia see Chapter 7.

Pharmacological management – fractures

(For information regarding analgesia to perform fracture reduction procedures see 'Dislocations'.)

Analgesia for mild to moderate pain including paracetamol and NSAIDs and oral opioids may be used (Therapeutic Guidelines Limited 2012b) (see Tables 5.11, 5.12 and 5.13).

For further information on pain and analgesia see Chapter 7.

Antibiotic prophylaxis for open fractures

The antibiotic selection and duration of therapy depend on the type and extent of tissue damage and the time to debridement (Therapeutic Guidelines Limited 2014e).

If there is severe tissue damage or clinical evidence of infection, empirical therapy is required for 7 days (see Table 5.9). If established bone infection is present, empirical therapy is required for >7 days followed by oral therapy.

The tetanus immunisation status of all patients with open fractures should be determined and tetanus toxoid vaccine or immunoglobulin should be given as indicated. The criteria for tetanus prophylaxis in the case of open fractures are highlighted in Table 5.10.

Dislocations

Definition

A joint dislocation is a complete separation of the surfaces of a joint, which in some instances may also be associated with a fracture or compound fracture and is frequently the result of injury. A dislocation may also be due to a congenital disorder, such as developmental dysplasia of the hip or associated with other pathologies such as stroke.

Clinical significance

A dislocated joint is a significant injury that undiagnosed is likely to lead to marked dysfunction and pain. The shoulder is the most commonly dislocated joint with a re-dislocation rate of anywhere between 17% and 96% (Whelan et al. 2014).

---

[8]Further information on wound management is beyond the scope of this handbook.

TABLE 5.9 Antibiotic prophylaxis for open fracture

	Empirical therapy	Antibiotic prophylaxis	Presumptive therapy
Criteria	If there is severe tissue damage or clinical evidence of infection	No tissue damage or clinical evidence of infection and debridement has occurred within 8 hours	No tissue damage or clinical evidence of infection and debridement has NOT occurred within 8 hours
Duration of therapy	7 days; however, if established bone infection is evident, treatment is prolonged and followed up with oral therapy	24–72 hours	7 days
	IV	Oral	
First line	Piperacillin + tazobactam *or* Ticarcillin + clavulanate	Amoxycillin + clavulanate	Cephazolin IV
Patients with penicillin hypersensitivity	Cephazolin *plus* metronidazole	Cephalexin *plus* metronidazole	
Patients with immediate hypersensitivity to penicillins	Ciprofloxacin *plus* clindamycin	Ciprofloxacin *plus* clindamycin	Clindamycin IV or oral

Adapted from: Therapeutic Guidelines Limited, 2014e. Open fractures. In: eTG complete [Internet]. Therapeutic Guidelines Limited, Melbourne.

TABLE 5.10 Tetanus prophylaxis criteria

	Time since vaccination	Type of wound	Tetanus vaccine required	Tetanus immunoglobulin required
History of 3 or more doses of tetanus toxoid vaccine	<5 years	All wounds	No	No
	5–10 years	Clean minor wounds	No	No
		All other wounds	Yes	No
	>10 years	All wounds	Yes	No
Uncertain vaccination history or <3 doses of tetanus toxoid		Clean minor wounds	Yes	No
		All other wounds	Yes	Yes

Adapted from: Therapeutic Guidelines Limited, 2014. Open fractures. In: eTG complete [Internet]. Therapeutic Guidelines Limited, Melbourne.

Pharmacological management

Procedure-related sedation and analgesia are recommended for the reduction of dislocations and fractures (Therapeutic Guidelines Limited 2012c). Strategies to minimise pain during procedures not requiring sedation include:

+ non-sedating oral analgesics (e.g. paracetamol, non-steroidal anti-inflammatory medications)
+ local anaesthetic infiltration
+ nerve or plexus block
+ regional intravenous anaesthesia.

However, most patients will also require sedation for reduction of dislocation of large joints (e.g. shoulders, hips, knees and elbows) and reduction and splinting of long bone fractures (see Table 5.16).

Agents used to achieve *minimal sedation* include:

+ inhaled analgesics are useful when minimal to moderate analgesia is required rapidly for short procedures, including:
  - nitrous oxide [50% to 70% in oxygen]
  - methoxyflurane
+ oral opiates can be used for planned procedures requiring minimal sedation and analgesia
  - oxycodone immediate release.

Agents used to achieve *moderate* sedation include:

+ intravenous opioids in titrated small doses
  - fentanyl
  - morphine – slower onset of action than fentanyl but may be used if post-procedural pain is expected
+ benzodiazepines
  - midazolam
+ others may be used to provide deeper levels of sedation
  - ketamine
  - propofol.

■ Miscellaneous

There are multiple conditions that present with musculoskeletal symptoms; these include, but are not limited to:

+ haematological conditions such as haemophilia (see Chapter 9)
+ metabolic disorders such as diabetes and hyperthyroidism (see Chapter 8)
+ endocrine osteoporosis (see Chapter 8).

Musculoskeletal physiotherapists need to be cognisant of systemic conditions that mimic musculoskeletal disorders and refer to the relevant health professionals as required.

Tables 5.11 to 5.19 provide a more detailed description of the medications discussed in this chapter, including mechanisms of action, indications for use,

Text continued on p. 162

TABLE 5.11 Detailed description of paracetamol

Medication	Mechanism of action	Indications for therapeutic use	Common side effects	Practice points	Common adult, child dosage ranges
Paracetamol (Therapeutic Guidelines Limited 2010a, 2012a)	Inhibits synthesis of prostaglandins in the hypothalamus and spine and inhibits inducible nitric oxide synthesis in macrophages	Treatment of mild to moderate pain, particularly pain originating in soft tissue and musculoskeletal systems May also be used in conjunction to reduce the overall daily doses of NSAIDs or opioids required, and thus the risk of their adverse effects	Raised aminotransferases Hepatotoxicity hypersensitivity reactions, neutropenia, thrombocytopenia, pancytopenia, acute hepatitis	If paracetamol alone is inadequate for treating pain, adding an NSAID may provide additional analgesia and allow use of lower or intermittent doses of NSAID Available in many different forms and in combination with many other analgesics Always take care not to duplicate therapy or exceed maximum recommended daily dose of paracetamol	*Adult, child >12 years, oral/rectal:* 0.5–1 g every 4–6 hours (maximum 4 g daily) Controlled release 1330 mg every 6–8 hours (maximum 3990 mg/day) *Children, oral/rectal:* 15 mg/kg every 4–6 hours *Note:* Also available as IV preparation – dosed at the same dose Onset of pain relief is: • 30 minutes after oral dosing • 5–10 minutes after starting IV infusion Rectal absorption can be variable

NSAID, non-steroidal anti-inflammatory.
Adapted from: Australian Medicines Handbook (online). 2015. Australian Medicines Handbook Pty Ltd, Adelaide. <http://amhonline.amh. net.au/>.

TABLE 5.12 Detailed description of non-steroidal anti-inflammatories (NSAIDS)

Medication	Mechanism of action	Indications for therapeutic use	Common side effects	Practice points	Common adult, child dosage ranges
CLASS: Non-steroidal anti-inflammatory (NSAIDs) (Therapeutic Guidelines Limited 2010a) **Non-selective NSAIDs** Diclofenac Ibuprofen Indomethacin Ketoprofen Ketorolac Mefenamic acid Naproxen Piroxicam Sulindac **Selective NSAIDs (COX-2 inhibitors)** Celecoxib Etoricoxib Meloxicam Parecoxib	Prevent production of prostaglandins by inhibiting cyclo-oxygenase (COX) to produce anti-inflammatory, analgesic and antipyretic functions COX is present as COX-1 and COX-2 COX-1 inhibition causes impaired gastric protection and antiplatelet effects COX-2 inhibition causes anti-inflammatory and analgesic action A reduction in renal function occurs with both COX-1 and COX-2 inhibition Most NSAIDs are non-selective (inhibiting both COX-1 and COX-2)	Pain due to inflammation, tissue injury and inflammatory arthropathies	Nausea, dyspepsia, GI ulceration or bleeding, raised liver enzymes (especially diclofenac), diarrhoea, headache, dizziness, salt and fluid retention, hypertension	Use precaution in patients with the following: • cardio or cerebrovascular disease • active GIT disease • history of NSAID-induced hypersensitivity reactions • pre-existing renal disease, or concurrent use of nephrotoxic medications • hepatic • elderly • dehydration • asthma • coagulation disorders or concurrent anticoagulant or antiplatelet medications • pregnancy and breastfeeding Dose reduction may be required in: • renal disease • hepatic disease • elderly Very little difference in anti-inflammatory response between different NSAIDs, so choice of agent depends on individual response and tolerance There is no rationale for using more than one NSAID at a time (excluding low-dose aspirin)	**Celecoxib** *Adult oral:* 200–300 mg daily in 1–2 doses Do not use >200 mg daily long term Half-life: 4–15 hours **Diclofenac** *Adult oral/rectal:* 75–150 mg daily in 2 or 3 doses (maximum 200 mg daily) *Child >1 year oral/rectal:* 0.5–1 mg/kg (maximum 50 mg) 2 or 3 times daily *Topical:* 1% gel, rub into the affected area 3 or 4 times daily Half-life:1–2 hours **Etoricoxib** *Adult oral:* 30–120 mg once daily Half-life: 22 hours **Ibuprofen** *Adult oral:* 200–400 mg 3 or 4 times a day (maximum 2.4 g daily) *Child >3 months, oral:* 5–10 mg/kg (maximum 400 mg) 3 or 4 times a day. *Topical adult, child >12 years:* rub 4–10 cm into the affected area if needed, up to 4 times daily

COX-2 selective inhibitors have minimal effect on COX-1, but they are still associated with GI side effects at therapeutic doses	About 60% of patients will respond to any NSAID; those who do not respond to one may respond to another To reduce complications: • try a topical NSAID before using one orally • use the lowest effective dose for the shortest period of time • use paracetamol to enable lower doses of NSAID	Half-life :2–2.5 hours **Indomethacin** *Adult oral:* 25–50 mg 2–4 times daily *Adult rectal:* 100 mg once or twice daily *Child oral:* Initially 0.5–1 mg/kg twice daily (maximum of 4 mg/kg) Half-life: 4.5–6 hours **Ketoprofen** *Adult, oral:* 200 mg once daily *Adult, rectal:* 100 mg at bedtime *Topical:* Apply to the affected area 2–4 times daily Half-life: 1.5–2 hours **Ketoralac** *Adult, IM/IV:* 10 mg followed by 10–30 mg every 4–6 hours (maximum 90 mg daily) *Adult, oral:* 10 mg every 4–6 hours (maximum 40 mg daily) Half-life: 4–6 hours **Mefenamic acid** *Adult, oral:* Up to 500 mg 3 times daily Half-life: 3–4 hours

Continued

TABLE 5.12 Detailed description of non-steroidal anti-inflammatories (NSAIDS)—cont'd

Medication	Mechanism of action	Indications for therapeutic use	Common side effects	Practice points	Common adult, child dosage ranges
					Meloxicam *Adult, oral:* 7.5–15 mg once daily Half-life: 20 hours **Naproxen** *Adult, oral:* Conventional product, 250–500 mg twice daily Controlled release product, 750–1000 mg once daily (up to a maximum of 1250 mg daily) *Child >2 years, oral:* 5–7.5 mg/kg (maximum 500 mg) twice daily Half-life: 12–15 hours **Parecoxib** *Adult, IM/IV:* 40 mg single dose Half-life: 6.5–7 hours (active metabolite) **Piroxicam** *Adult, oral:* 10–20 mg once daily, usually for no more than 14 days *Topical:* Apply to the affected area 3 or 4 times daily. Half-life: 30–50 hours **Sulindac** *Adult, oral:* 200–400 mg daily in 1 or 2 doses Half-life:16 hours (active metabolite)

Adapted from: Australian Medicines Handbook Pty Ltd, 2015. Australian Medicines Handbook (online). Australian Medicines Handbook Pty Ltd, Adelaide. <*http://amhonline.amh. net.au/*>.

TABLE 5.13 Detailed description of opioids

Medication	Mechanism of action	Indications for therapeutic use	Common side effects	Practice points	Common adult, child dosage ranges
CLASS: Opioids **Opioids used in MSK conditions:** Codeine Dextropropoxyphene Fentanyl Morphine Oxycodone Tramadol	Activate opioid receptors in the central and peripheral nervous systems to produce analgesia, respiratory depression, sedation and constipation	Acute or chronic pain	Nausea and vomiting, dyspepsia, drowsiness, dizziness, headache, orthostatic hypotension, itch, dry mouth, miosis, urinary retention, constipation	Use with caution in the following patient groups: • uncorrected endocrine abnormalities, hypothyroidism, adrenocortical insufficiency, acute alcoholism, myasthenia gravis, CNS depression • epilepsy or a recognised risk for seizure • raised intracranial pressure • hypotension, shock • phaeochromocytoma • gastrointestinal ileus • respiratory depression • renal impairment • hepatic impairment • elderly • pregnancy and breastfeeding Available in many different dose forms (immediate release, slow release, mixtures, tablets, sachets, capsules); take care to always select the correct dose form Always use a regular laxative for people requiring regular opioids to prevent constipation Physical dependence is common Recommended doses are for those that are opioid naive Patients with a history of opioid use may require higher doses	**Codeine** *Adult, oral:* 30–60 mg every 4 hours if needed (maximum 240 mg in 24 hours) *Child >1 year, oral:* 0.5–1 mg/kg every 4–6 hours if needed (maximum 240 mg in 24 hours) Duration of action: 3–4 hours Practice points: • available in fixed dose combinations with aspirin, ibuprofen and paracetamol • codeine (a prodrug) is metabolised to morphine; people with normal codeine metabolism metabolise 30 mg of codeine to approximately 4.5 mg of morphine • metabolised by CYP2D6 which has genetic variation, resulting in some patients being ultra-rapid metabolisers increasing their risk of toxicity and some being slow metabolisers who do not metabolise sufficient codeine to have a beneficial effect

Continued

TABLE 5.13 Detailed description of opioids—cont'd

Medication	Mechanism of action	Indications for therapeutic use	Common side effects	Practice points	Common adult, child dosage ranges
				Dextropropoxyphene practice points Do not use because: • evidence for use is lacking; no benefit over regular paracetamol when used in combination with regular paracetamol • regular use may lead to accumulation of and the cardiotoxic nordextropropoxyphene • very toxic in acute overdosage • regular monitoring of renal function and ECGs must be performed	**Dextropropoxyphene:** *Adult, oral:* 100 mg every 4 hours when necessary (maximum 600 mg daily) All products have been withdrawn from the market in several countries due to safety concerns; it is still available in Australia, but restrictions for prescribing exist (http://www.tga.gov.au.atlantis2.anu.edu.au:2048/alert/dextropropoxyphene-pain-killers-containing-dextropropoxyphene-di-gesic-and-doloxene-10-october-2013)
				Fentanyl practice points Also available in patch and lozenge form, which are used in chronic pain	**Fentanyl – acute pain:** For use in chronic pain (see Chapter 7) *Adult, subcutaneous:* | Age (years)	Initial dose (in mcg) every 4 hours as required
---	---
<39	100–200
40–59	75–150
60–69	40–100
70–85	40–75
>85 years	30–50	 *Intranasal, child 1–12 years:* 1.5 mcg/kg (maximum 100 mcg); if needed, a second dose of 0.75–1.5 mcg/kg (maximum 100 mcg) may be given after 5–10 minutes Duration of action: 0.5–2 hours

Morphine practice points
Peak analgesia following a dose of morphine occurs within:
• 60 minutes after conventional oral liquid
• 50–90 minutes after SC injection (30–60 minutes after IM)
• 20 minutes after IV injection
Do not use controlled release products for acute pain management
Avoid use in renal impairment due to accumulation of toxic metabolite

Morphine – acute pain:
For use in chronic pain (see Chapter 7)
Adult, child >50 kg, IV:
Initially, 0.5–2 mg; repeat every 3–5 minutes and titrate as above
Adult, child >50 kg, SC/IM:

Age (years)	Initial dose (in mg) every 2 hours as required
<39	7.5–12.5
40–59	5–10
60–69	2.5–7.5
70–85	2.5–5
>85 years	2–3

Adult, oral:
Do not use controlled release products for treatment of acute pain
Conventional oral product, initially 5–15 mg every 4 hours
Child (1–12 years and <50 kg):
IV infusion: initially 0.02–0.04 mg/kg/hour
IV bolus: initially 0.05 mg/kg (over at least 5 minutes) every 2 hours
Subcutaneous: 0.1–0.2 mg/kg every 4 hours
Duration of action:
2–4 hours (injection, immediate release tablet and liquid)
12–24 hours (modified release tablets and suspension)

Continued

TABLE 5.13 Detailed description of opioids—cont'd

Medication	Mechanism of action	Indications for therapeutic use	Common side effects	Practice points	Common adult, child dosage ranges
				Oxycodone practice points May be tried as an alternative opioid for patients intolerant of morphine Do not use controlled release tablets for acute pain as slow onset and offset make rapid, safe titration impossible	**Oxycodone – acute pain:** (For use in chronic pain see Chapter 7) *Adult IV:* 0.5–2 mg; repeat every 3–5 minutes *Adult, subcutaneous:* *Adult, oral:* Do not use controlled release tablets for treatment of acute pain *Conventional oral product:* initially 5–15 mg every 4 hours *Acute pain: child >1 year,* *Conventional oral product:* initially 0.1–0.2 mg/kg (maximum 5 mg) every 4–6 hours Duration of action: 3–4 hours (injection, immediate release tablets, capsules and oral liquid) 12 hours modified release products

Age (years)	Initial dose (in mg) every 2 hours
<39	7.5–12.5
40–59	5–10
60–69	2.5–7.5
70–85	2.5–5
>85 years	2–3

	Tramadol practice points	Tramadol
	Analgesic effect starts within 1 hour of oral administration and peaks at 2–4 hours Do not use controlled release products for acute pain management 6–10% of Caucasians and 1–2% of Asians lack the enzyme CYP2D6; these people may obtain reduced analgesia with tramadol Reduce dose in renal, hepatic impairment and the elderly	*Adult, IV/IM:* 50–100 mg every 4–6 hours, up to a total daily dose of 600 mg Adult, oral (conventional product): 50–100 mg every 4–6 hours when necessary (maximum 400 mg daily or 300 mg daily if >75 years) *Adult, oral (12-hour controlled release product):* 50–200 mg every 12 hours (maximum 400 mg) *Child >1 year, oral (conventional product:* **Only used in children under specialist supervision** 1–2 mg/kg every 4 hours when necessary (maximum 400 mg) Duration of action: 3–6 hours (immediate release capsules and injections) 12–24 hours modified release tablets

CNS, central nervous system; MSK, musculoskeletal.
Adapted from: Australian Medicines Handbook (online). Australian Medicines Handbook Pty Ltd, 2015. Australian Medicines Handbook Pty Ltd, Adelaide. <*http://amhonline.amh.net.au/*>.

TABLE 5.14 Detailed description of supplementary medicines

Medication	Mechanism of action	Indications for therapeutic use	Common side effects	Practice points				Common adult, child dosage ranges
Capsaicin (Link Medical Products Pty Ltd 1995)	Produces analgesia by interfering with the synthesis, storage, transport and release of substance P, a neurotransmitter of pain impulses from the periphery to the central nervous system and an important mediator of inflammation	Used as an adjunct for pain relief in arthritis, diabetic nephropathy and post-herpetic neuralgia	Mild to moderate burning sensation after application, effect is usually temporary	Capsaicin selectively relieves pain without interfering with sensory perception from the treated area The cream may cause temporary burning upon application It is more frequent if the cream is used less than 3 times per day Unless treating the hands, wash hands thoroughly with soap and water after application If found to irritate the fingers, use a glove when applying				Available as 0.025% or 0.075% creams Applied to affected area up to 3 or 4 times per day
Fish Oil (Therapeutic Guidelines Limited 2010e)	When long-chain omega-3 fatty acids, eicosapentaenoic acid (EPA) and docosahexaenoic acid (DHA), are taken in doses greater than 2.7 g daily, they have anti-inflammatory properties, after 2–3 months of treatment	Use can reduce the doses of NSAIDs, DMARDs and corticosteroids required to manage inflammatory conditions	The cost of the capsules and the number required to take an effective dose can be prohibitive to ongoing treatment	Content of selected commercial fish oil products				
				Fish oil (total)	Omega-3 (total)	EPA	DHA	Minimum daily dose needed to give anti-inflammatory effect
				1 g capsules	300 mg	180 mg	120 mg	9 capsules
				1.5 g capsules	450 mg	270 mg	180 mg	6 capsules
				Standard fish oil liquid	2.7 g/15 mL	18%	12%	15 mL
				Concentrated fish oil liquid (4.6 g/5 mL)	2.7 g/5 mL	1.9 g/5 mL	927 mg/5 mL	5 mL

Glucosamine and chondroitin (Therapeutic Guidelines Limited 2010l)	Glucosamine sulfate and chondroitin sulfate are derivatives of glycosaminoglycans, and are building blocks of the ground substance of the articular cartilage proteoglycans The rationale for using glucosamine sulfate is based on animal models of osteoarthritis, in which there has been normalisation of cartilage metabolism, some anti-inflammatory effect and a rebuilding of experimentally damaged cartilage	Use in osteoarthritis is only supported by evidence in OA of the knee, and long-term efficacy and toxicity have not been determined, but a trial of 3–6 months may be reasonable in patients wanting to try alternate therapies	Most formulations of glucosamine are prepared from shellfish, and so should not be used in patients with significant seafood allergy Glucosamine can affect glycaemic control and the INR, so vigilant monitoring of BGLs in diabetic patients and INR in those on warfarin is recommended	The doses usually used are glucosamine sulfate 1500–2000 mg daily and chondroitin sulfate 800–1200 mg daily Note that evidence supporting glucosamine and chondroitin use is not strong

BGLs, blood glucose levels; DMARDs, disease-modifying antirheumatic drugs; INR, international normalized ratio; NSAIDs, non-sedating anti-inflammatory drugs.
Adapted from: Australian Medicines Handbook Pty Ltd, 2015. Australian Medicines Handbook (online). Australian Medicines Handbook Pty Ltd, Adelaide. <http://amhonline.amh.net.au/>.

TABLE 5.15 Detailed description of corticosteroids

Medication	Mechanism of action	Indications for therapeutic use	Common side effects	Practice points	Common adult and children dosage ranges
CLASS: **Corticosteroids** (Therapeutic Guidelines Limited 2010b, 2010d) **Corticosteroids used in MSK conditions** *Oral:* Prednisolone/prednisone Hydrocortisone *Parenteral:* Betamethasone Cortisone Dexamethasone Hydrocortisone Methylprednisolone Triamcinolone Hydrocortisone	Regulate gene expression, which results in: • glucocorticoid effects, e.g. gluconeogenesis, proteolysis, lipolysis, suppression of inflammation and immune responses • mineralocorticoid effects, e.g. hypertension, sodium and water retention, potassium loss	Used in a wide range of conditions for their anti-inflammatory and immunosuppressant effects Intraarticular injection, or injection into soft tissue, of long-acting or depot corticosteroid may provide pain relief in musculoskeletal disorders	Adrenal suppression, increased susceptibility to infection, masking of signs of infection, sodium and water retention, oedema, hypertension, hypokalaemia, hyperglycaemia, dyslipidaemia, osteoporosis, fractures, increased appetite, dyspepsia, delayed wound healing, skin atrophy, bruising, acne, facial flushing, hirsutism, growth retardation in children, myopathy, muscle weakness and wasting, fat redistribution (producing cushingoid appearance), weight gain, menstrual irregularity, amenorrhoea, psychiatric effects, posterior subcapsular cataracts	Corticosteroids may have predominantly glucocorticoid effects (e.g. dexamethasone), mineralocorticoid effects (fludrocortisone) or a combination of both (e.g. hydrocortisone) Use in with caution in the following patients: • latent TB • peptic ulcer disease • diabetes • hypertension • psychiatric disorders • glaucoma • osteoporosis • myasthenia gravis • infection • surgery • pregnancy Prednisone is converted to the pharmacologically active prednisolone and vice versa	See Table 5.5 in 'Arthritis' section for usual doses of local corticosteroid injections **Prednisolone/prednisolone** *Adult, oral autoimmune or inflammatory dose:* Initially 5–60 mg once daily Taper dose according to response; usual maintenance dose 2.5–15 mg once daily (higher doses may be needed) *Child >1 month, autoimmune or inflammatory disease:* Initially 1–2 mg/kg (usual maximum 60 mg); taper dose according to response **Hydrocortisone** *Adult, initial control of autoimmune or inflammatory disease, IV/IM:* 100–500 mg 3 or 4 times daily according to severity of condition

Intra- or periarticular injection: post-injection flare of pain, injection site periarticular calcifications, skin and subcutaneous tissue atrophy at injection site	Considerations for intra- articular injections: • do not give >4 injections/year into any single joint as this may increase the risk of cartilage damage • avoid further intraarticular injections if there is no response after 2 consecutive injections • giving an intraarticular injection to a big toe affected by gout is generally not recommended because the procedure is very painful • some practitioners use a mixture of local anaesthetic and corticosteroid to reduce discomfort following intraarticular injection	*Child, initial control of autoimmune or inflammatory disease, IV/IM*: 2–4 mg/kg (maximum 100 mg) every 6 hours for 24 hours, then reduce over subsequent 24 hours; or change to oral prednisolone

MSK, musculoskeletal; TB, tuberculosis.
Adapted from: Australian Medicines Handbook (online). Australian Medicines Handbook Pty Ltd, 2015. Australian Medicines Handbook Pty Ltd, Adelaide. <http://amhonline.amh. net.au/>.

TABLE 5.16 Detailed description of muscle relaxants and sedating agents[9]

Medication	Mechanism of action	Indications for therapeutic use	Common side effects	Practice points	Common adult, child dosage ranges
CLASS: Benzodiazepines Diazepam (Australian Medicines Handbook Pty Ltd 2015b) Midazolam	Potentiate the inhibitory effects of GABA in the CNS, causing anxiolytic, sedative, hypnotic, muscle relaxant and antiepileptic effects	MSK indications: muscle relaxants (diazepam) Conscious sedation (midazolam)	Drowsiness, over-sedation, light-headedness, memory loss, hypersalivation, ataxia, slurred speech, dependence, effects on vision (e.g. blurred vision), impaired tracking	Use caution in the following patients: • respiratory depression • mysathenia gravis • those at risk of dependence • renal or hepatic impairment • elderly and children • pregnancy and breastfeeding	**Diazepam – muscle spasm:** *Adult:* 2–5 mg orally, up to 3 times daily **Midazolam – conscious sedation:** *Adult IV:* Initial dose 2–2.5 mg; if elderly or debilitated, 1–1.5 mg initially
CLASS: Inhaled anaesthetics (Therapeutic Guidelines Limited 2012c) Nitrous oxide Methoxyflurane	Thought to enhance inhibitory ion channel activity and inhibit excitatory activity in the brain to induce hypnosis and amnesia, and in the spinal cord to cause immobility in response to painful stimuli	Analgesia (in subanaesthetic concentrations) Weak anaesthetics, but strong analgesic activity, so used in subanaesthetic concentrations in obstetrics, emergency care and procedures not requiring loss of consciousness	Shivering (independent of temperature), nausea, vomiting	Use with caution in the following patients: • cardiovascular disease • vitamin B12 deficiency • elderly • children Methoxyflurane practice points: • usually used for immediate, short-term pain relief in the pre-hospital setting (e.g. by ambulance personnel) • onset of pain relief after 6–8 breaths; continues for several minutes after use 3 mL of methoxyflurane used intermittently provides analgesia for approximately 20–30 minutes	**Nitrous oxide** *Adult, child:* 25–50% with oxygen **Methoxyflurane** *Adult:* 0.2–0.7%; up to 6 mL daily (maximum 15 mL per week) Do not use on consecutive days

| Ketamine | Antagonises N-methyl-D-aspartate (NMDA) receptors; also interacts with muscarinic receptors, descending monoaminergic pain pathways, voltage-sensitive calcium channels and opioid receptors in brain and spinal cord | Procedural sedation and analgesia Useful as sole agent for short painful procedures, as there is minimal delay in resuming eating | Elevated BP and pulse rate, increased muscle tone, lacrimation, hypersalivation, nausea and vomiting, raised intracranial pressure, raised intraocular pressure, emergence reactions | Use with caution in the following patient groups: • conditions that may be worsened by an increase in BP and/or heart rate • psychiatric disorders • raised intracranial or intraocular pressure • penetrating eye injury • pregnancy and breastfeeding Illicit/recreational use of ketamine occurs (known as 'special K' or 'vitamin K') | *Adults and children, IV:* Up to 1–1.5 mg/kg slowly titrated to effect over 2–5 minutes; then give half dose every 10 minutes if required *Adults and children, IM:* 3–4 mg/kg; give half dose after 10 minutes if required After a single dose, analgesic effects last about 40 minutes and amnesia lasts 1–2 hours |
| Propofol | Uncertain, but its main CNS depressant action is thought to be via the GABA receptor May also shorten channel opening times at nicotinic acetylcholine receptors and sodium channels in the cerebral cortex | Conscious sedation | Pain on injection, bradycardia, hypotension, apnoea, flushed skin or rash, cough | Formulation has a high lipid content | *Adult, IV:* 0.5–1 mg/kg over 1–5 minutes, then infuse 1.5–3 mg/kg/hour Unconsciousness occurs approximately 30 seconds after injection, with recovery taking 3–5 minutes after infusion is ceased |

BP, blood pressure; CNS, central nervous system; GABA, gamma-aminobutyric acid.
Adapted from: Australian Medicines Handbook (online). Australian Medicines Handbook Pty Ltd, 2015. Australian Medicines Handbook Pty Ltd, Adelaide. <http://amhonline.amh.net.au/>.

ᵃSee also Chapters 6 and 10.

TABLE 5.17 Detailed description of gout medication

Medication	Mechanism of action	Indications for therapeutic use	Common side effects	Practice points	Common adult, child dosage ranges
Allopurinol (Therapeutic Guidelines Limited 2010g)	Reduces uric acid production by inhibiting xanthine oxidase, and lowers plasma and urinary urate concentrations	Gout Hyperuricaemia	Maculopapular or itchy rash	Use with caution in the following patients: • allergy to allopurinol • acute attack of gout • Asian ancestry (increases risk of hypersensitivity reactions) • renal impairment • pregnancy and breastfeeding • concurrent mercaptopurine or azathioprine therapy	*Initial therapy:* Start with a low dose (50–100 mg daily) and slowly increase at monthly intervals (e.g. by 50–100 mg daily) according to response; aim for plasma urate concentration <0.36 mmol/L *Maintenance:* Usual range 300–600 mg daily – this is reduced in renal impairment (maximum 900 mg daily)
Probenicid (Therapeutic Guidelines Limited 2010g)	Increases renal excretion of uric acid by blocking its renal tubular reabsorption	Gout Also used to prolong effects of beta-lactam antibiotics	Rash, nausea, vomiting	Use with caution in the following patients: • allergy to probenicid • history of blood dyscrasias • G6PD deficiency • renal impairment • pregnancy and breastfeeding Ensure adequate fluid intake during the first few months of treatment to reduce the risk of uric acid kidney stones	*Adult:* 250 mg twice daily for 1 week *Maintenance:* 500 mg twice daily, increasing if necessary every 4 weeks (by increments of 500 mg) up to 2 g daily in divided doses Titrate doses according to plasma urate concentration, aiming for <0.36 mmol/L

| Colchicine (Therapeutic Guidelines Limited 2010g) | Inhibits neutrophil migration, chemotaxis, adhesion and phagocytosis in the inflamed area; reduces the inflammatory reaction to urate crystals but has no effect on uric acid production or excretion | Relief of pain in acute gout Prophylaxis of recurrent gout attacks including when starting urate-lowering treatment | Diarrhoea, nausea, abdominal discomfort, vomiting, pharyngolaryngeal pain | Use with caution in the following patients:
• history of blood dyscrasias
• severe GI disease
• corneal wounds or ulcer
• other medications (many interactions)
• renal and hepatic impairment
• breastfeeding
Joint inflammation subsides within 48 hours in most patients
If the dose is too high, colchicines may accumulate, and significant toxicity can result; regular monitoring of complete blood count and renal function is important | *Acute attack, adult:*
1 mg as soon as possible, then 0.5 mg 1 hour later (maximum 1.5 mg per course); do not repeat the course within 3 days
Prophylaxis including when starting urate-lowering treatment, adult:
500 mcg once or twice daily, according to response and GI symptoms
Dose always reduced in renal impairment |

Adapted from: Australian Medicines Handbook Pty Ltd, 2015. Australian Medicines Handbook (online), Australian Medicines Handbook Pty Ltd, Adelaide. <http://amhonline.amh.net.au/>.

TABLE 5.18 Detailed description of disease-modifying anti-rheumatic drugs (DMARDs)

Medication	Mechanism of action	Indications for therapeutic use	Common side effects	Practice points	Common adult dosage ranges
Class: DMARDs (Therapeutic Guidelines Limited 2010d, 2010f, 2014b) Methotrexate (MTX)	Folic acid antagonist Inhibits DNA synthesis and cell replication by competitively inhibiting the conversion of folic acid to folinic acid, with cytotoxic, immunosuppressive and anti-inflammatory action	MSK indications include: rheumatoid arthritis and psoriatic arthritis	Myelosuppression, nausea and vomiting (more frequent with high doses), oral mucositis, pulmonary toxicity, hepatotoxicity, rash, itch, urticaria, photosensitivity; neurotoxicity (e.g. aseptic meningitis, encephalopathy, leucoencephalopathy) with high dose or intrathecal use	Contraindicated in: • immunodeficiency • myelosuppression • blood disorders • peptic ulceration • ulcerative colitis • poor nutritional status • serious or untreated infection Use with caution in: • renal, hepatic disease • pregnancy and breastfeeding	5–10 mg orally, on one specified day per week, increasing up to a maximum dose of 25 mg orally, SC or IM, on one specified day per week depending on clinical response and adverse effects Folic acid 5–10 mg orally, once weekly (preferably not on the day that the methotrexate is taken) or 1 mg on the 6 other days MTX is not taken
Hydroxychloroquine	Anti-inflammatory May also have immunosuppressive effects	Rheumatoid arthritis (RA) Systemic lupus erythematosus (SLE)	Nausea, vomiting, diarrhoea, anorexia, abdominal cramps, rash, itch, alopecia, headache, blurred vision	Contraindicated in: • retinopathy • allergy to chloroquine or hydroxychloroquine Use with caution in: • diabetes • haematological disorders • psoriasis • G6PD deficiency • pregnancy and breastfeeding Regular ophthalmological review is recommended May take approximately 2–6 months of treatment before benefit is seen in rheumatoid arthritis Hydroxychloroquine has a long half-life (>30 days); consider this when changing dose or stopping treatment (e.g. due to adverse effects)	200–400 mg orally, daily

Sulfasalazine	Anti-inflammatory, immunosuppressant	Rheumatoid arthritis Psoriatic arthritis	Vomiting, reversible male infertility (oligospermia), haemolysis (not usually severe), Stevens–Johnson syndrome (rare)	Contraindicated in thrombocytopenia Use with caution in: • hepatic impairment • children • allergy to sulfonamides • asthma • pregnancy and breastfeeding May take 1–3 months of treatment before benefit is seen	500 mg orally (enteric-coated), twice daily, increasing gradually up to 1.5 g orally, twice daily
Leflunomide	Inhibits pyrimidine synthesis in leucocytes and other rapidly dividing cells by inhibiting activity of dihydro-orotate dehydrogenase Has immunosuppressive, immunomodulating and antiproliferative properties Also has uricosuric effects	Rheumatoid arthritis Psoriatic arthritis	Abdominal pain, diarrhoea, nausea, vomiting, cholelithiasis, raised liver enzymes, hair loss, mild allergic reactions (e.g. rash), itch, eczema, weight loss, weakness, synovitis, tenosynovitis, headache, dizziness, paraesthesia, peripheral neuropathy, bronchitis, pharyngitis, dyspnoea, pneumonia, hypertension	Contraindicated in: • allergy to leflunomide or teriflunomide • history of Stevens–Johnson syndrome, toxic epidermal necrolysis, erythema multiforme • severe immunodeficiency states or bone marrow depression • lymphoproliferative disease within the last 5 years or myelodysplasia • history of interstitial lung disease • pregnancy Use with caution in the following patients: • infection • hepatic impairment • children • women of childbearing age • breastfeeding Adverse effects may be prolonged after stopping leflunomide as it has an active metabolite with a long half-life (2–4 weeks); clinical improvement usually starts after about 4 weeks of treatment and stabilises within 4–6 months	10–20 mg orally, daily

Continued

TABLE 5.18 Detailed description of disease-modifying anti-rheumatic drugs (DMARDs)—cont'd

Medication	Mechanism of action	Indications for therapeutic use	Common side effects	Practice points	Common adult dosage ranges
Cyclosporin	Complexes with cytoplasmic immunophilins (cyclophilin and FKBP-12 respectively), which block the action of calcineurin in activated T cells	Rheumatoid arthritis Psoriatic arthritis	Gingival hyperplasia (more common in children and adolescents), hirsutism, nephrotoxicity, hypertension, hypercholesterolaemia, neurotoxicity, raised bilirubin, raised aminotransferases, hypomagnesaemia, hyperkalaemia, opportunistic infection, diarrhoea, hyperglycaemia, diabetes	Use with caution in the following patients: • uncontrolled hypertension • renal impairment • children • breastfeeding • concurrent use of nephrotoxic medications • infection • pregnancy Benefit may not be seen until after approximately 2–4 months of treatment; stop cyclosporin treatment if response is insufficient after 6 months Regular monitoring of renal function and FBC is required	1 mg/kg orally, twice daily, with gradual titration up to a maximum of 2.5 mg/kg orally, twice daily

FBC, full blood count; MSK, musculoskeletal.
Adapted from: Australian Medicines Handbook Pty Ltd, 2015. Australian Medicines Handbook (online). Australian Medicines Handbook Pty Ltd, Adelaide. <http://amhonline.amh.net.au/>.

TABLE 5.19 Detailed description of biological DMARDs

Medication	Mechanism of action	Indications for therapeutic use	Common side effects	Practice points	Common adult dosage ranges
Abatacept (Therapeutic Guidelines Limited 2010d)	Co-stimulation modulator; binds to CD80 and CD86 on antigen-presenting cells, which prevents full activation of CD28 T lymphocytes, thus reducing cytokine production and inflammation	Moderate-to-severe rheumatoid arthritis; use with methotrexate	Infections, autoimmune disorders (e.g. psoriasis), headache, dizziness, paraesthesia, hypertension, increased liver enzymes, leucopenia, infusion-related reactions (below), injection site reactions (e.g. haematoma, erythema, itch), alopecia, rash, nausea, diarrhoea, dyspepsia, mouth ulcers, weakness	Use with caution in the following patients: • infection • COPD • surgery • pregnancy and breastfeeding Regular monitoring of renal and liver function is required Response may be seen within 14 days and improvement may continue for >1 year Consider stopping if there is no effect after 3–4 months	500–1000 mg IV, as a single dose at 0, 2 and 4 weeks, and thereafter every 4 weeks
CLASS: TNF-alpha antagonists (Therapeutic Guidelines Limited 2010d, 2010f) Adalimumab Certolizumab Etanercept Golimumab Infliximab	Bind to TNF-alpha and inhibit its activity TNF-alpha is a cytokine involved in inflammatory and immune responses and in the pathogenesis of rheumatoid arthritis, psoriasis and inflammatory bowel disease	Moderate-to-severe active rheumatoid arthritis Psoriatic arthritis	Infections, rash, itch, headache, autoantibodies **Adalimumab** Nausea, weakness, flu-like syndrome, injection site reaction, antibodies to adalimumab, allergy, hyperlipidaemia **Etanercept** Injection site reaction, allergic reactions, fever, antibodies to etanercept (non-neutralising), abdominal pain, dyspepsia	Contraindicated in: • demyelinating disorders (e.g. MS) • heart failure • treatment with another cytokine modulator Use with caution in the following patients: • history of blood dyscrasia • respiratory disease • psoriasis • infection • malignancy • surgery • pregnancy and breastfeeding	**Adalimumab:** 40 mg SC, every 2 weeks Practice points: • initial response occurs within 1–2 weeks, with maximum response by 12–16 weeks • poorer response in patients who develop antibodies against adalimumab **Certolizumab:** 400 mg SC, as a single dose at 0, 2 and 4 weeks, and thereafter 200 mg SC, every 2 weeksor certolizumab 400 mg SC, every 4 weeks

Continued

TABLE 5.19 Detailed description of biological DMARDs—cont'd

Medication	Mechanism of action	Indications for therapeutic use	Common side effects	Practice points	Common adult dosage ranges
			Golimumab Injection site reactions, antibodies to golimumab, hypertension, increased hepatic aminotransferases, abdominal pain, nausea, dizziness, weakness **Infliximab** Infusion-related effects, nausea, abdominal pain, vomiting, fever, cough, fatigue, vertigo, dizziness, flushing, serum sickness-like reaction, antibodies to infliximab	Consider need for immunisation before starting treatment Continue monitoring for adverse effects, including infections, for 5 months after stopping treatment, due to their long half-life (may be less for etanercept)	Practice points: response occurs within 12 weeks of treatment, may be reduced in patients who develop antibodies against certolizumab **Etanercept**: 25 mg SC, twice weekly or 50 mg SC, once weekly Practice points: benefit may be seen after approximately 1–12 weeks of treatment **Golimumab**: 50 mg SC, every 4 weeks Practice points: benefit may be seen within 12 weeks of treatment **Infliximab**: 3 mg/kg IV, as a single dose at 0, 2 and 6 weeks, and thereafter every 8 weeks Practice points: benefit is usually seen within 12 weeks

| Tociluzimab | Inhibits the activity of interleukin-6 (IL-6), a cytokine involved in the pathogenesis of rheumatoid arthritis (RA) and systemic juvenile idiopathic arthritis (JIA), by binding to its receptors | Moderate-to-severe RA with poor prognostic factors or after inadequate response, or intolerance, to another antirheumatic medication Use with methotrexate or another antirheumatic if possible | Infections (including opportunistic), neutropenia, increased liver enzymes, gastritis, mouth ulcers, diarrhoea, nausea, increased lipids (largely LDL), hypertension, infusion-related reactions, antibodies to tocilizumab, rash, itch, headache, dizziness | Use with caution in the following patients:
• low neutrophils or platelets
• previous TNF-alpha antagonist treatment
• history of diverticulitis or GI ulceration
• infection
• hepatic impairment
• surgery
• pregnancy and breastfeeding | 8 mg/kg IV, every 4 weeks Effect may be seen within 2 weeks in RA |

GI, gastrointestinal; LDL, low-density lipoprotein; MS, multiple sclerosis; TNF, tumour necrosis factor.
Adapted from: Australian Medicines Handbook Pty Ltd, 2015. Australian Medicines Handbook (online). Australian Medicines Handbook Pty Ltd, Adelaide. <*http://amhonline.amh. net.au/*>.

side effects and relevant practice points and dosing information. The purpose of the information in these tables is to assist physiotherapists in enhancing patient management and monitoring for potential medication side effects. The information in these tables has been adapted from the *Australian Medicines Handbook* (Australian Medicines Handbook Pty Ltd 2015a) and the relevant Therapeutic Guidelines.

■ References

Ahmed, N., Poate, T., Nacher-Garcia, C., et al., 2014. Temporomandibular joint multidisciplinary team clinic. British Journal of Oral and Maxillofacial Surgery 52, 827–830.

Anderson, R.J., Todd, D.J., 2015. Bursitis: an overview of clinical manifestations, diagnosis, and management. UpToDate [Internet]. <http://www.uptodate.com/contents/bursitis-an-overview-of-clinical-manifestations-diagnosis-and-management?source=search_result&search=Bursitis&selectedTitle=1~94> (accessed 12.04.16).

Apostolopoulos, D., Hoi, A.Y., 2013. Systemic lupus erythmatosus: when to consider and management options. Australian Family Physician 42 (10), 696–700.

Arif, T., Masood, Q., Singh, J., et al., 2015. Assessment of esophageal involvement in systemic sclerosis and morphea (localized scleroderma) by clinical, endoscopic, manometric and pH metric features: a prospective comparative hospital based study. BMC Gastroenterology 15 (24), 1–9.

Australian Institute of Health and Welfare (AIHW), 2009. Department of Health and Ageing, A picture of rheumatoid arthritis [Internet]. <http://www.aihw.gov.au/workarea/downloadasset.aspx?id=6442459857> (accessed 08.06.15).

Australian Institute of Health and Welfare (AIHW), 2015. Arthritis, osteoporosis and other musculoskeletal conditions [Internet]. <http://www.aihw.gov.au/arthritis-and-musculoskeletal-conditions/> (accessed 12.09.15).

Australian Medicines Handbook Pty Ltd, 2015a. *Australian Medicines Handbook* (online). Adelaide: Australian Medicines Handbook Pty Ltd. <http://amhonline.amh.net.au/>.

Australian Medicines Handbook Pty Ltd, 2015b. Diazepam (neurology). *Australian Medications Handbook* (online). Adelaide: Australian Medicines Handbook Pty Ltd. <https://amhonline-amh-net-au>.

Australian Rheumatology Association, 2011. *Biological Recommendations*. <http://rheumatology.org.au/otherpages/biological-guidelines.asp>.

Australian Rheumatology Association, 2015. *Scleroderma Special Interest Group*. <http://rheumatology.org.au/rheumatologists/asig-public.asp> (accessed 12.04.16).

Barile, M.F., Wu, J.S., McMahon, C.J., 2014. Femoral head avascular necrosis: a frequently missed incidental finding on multidetector CT. Clinical Radiology 69, 280–285.

Baumbach, S.F., Lobo, C.M., Badyine, I., et al., 2014. Prepatellar and olecranon bursitis: literature review and development of a treatment algorithm. Archives of Orthopaedic & Trauma Surgery 134, 359–370.

Baumbach, S.F., Wyen, H., Perez, C., et al., 2013. Evaluation of current treatment regimens for prepatellar and olecranon bursitis in Switzerland. European Journal of Trauma and Emergency Surgery 39, 65–72.

Breedland, I., van Scheppingen, C., Leijsma, M., et al., 2011. Effects of a group-based exercise and educational program on physical performance and disease self-management in rheumatoid arthritis: a randomized controlled study. Physical Therapy 91 (6), 879–893.

Brukner, P., Khan, K., 2012. Clinical Sports Medicine, 4th ed. McGraw-Hill Education (Australia) Pty Ltd, Australia.

Buono, A.D., Franceschi, F., Palumbo, A., et al., 2012. Diagnosis and management of olecranon bursitis. Surgeon, Journal of the Royal Colleges of Surgeons of Edinburgh and Ireland 10, 297–300.

Cardoso, J.R., Teixeira, E.C., Moreira, M.D., et al., 2008. Effects of exercises on Bell's palsy: systematic review of randomized controlled trials. Otology and Neurotology 29 (4), 557–560.

Carpenter, C.R., Schuur, J.D., Everett, W.W., et al., 2011. Evidence-based diagnostics: adult septic arthritis. Academic Emergency Medicine : Official Journal of the Society for Academic Emergency Medicine 18 (8), 781–796.

Cinar, N., Bodur, H., Eser, F., et al., 2015. The prevalence and characteristics of psoriatic arthritis in patients with psoriasis in a tertiary hospital. Archives of Rheumatology 30 (1), 23–27.

Connelly, K., Morand, E.F., Hoi, A.Y., 2013. Asian ethnicity in systemic lupus erythematosus: an Australian perspective. Internal Medicine Journal 43, 618–624.

Conterno, L.O., Turchi, M.D., 2013. Antibiotics for treating chronic osteomyelitis in adults. The Cochrane Database of Systematic Reviews 6 (9), doi:10.1002/14651858.CD004439 .pub3.

Cook, J.L., Purdam, C.R., 2009. Is tendon pathology a continuum? A pathology model to explain the clinical presentation of load-induced tendinopathy. British Journal of Sports Medicine 43 (6), 409–416.

Cook, J.L., Purdam, C.R., 2014. The challenge of managing tendinopathy in competing athletes. British Journal of Sports Medicine 48, 506–509.

Cross, M., Smith, E., Hoy, D., et al., 2014. The global burden of hip and knee osteoarthritis: estimates from the Global Burden of Disease 2010 study. Annals of the Rheumatic Diseases 73 (7), 1323–1330.

da Costa, B.R., Reichenbach, S., Keller, N., et al., 2016. Effectiveness of non-steroidal anti-inflammatory drugs for the treatment of pain in knee and hip osteoarthritis: a network meta-analysis. Lancet [Internet]. <http://dx.doi.org/10.1016/S0140-6736(16)30002-2> (accessed 12.04.16.); [Epub ahead of print].

Dagfinrud, H., Kvien, T.K., Hagen, K.B., 2008. Physiotherapy interventions for ankylosing spondylitis. The Cochrane Database of Systematic Reviews (1), CD002822, doi:10.1002/14651858.CD002822.pub3.

Devor, M., Amir, R., Rappaport, Z.H., 2002. Pathophysiology of trigeminal neuralgia: the ignition hypothesis. The Clinical Journal of Pain 18, 4–13.

Gibson, J.N.A., Waddell, G., 2005. Surgery for degenerative lumbar spondylosis (review). The Cochrane Database of Systematic Reviews (4), CD001352, doi:10.1002/14651858.CD001352. pub3.

French, H.P., Cusack, T., Brennan, A., et al., 2013. Exercise and Manual Physiotherapy Arthritis Research Trial (EMPART) for osteoarthritis of the hip: a multicenter randomized controlled trial. Archives of Physical Medicine and Rehabilitation 94, 302–314.

Fu, S.-C., Rolf, C., Cheuk, Y.-C., et al., 2010. Deciphering the pathogenesis of tendinopathy: a three-stage process. Sports Medicine, Arthroscopy, Therapy & Technology 30 (2), 1–12.

Gibson, J.N.A., Waddell, G., 2005. Surgery for degenerative lumbar spondylosis (review). The Cochrane Database of Systematic Reviews (4), CD001352, doi:10.1002/14651858.CD001352. pub3.

Hawkins, K., Ghazi, F., 2012. The addition of a supervised exercise class to a home exercise programme in the treatment of patients with knee osteoarthritis following corticosteroid injection: a pilot study. International Musculoskeletal Medicine 34 (4), 159–165.

Huisstede, B.M., Friden, J., Coert, J.H., et al., 2014. Carpal tunnel syndrome: hand surgeons, hand therapists, and physical medicine and rehabilitation physicians agree on a multidisciplinary treatment guideline – results from the European HANDGUIDE study. Archives of Physical Medicine and Rehabilitation 95, 2253–2263.

Iversen, M.D., Chhabriya, R.K., Shadick, N., 2011. Predictors of the use of physical therapy services among patients with rheumatoid arthritis. Physical Therapy 91 (1), 65–76.

Jain, T.K., Sharma, N.K., 2014. The effectiveness of physiotherapeutic interventions in treatment of frozen shoulder/adhesive capsulitis: a systematic review. Journal of Back and Musculoskeletal Rehabilitation 27, 247–273.

Jowett, S., Crawshaw, D.P., Helliwell, P.S., et al., 2013. Cost-effectiveness of exercise therapy after corticosteroid injection for moderate to severe shoulder pain due to subacromial impingement syndrome: a trial-based analysis. Rheumatology 52, 1485–1491.

Jüni, P., Hari, R., Rutjes, A.W.S., et al., 2015. Intra-articular corticosteroid for knee osteoarthritis. The Cochrane Database of Systematic Reviews (10), CD005328, doi:10.1002/14651858. CD005328.pub3.

Kanis, J.A., Oden, A., McCloskey, E.V., et al., 2012. A systematic review of hip fracture incidence and probability of fracture worldwide. Osteoporosis International Feb (23), 2239–2256.

Kearney, R.S., Parsons, N., Metcalfe, D., et al., 2015. Injection therapies for Achilles tendinopathy. The Cochrane Database of Systematic Reviews (5), CD010960, doi:10.1002/14651858. CD010960.pub2.

Kelley, M.J., Shaffer, M.A., Kuhn, J.E., et al., 2013. Shoulder pain and mobility deficits: adhesive capsulitis. Journal of Orthopaedic Sports Physical Therapy 43 (5), A1–A31.

Khanna, P.P., Gladue, H.S., Singh, M.K., et al., 2014. Treatment of gout: a systematic review. Seminars in Arthritis and Rheumatism 44, 31–38.

Levin, K. Lumbar spinal stenosis: treatment and prognosis, 2015. UpToDate [Internet]. <http://www.uptodate.com/contents/lumbar-spinal-stenosis-treatment-and-prognosis?source=search_result&search=Lumbar+spinal+stenosis%3A+treatment+and+prognosis&selectedTitle=1~26> (accessed 12.04.16).

Link Medical Products Pty Ltd, 1995, *Zostrix cream (capsacian) Australian approved product information*. NSW: Link Medical Products Pty Ltd.

Malliaras, P., Barton, C.J., Reeves, N.D., et al., 2013. Achilles and patellar tendinopathy loading programmes. A systematic review comparing clinical outcomes and identifying potential mechanisms for effectiveness. Sports Medicine 43, 267–286.

McCreesh, K., Lewis, J., 2013. Continuum model of tendon pathology – where are we now? International Journal of Experimental Pathology 94, 242–247.

Mease, P.J., Armstrong, A.W., 2014. Managing patients with psoriatic disease: the diagnosis and pharmacologic treatment of psoriatic arthritis in patients with psoriasis. Drugs 74, 423–441.

Muraki, S., Akune, T., Oka, H., et al., 2012. Incidence and risk factors for radiographic lumbar spondylosis and lower back pain in Japanese men and women: the ROAD study. Osteoarthritis and Cartilage 20, 712–718.

National Institute for Health and Care Excellence (NICE), 2009. *Low Back Pain: Early Management of Persistent Non-specific Low Back Pain*. [Internet] <http://www.nice.org.uk/guidance/cg88/chapter/1-guidance#pharmacological-therapies> (accessed 10.04.16).

National Institute for Health and Care Excellence (NICE), 2015. *Musculoskeletal Conditions Overview*. [Internet] <http://pathways.nice.org.uk/pathways/musculoskeletal-conditions> (accessed 12.09.15).

Ofir, C., Oleg, D., Gavriel, M., et al., 2014. Timing matters: NSAIDs interfere with the late proliferation stage of a repaired rotator cuff tendon healing in rats. Archives of Orthopaedic & Trauma Surgery 134 (4), 515–520.

Otoo, S.K.W., Hendrick, P., Ribeiro, D.C., 2015. The comparative effectiveness of advice/education compared to active physiotherapy (manual therapy and exercise) in the management of chronic non-specific low back pain. Physical Therapy Reviews 20 (1), 16–28.

Pons-Estel, G.J., Alarcón, G.S., Scofield, L., et al., 2010. Understanding the epidemiology and progression of systemic lupus erythematosus. Seminars in Arthritis and Rheumatism 39, 257–268.

Pratelli, E., Pintucci, M., Cultrera, P., et al., 2015. Conservative treatment of carpal tunnel syndrome: comparison between laser therapy and fascial manipulation. Journal of Bodywork and Movement Therapies 19, 113–118.

Prince, D.S., McGuigan, L.E., McGirr, E.E., 2014. Working life and physical activity in ankylosing spondylitis pre and post anti-tumor necrosis factor-alpha therapy. International Journal of Rheumatic Diseases 2 (17), 165–172.

Punzi, L., Scanu, A., Ramonda, R., et al., 2012. Gout as autoinflammatory disease: new mechanisms for more appropriated treatment targets. Autoimmunity Reviews 12, 66–71.

Ranalletta, M., Rossi, L.A., Bongiovanni, S.L., et al., 2016. Corticosteroid injections accelerate pain relief and recovery of function compared with oral NSAIDs in patients with adhesive capsulitis: a randomized controlled trial. American Journal of Sports Medicine 44, 474–481.

Rashid, A., Matthews, N.S., Cowgill, H., 2013. Physiotherapy in the management of disorders of the temporomandibular joint – perceived effectiveness and access to services: a national United Kingdom survey. Surgery 51 (1), 52–57.

Reid, D.A., Potts, G., Burnett, M., et al., 2014. Physiotherapy management of knee and hip osteoarthritis: a survey of patient and medical practitioners' expectations, experiences and perceptions of effectiveness of treatment. New Zealand Journal of Physiotherapy 42 (2), 118–125.

Resteghini, P., Yeoh, J., 2012. High-volume injection in the management of recalcitrant mid-body Achilles tendinopathy: a prospective case series assessing the influence of neovascularity and outcome. International Musculoskeletal Medicine 34 (2), 92–100.

Robinson, P.C., Horsburgh, S., 2014. Gout: joints and beyond, epidemiology, clinical features, treatment and co-morbidities. Maturitas 78, 245–251.

Roddy, E., Zwierska, I., Hay, E.M., et al., 2014. Subacromial impingement syndrome and pain: protocol for a randomised controlled trial of exercise and corticosteroid injection (the SUPPORT trial). BMC Musculoskeletal Disorders 15 (81), 1–10.

Salinas, R.A., Alvarez, G., Daly, F., et al., 2010. Corticosteroids for Bell's palsy (idiopathic facial paralysis). The Cochrane Database of Systematic Reviews (3), CD001942.

Sarlani, E., Balciunas, B.A., Grace, E.G., 2005. Orofacial pain – part I: assessment and management of musculoskeletal and neuropathic causes. AACN Advanced Critical Care 16, 333–346.

Sayegh, E.T., Strauch, R.J., 2014. Treatment of olecranon bursitis: a systematic review. Archives of Orthopaedic and Trauma Surgery 134, 1517–1536.

Scott, A., Backman, L.J., Speed, C., 2015. Tendinopathy: update on pathophysiology. Journal of Orthopaedic and Sports Physical Therapy 45 (11), 833–841.

Singh, J.A., Furst, D.E., Bharat, A., et al., 2012. 2012 update of the 2008 American College of Rheumatology (ACR) Recommendations for the Use of Disease-modifying Anti-rheumatic Drugs and Biologics in the Treatment of Rheumatoid Arthritis (RA). Arthritis Care and Research 64 (5), 625–639.

Slipman, C.W., Patel, R.K., Botwin, K., et al., 2003. Epidemiology of spine tumors presenting to musculoskeletal physiatrists. Archives of Physical Medicine and Rehabilitation 84, 492–495.

Stockdale, J., Selfe, J., Roddam, H., 2014. An exploration of the impact of anti-TNF(medication on exercise behaviour in patients with ankylosing spondylitis. Musculoskeletal Care 12, 150–159.

Su, B., O'Connor, P., 2013. NSAID therapy effects on healing of bone, tendon, and the enthesis. Journal of Applied Physiology 115, 892–899.

Tarr, T., Dérfalvi, B., Győri, N., et al., 2015. Similarities and differences between pediatric and adult patients with systemic lupus erythematosus. Lupus 24, 796–803.

The Gale Group, Inc., 2008. Gale Encyclopedia of Medicine. The Gale Group, Farmington Hills, Michigan.

Therapeutic Guidelines Limited, 2010a. Osteoarthritis: pharmacological treatment. In: eTG complete [Internet]. Therapeutic Guidelines Limited, Melbourne.

Therapeutic Guidelines Limited, 2010b. Joint aspiration and injection. In: eTG complete [Internet]. Therapeutic Guidelines Limited, Melbourne.

Therapeutic Guidelines Limited, 2010c. Septic arthritis. In: eTG complete [Internet]. Therapeutic Guidelines Limited, Melbourne.

Therapeutic Guidelines Limited, 2010d. Rheumatoid arthritis. In: eTG complete [Internet]. Therapeutic Guidelines Limited, Melbourne.

Therapeutic Guidelines Limited, 2010e. Fish oil (omega-3 long chain polyunsaturated fatty acids). In: eTG complete [Internet]. Therapeutic Guidelines Limited, Melbourne. 2015 Nov.

Therapeutic Guidelines Limited, 2010f. Psoriatic arthritis. In: eTG complete [Internet]. Therapeutic Guidelines Limited, Melbourne.

Therapeutic Guidelines Limited, 2010g. Gout. In: eTG complete [Internet]. Therapeutic Guidelines Limited, Melbourne.

Therapeutic Guidelines Limited, 2010h. Adhesive capsulitis (frozen shoulder). In: eTG complete [Internet]. Therapeutic Guidelines Limited, Melbourne.

Therapeutic Guidelines Limited, 2010i. General management of tendonopathies. In: eTG complete [Internet]. Therapeutic Guidelines Limited, Melbourne.

Therapeutic Guidelines Limited, 2010j. Carpel tunnel syndrome. In: eTG complete [Internet]. Therapeutic Guidelines Limited, Melbourne.

Therapeutic Guidelines Limited, 2010k. Ankylosing spondylitis: pharmacological management. In: eTG complete [Internet]. Therapeutic Guidelines Limited, Melbourne.

Therapeutic Guidelines Limited, 2010l. Complementary medicine: use in rheumatology. In: eTG complete [Internet]. Therapeutic Guidelines Limited, Melbourne.

Therapeutic Guidelines Limited, 2012a. Sprains and strains. In: eTG complete [Internet]. Therapeutic Guidelines Limited, Melbourne.

Therapeutic Guidelines Limited, 2012b. Acute pain: minor trauma. In: eTG complete [Internet]. Therapeutic Guidelines Limited, Melbourne.

Therapeutic Guidelines Limited, 2012c. Procedure-related pain in adults: procedures with sedation. In: eTG complete [Internet]. Therapeutic Guidelines Limited, Melbourne.

Therapeutic Guidelines Limited, 2014a. Osteomyelitis. In: eTG complete [Internet]. Therapeutic Guidelines Limited, Melbourne.

Therapeutic Guidelines Limited, 2014b. Septic bursitis. In: eTG complete [Internet]. Therapeutic Guidelines Limited, Melbourne.

Therapeutic Guidelines Limited, 2014c. Systemic lupus erythematosus. In: eTG complete [Internet]. Therapeutic Guidelines Limited, Melbourne.

Therapeutic Guidelines Limited, 2014d. Inflammatory connective tissue diseases: scleroderma. In: eTG complete [Internet]. Therapeutic Guidelines Limited, Melbourne.

Therapeutic Guidelines Limited, 2014e. Open fractures. In: eTG complete [Internet]. Therapeutic Guidelines Limited, Melbourne.

Towheed, T.E., Maxwell, L., Anastassiades, T.P., et al., 2005. Glucosamine therapy for treating osteoarthritis. The Cochrane Database of Systematic Reviews (2), CD002946.

Trobisch, P.D., Bauman, M., Weise, K., et al., 2010. Histologic analysis of ruptured quadriceps tendons. Knee Surgery, Sports Traumatology, Arthroscopy 18, 85–88.

Walmsley, S., Osmotherly, P.G., Rivett, D.A., 2014. Clinical identifiers for early-stage primary/idiopathic adhesive capsulitis: are we seeing the real picture? Physical Therapy 94 (7), 968–976.

Wani, S., Raka, N., Jethwa, J., et al., 2013. Comparative efficacy of cervical retraction exercises (McKenzie) with and without using pressure biofeedback in cervical spondylosis. International Journal of Therapy and Rehabilitation 20 (10), 501–508.

Whelan, D.B., Litchfield, R., Wambolt, E., et al., 2014. External rotation immobilization for primary shoulder dislocation: a randomized controlled trial. Clinical Orthopaedics and Related Research 472 (8), 2380–2386.

Wiegand, N., Vámhidy, L., Lörinczy, D., 2010. Differential scanning calorimetric examination of ruptured lower limb tendons in human. Journal of Thermal Analysis and Calorimetry 101, 487–492.

Woolf, A.D., Pfleger, B., 2003. Burden of major musculoskeletal conditions. Bulletin of the World Health Organization 81, 646–656.

Yeun, H.K., Cunningham, M.A., 2014. Optimal management of fatigue in patients with systematic lupus erythematosus: a systematic review. Therapeutics and Clinical Risk Management 10, 775–786.

Neurological system

Jacqueline Reznik, Ofer Keren, Iftah Biran, Ilana Schumacher

This chapter will discuss the role that medications have in the supplementary management of the most common neurological conditions treated by physiotherapists. By the end of this chapter (including cross-referencing with other relevant chapters) the reader should have an understanding of:

+ the major classification of neurological disorders according to structure, location, signs and symptoms
+ pharmacotherapy options for the major neurological disorders
+ usual dosages, routes of administration and major contraindications and precautions of these medications
+ potential impacts of these medications on physiotherapeutic management.

Pharmacological interventions for major symptoms seen in neurological disorders

Extrapyramidal (Parkinsonism)

Involuntary movements

Spasticity

Cognitive decline (dementia)

Seizures (epilepsy)

Specialised drugs used for specific neurological conditions

Multiple sclerosis

Amyotrophic lateral sclerosis/motor neurone disease

◼ Introduction

Neurological disorders, along with mental and substance use disorders, account for a substantial proportion of the world's disease burden (Global Burden of Disease Study 2013 Collaborators 2015; Whiteford et al. 2015). The Global Burden of Disease (GBD) Studies and, in particular, the most recent versions (GBD 2010, GBD 2013) clearly show that neurological disorders have large and widespread consequences (Stovner et al. 2014).

Under the heading of neurological disorders in GBD 2013 are listed Alzheimer's disease (AD), Parkinson's disease (PD), epilepsy, multiple sclerosis (MS) and headache disorders. Cerebrovascular disease/stroke and peripheral neuropathies are listed elsewhere in GBD 2013. This chapter includes the drug regimens for the above-mentioned disorders excluding headache disorders, which are beyond the scope of the chapter. Regarding cardiovascular disorders, general drug therapy will be dealt with in the chapter on the cardiovascular system (Chapter 2). However, specific issues for cerebrovascular disorders relating to residual signs and symptoms such as spasticity, which are of importance to neurological physiotherapists, will be dealt with in this chapter. The American Academy of Neurology (AAN) provides guidelines to help make decisions related to the diagnosis and treatment of neurological diseases (https://www.aan.com). References with specific guidelines for a number of neurological disorders are also available at the end of this chapter (Goldstein 2011; Miller et al. 2009; National Institute for Health and Care Excellence (NICE) 2013, 2014; Sellbach & Silburn 2012; NHMRC Partnership on Dealing with Dementia and Related Functional Decline in Older People (CDPC) 2015).

This chapter follows the AAN diagnostic nomenclature and guidelines (AAN guidelines available at https://www.aan.com) and the Australian approved indications as specified on the MIMS registry (available on the MIMS website, http://www.mims.com.au). Emphasis will be placed on those signs and symptoms and conditions most frequently treated by physiotherapists, and where the physiotherapists' input is vital in monitoring the effects of the prescribed medications. The focus of this chapter is on the major drugs prescribed for specific neurological disorders and their relevance for the physiotherapist (Table 6.1). As indicated in Table 6.1 many of the drugs prescribed for neurological disorders are discussed in other chapters of this handbook, to which the reader is directed.

The autonomic nervous system (ANS) and its importance in the field of pharmacotherapy are discussed in Chapter 1.

Major drug groups

Each category and the specific subgroup of drugs will be reviewed in terms of mechanism of action, route of administration, effects and adverse effects. Examples are provided for the different clinical situations in which particular drugs would be used. A range of options is available for the treatment and/or management of neurological disorders and, although physiotherapists caring for individuals with neurological disorders are primarily interested in treating or managing the signs and symptoms of specific neurological conditions, it is critical that all patients are carefully assessed. Although a definitive diagnosis

TABLE 6.1 Drugs used in neurological disorders

General category	Specific group	Relevance for physiotherapist	Where addressed
Drugs that act solely on the nervous system – symptom-oriented	Drugs used in movement disorders	+++	This chapter
	Drugs used for spasticity	+++	This chapter
	Antiepileptic drugs	+	This chapter
	Drugs used in dementias	+	This chapter
	Psychotropic drugs	+	Chapter 10
Drugs that act solely on the nervous system – disease-oriented	Drugs for MS	+++	This chapter
	Drugs for ALS/MND	++	This chapter
	Drugs used in dementias (some are symptom-oriented)	+	This chapter
Adjuvant drugs that are used to treat neurological disorders	Vascular	+	Chapter 2
	Pain	+++	Chapter 7
	Anti-inflammatory	+	Chapter 5

ALS, amyotrophic lateral sclerosis; MND, motor neurone disease; MS, multiple sclerosis.

may not be possible, relevant clinical outcome measures must be carefully documented (Hill et al. 2010). In addition to the impact of the physiotherapy intervention on the patient the treating physiotherapist can also monitor the impact of the drug intervention using the appropriate measures. The signs and symptoms observed in these patient groups are largely due to the affected structures and their locations.

The structure and function of the neurological system can be approached in various ways: anatomic (structure and location); sensory and motor; central and peripheral; cognitive; behavioural and emotional; general and autonomic. In this chapter common neurological signs and symptoms will be reviewed from both the sensory/motor and the central/peripheral perspectives.

Neurological localisation of signs and symptoms

Table 6.2 outlines the main structures, location and most common neurological signs and symptoms. As indicated some signs and symptoms will be contralateral or ipsilateral, whereas others may be unilateral or bilateral. This will depend upon the location of the lesion.

Depending upon the structure(s) affected the neurological signs and symptoms will vary. In many neurological disorders multiple structures are

TABLE 6.2 Structure, location, signs and symptoms

Structure	Location	Signs and symptoms (S&S)[a]
Central nervous system (CNS)	Cortex	Spasticity, weakness (plegia/paresis), sensory disturbances (neglect), apraxia, cognitive disturbances, psychiatric manifestations Seizures (Contralateral S&S)
	Basal ganglia	Bradykinesia, rigidity, resting tremor (Unilateral – progressing to bilateral)
	Tracts (white matter)	All CNS signs
Spinal (motor) Spinal (sensory)	Brain stem	Spasticity, weakness, sensory disturbances (Contralateral or ipsilateral S&S)
	Spinal cord	Spasticity, weakness, sensory disturbances (Contralateral and/or ipsilateral S&S)
	Anterior horn	Weakness, hypotonus and reduced reflex responses
	Dorsal horn	Pain[1], sensory loss
	Cerebellum	Ataxia, intention tremor (Ipsilateral S&S)
Peripheral nervous system (PNS)	Peripheral nerves	Hypotonicity, weakness, atrophy, sensory disturbances (Ipsilateral S&S)
Neuromuscular junction (NMJ)	Neuromuscular junction	Weakness (with fatigue), no sensory disturbances (Ipsilateral S&S)
Muscles	Muscle	Hypotonicity, weakness, atrophy (Ipsilateral S&S)

[a]See Table 6.3 for a description of the various signs and symptoms.

affected leading to multiple signs and symptoms. Listed in Table 6.2 are the most common signs and symptoms on which physiotherapy interventions may have an effect.

The structures described in Table 6.2 are all linked to specific systems: motor and/or sensory; cognitive and/or behavioural. The motor and sensory signs and symptoms can be further divided into central (upper motor neurone syndrome) or peripheral (lower motor neurone syndrome).

Table 6.3 outlines the definitions and clinical features of the major signs and symptoms, motor and sensory, cognitive and behavioural, as seen in neurological disorders.

Disease mechanisms

All diseases, including neurological diseases, can be attributed to specific disease mechanisms. The underlying disease mechanism will in many cases dictate the

Text continued on p. 174

---

[1]For further details see Chapter 7.

TABLE 6.3 Definitions and clinical features of the major signs and symptoms seen in neurological disorders

Affected system	Signs/symptoms	Clinical characteristics	Anatomic location
Motor	Weakness	Loss of muscle strength; true weakness results only when part of the motor pathway is damaged or diseased Weakness may appear gradually or suddenly; it may affect all muscles in the body (generalised weakness) or only a specific part of the body (monoplegia, hemiplegia, paraplegia, tetraplegia etc)	UMN LMN NMJ Muscle
	Spasticity	Classically defined as a velocity-dependent increase in resistance to passive stretch of a muscle with exaggerated tendon reflexes (Lance 1980) It is one of several components of the UMNS (Trompetto et al. 2014) Recognised clinically by: 1 the characteristic pattern of involvement of certain muscle groups (primarily anti-gravity muscles) 2 the increased responsiveness of muscles to stretch (dependent upon stretch velocity), the 'clasp-knife phenomenon' 3 markedly increased tendon reflexes 4 clonus	UMN
	Apraxia	Inability to execute learned purposeful (functional) movements despite having capacity to perform movements (Bickerton et al. 2012; Heilman & Rothi 1997)	Premotor or supplementary motor areas or the inferior parietal lobe Usually occurs following (L) hemisphere lesions (Zwinkels et al. 2004)
	Bradykinesia	Slowness of all voluntary movement and speech	
	Hypokinesia	Characterised by reduced or complete loss of muscle movement	Due to a disruption in the basal ganglia (Ling et al. 2012; Mazzoni, Shabbott & Cortés 2012)

Continued

TABLE 6.3 Definitions and clinical features of the major signs and symptoms seen in neurological disorders—cont'd

Affected system	Signs/symptoms	Clinical characteristics	Anatomic location
Motor—cont'd	Rigidity	Muscle rigidity is a state of continuous firm, tense muscles with marked resistance to passive movement and is characterised by an evenly distributed increase in muscle tone in flexor and extensor muscle groups; it is not velocity dependent and tendon jerks are usually within normal limits Two types of rigidity: 1 plastic 2 cogwheel	
	Hyperkinesia/ involuntary movements	Excessive involuntary movements (Sanger et al. 2010)	A result of improper regulation of the basal ganglia–thalamo–cortical circuitry (Den Dunnen 2013)
	Tremor	Physiological tremors: 1 resting 2 postural 3 essential Pathological tremors: 1 Parkinsonian (resting) 2 cerebellar (intention) 3 primary orthostatic (McAuley et al. 2000)	
	Muscle atrophy	Wasting or loss of muscle tissue: 1 disuse atrophy, which occurs from a lack of physical activity or 2 neurogenic atrophy, which occurs when there is an injury/disease to the nerve, muscle or NMJ Both cause some loss of movement or strength	UMN LMN

Motor—cont'd	Hypotonia/flaccidity	State of low muscle tone (less than normal tension and resistance during flexion or extension of a muscle group) Found initially post severe CNS damage such as spinal shock and cerebral shock (or flaccidity) post acute stroke	UMN LMN
	Ataxia	From the Greek meaning 'lack of order' – reduced muscle coordination during voluntary movements. Three main types of ataxia (Burke & Hammans 2008, 2012): 1 cerebellar ataxia 2 sensory ataxia 3 vestibular ataxia	1 Impairment of cerebellum by trauma/disease 2 Disruption of sensory nerve fibres particularly in the dorsal columns of the spinal cord 3 Result of peripheral or central diseases of the vestibular nuclei and connections to and from the vestibular nuclei
	Balance disorders	Disturbances of static or dynamic stability depending upon whether or not movement is involved	May occur as a result of altered signalling to and/or from the visual, vestibular and/or proprioceptive pathways (Horak 2006)
Sensory	Paraesthesia/ dysaesthesia	A sensation of burning, numbness, tingling, itching or prickling in the absence of noxious stimuli May be transient or chronic (Mogyoros, Bostock & Burke 2000; Sharif-Alhoseini, Rahimi-Movaghar & Vaccaro 2012)	UMN LMN Possibly due to ectopic impulse activity in cutaneous afferents or their central projections
	Hypoaesthesia	Abnormally decreased sensitivity to stimuli, particularly to touch	UMN LMN
Cognitive	Dementia		UMN
	Aphasia		UMN
Behavioural	See Chapter 10		UMN
Urogenital	See Chapter 4		UMN LMN

CNS, central nervous system; LMN, lower motor neurone; NMJ, neuromuscular junction; UMN(S), upper motor neurone syndrome.

TABLE 6.4 Disease mechanisms in neurological disorders and examples of disease states for each category

Mechanism	Disorder(s)
Vascular	Cerebrovascular disease (CVA) – stroke (haemorrhagic/embolic) (CNS) AVM/aneurism
Inflammatory/ autoimmune	Multiple sclerosis – diffuse inflammatory lesions in CNS Acute disseminated encephalomyelitis (ADEM) Guillain Barré syndrome (GBS) – acute inflammatory peripheral nerve damage Vasculitis (CNS + PNS)
Infections	All areas can be involved: • encephalitis – infectious disorder affecting CNS • CMV-induced neuropathy, HIV-induced neuropathy • poliomyelitis
Degenerative/genetic	Parkinson's disease (including Parkinson's plus) Huntington's disease Alzheimer's disease – degenerative disorder affecting cortical structures
Neoplastic	All areas can be involved in a neoplastic process: • primary malignancy in CNS • metastases to CNS • schwannoma – benign neoplasms involving peripheral nerves
Trauma	Traumatic brain injury (cortex/BS/BG/cerebellum) Cranial nerves – different sensory loss, i.e. vision, auditory, taste and smell Traumatic spinal cord injury Peripheral nerve injury
Metabolic/nutritious/toxic	B12 deficiency – involving both PNS and CNS – cognitive impairment, motor impairment, peripheral neuropathy

AVM, arteriovenous malformation; BG, basal ganglia; BS, brain stem; CMV, cytomegalovirus; CNS, central nervous system; PNS, peripheral nervous system.

pharmacotherapy and it is therefore important that physiotherapists have an understanding into which group the most commonly treated conditions fall. Table 6.4 lists the most common disease mechanisms for neurological disorders and examples of diseases in each category are given.

■ Pharmacological interventions for major symptoms seen in neurological disorders

This section outlines the major drug interventions in neurological disorders, listing the drugs by their major groups; that is, those acting upon the symptoms or on the disease or adjuvant drugs that are used to treat neurological disorders. The two most important drug groups for physiotherapists that act solely on the nervous system are those used in movement disorders and for spasticity. Since physiotherapists are the most likely persons to be monitoring these patients it is extremely important that they are aware of the mechanisms, special considerations, indications and dosages in these particular groups. Special consideration has therefore been given to these groups.

Monitoring the effects of pharmacotherapy can best be achieved by employing accurate continuing motor, sensory and behavioural clinical outcome measurements. Clinical outcome measurements may be either condition or symptom specific. In the clinical setting the appropriate measure should always answer the question: 'What am I trying to change?' (Hill et al. 2010).

Extrapyramidal (Parkinsonism)

Parkinson disease (PD), which is the example for most Parkinsonian disorders, is a progressive neurodegenerative disorder with typical motor symptoms:

♦ resting tremor
♦ bradykinesia
♦ rigidity
♦ gait impairment.

Late symptoms might include freezing, postural instability and falls as well as dysphagia (difficulty in swallowing). There are no routinely available medications that can modify and/or provide neuroprotection for the course of the disease. The goals of the treatments are to reduce impairment and disabilities (AlDakheel, Kalia & Lang 2014; Connolly & Lang 2014).

The pathogenesis of the disease is mainly associated with the progressive loss of dopaminergic neurons in the substantia nigra pars compacta (SNc). The main treatment strategies for PD consequently involve the dopamine system and improving the dopamine-dependent signs, particularly in the early stages of the disease (AlDakheel, Kalia & Lang 2014; Connolly & Lang 2014). Management concerning the recommendation of medication involves consideration of parameters such as age, time of onset, co-morbidities and severity of the motor symptoms and the non-motor symptoms, as well as the development of adverse reactions to the medications (such as dyskinesia). There are developed protocols for drug treatment depending upon the different signs and symptoms of the disease (Connolly & Lang 2014).

The major non-motor symptoms include hyposmia (loss of smell), fatigue, depression and constipation, and late symptoms might include psychiatric disturbances such as hallucinations and anxiety and autonomic disturbances such as orthostatic hypotension, sialorrhoea (hypersalivation) as well as cognitive impairments and, in severe cases, dementia.

The multidisciplinary approach to treatment of the Parkinsonian group of diseases is well established and is thought to be 'gold standard care' for PD. A multispecialty clinic brings together doctors and different allied health specialists, including physiotherapists, occupational therapists and speech and language therapists – and also includes support and advice from dieticians, social workers and sexologists – to complement standard medical treatment in the management of both motor and non-motor symptoms. While the neurologist determines disease severity and optimises medical treatment to reduce symptoms, allied health therapists work to minimise the impact of the disease process and improve the person's participation in everyday activities.

The most common rating scales used in the assessment of PD (that can also be adapted for the assessment of Parkinsonian disorders) are the Unified Parkinson Disease Rating Scale (UPDRS), Hoehn and Yahr staging and the

Schwab and England rating of activities of daily living. Although these scales are the most widely applied assessments of PD, they still present with considerable limitations that should be considered before using them for research (Perlmutter 2009).

Table 6.5 lists the major drug interventions for Parkinsonian disorders. Drugs from this group are used to treat Parkinson's disease as well as Parkinsonism related to other disorders such as drug-induced Parkinsonism.

PHYSIOTHERAPY PRACTICE POINTS: PARKINSONIAN DISORDERS

Physiotherapists involved in the treatment of PD patients must be aware of the '*on/off periods*' that may be considered a symptom of the disease or a side effect of the medications. The patient (or the patient's caregiver) should be advised to keep a diary in order to document these periods and physiotherapy treatment should ideally be given during the on periods. It is advisable, however, to assess the patient during both the on and off periods in order to be able to give advice to the patient (or the patient's caregiver) as to how to cope in these phases.

Some of the prescribed medications (see Table 6.5) will result in dyskinesias (and many patients actually prefer to be in the dyskinesic state). Again, it is important for the treating physiotherapist to be aware of this and be able to advise the patient how best to cope. Frequent falls are a common problem with PD patients and falls diaries should be implemented. This will allow all health professionals involved in the caregiving of these patients to have a better understanding of how to cope. Teaching the patient **how** to fall and get up again is an important strategy.

Other side effects of the medications include nausea, dizziness, reduced cardiac output and hypotension, all of which the physiotherapist must be aware of and take into consideration when drawing up a treatment plan.

Hallucinations, depression and suicidal tendencies may also be side effects of the disease process or the medications. Since physiotherapists are in a unique position to monitor these non-motor side effects they must document them carefully and communicate this information to the treating doctor.

Involuntary movements

Essential tremor (ET) is the most common adult involuntary movement disorder (IMD) and is characterised by tremor in different parts and on different sides of the body (hands, arms, head, voice, tongue, chin and, more rarely, legs). In contrast to the resting tremor of Parkinson's disease, ET is usually a postural and action tremor (Louis 2014). Some of the other involuntary movement disorders include athetosis, chorea and dyskinesia.

Assessment of involuntary movement disorders may be by clinical evaluation, surface electromyography, accelerometer and videotape recordings (Blond et al. 1992). The Abnormal Involuntary Movements Scale (AIMS) (Rush & Blacker 2008) was originally designed to aid early detection of tardive dyskinesias (TD) and provide a method for ongoing assessment.

Drugs used for involuntary movements

Disease processes involving the basal ganglia can manifest themselves not only in Parkinsonian symptoms but in multiple involuntary movement disorders

Text continued on p. 180

TABLE 6.5 Common anti-Parkinson drugs

Medication class/ drug group	Mechanism of action	Indications for therapeutic use	Common side effects	Practice points	Common adult dosage range
Levodopa-PDDI (peripheral dopa decarboxylase inhibitor) Levodopa–carbidopa Levodopa–benserazide	Since dopamine does not cross the blood–brain barrier (BBB), a precursor in the form of levodopa is administered, which crosses the BBB and is converted to dopamine in the brain where it reverses the depletion found in Parkinson's disease Carbidopa inhibits the decarboxylation of peripheral levodopa allowing more levodopa to cross the BBB	All motor symptoms Mainly for rigidity but may have an effect on other Parkinsonian signs (shakiness, stiffness, difficulty moving)	Dyskinesia, nausea, anorexia, dizziness, insomnia, chest pain, orthostatic hypotension, asthenia, muscle cramps or fatigue Possible discolouration of saliva, sweat or urine to a dark red, brown or black color Gastrointestinal effects in the form of increased motility	Concomitant administration of nonselective MAO-A inhibitors Possible symptoms of depression, suicidal behavior or psychotic behavior, including hallucinations Care if pre-morbid gastric ulcers as may precipitate gastrointestinal bleeding After long-term therapy (3–5 years) dyskinesia might develop	*Oral:* Usual dose carbidopa 25 mg orally given with first carbidopa–levodopa dose of the day; additional carbidopa 12.5–25 mg may be given during the day with each dose of carbidopa–levodopa (maximal total carbidopa dose 200 mg/day) Various combinations include: • carbidopa–levodopa 25–100, containing 25 mg of carbidopa and 100 mg of levodopa • carbidopa–levodopa 10–100, containing 10 mg of carbidopa and 100 mg of levodopa • carbidopa–levodopa 25–250, containing 25 mg of carbidopa and 250 mg of levodopa

Continued

TABLE 6.5 Common anti-Parkinson drugs—cont'd

Medication class/drug group	Mechanism of action	Indications for therapeutic use	Common side effects	Practice points	Common adult dosage range
Dopamine agonists Pramipexole	Treatment benefits are thought to be related to the stimulation of dopamine receptors in the striatum	All motor symptoms Because dopamine agonists are better tolerated and do not have the same risks of long-term complications as levodopa therapy, dopamine agonists are often the first choice of treatment for PD Pramipexole is also used to treat restless legs syndrome	Drowsiness, nausea, sweating, hallucinations, muscle pain, flu symptoms and dark coloured urine, chest pain, cough	Extended release form was approved by the FDA for Parkinson's disease in 2010	Dose range is 1.5–4.5 mg/day administered in equally divided doses every 8 hours
Monoamine oxidase (MAO-B) inhibitor Selegiline Rasagiline	MAO-B is an enzyme that breaks down dopamine MAO-B inhibitors prevent breakdown of dopamine	Reducing some of the motor symptoms associated with PD, early, mild motor symptoms	Mild nausea, dry mouth, light-headedness, constipation confusion, hallucinations May have interactions with certain foods, other medications, vitamins, herbal supplements	Two studies (LARGO and TEMPO) have shown that it can reduce wearing off in levodopa-treated patients	*Oral:* 5 mg bid 1 mg daily

Drug				Dosage
Catechol-O-methyl transferase (COMT) inhibitor Entacapone	COMT inhibitors prevent the breakdown of levodopa, prolonging the duration of action of a dose of levodopa Since COMT inhibitors do not contain levodopa, they must be taken with levodopa in order to have any benefit	COMT inhibitors may be prescribed when an individual experiences 'wearing off', particularly when dopamine agonists are not tolerated If involuntary movements (dyskinesias) develop after starting a COMT inhibitor, the dose of levodopa may need to be reduced	Drugs can increase the side effects caused by levodopa, notably dyskinesias, nausea and vomiting If these side effects increase after abdominal pain, diarrhoea and discoloured urine	200 mg with each dose of levodopa
Unspecified Amantadine	Amantadine acts presynaptically to enhance dopamine release or to inhibit its reuptake (Schneider et al. 1999) It can also act post-synaptically to increase the number, or alter the configuration of, dopamine receptors It is also a non-competitive NMDA receptor agonist and may provide protection against possible glutamate-mediated excitotoxicity in the context of TBI (Kraus & Maki 1997)	Used to alleviate tremors, slow movements and severe fatigue	May cause anticholinergic symptoms, including orthostatic hypotension, peripheral oedema, diarrhoea, loss of appetite, nausea, confusion, headache, insomnia, agitation, anxiety, depression, dream disorders, hallucinations, irritability, nervousness, fatigue or exacerbation of mental disorders Following abrupt dosage withdrawal, possible signs and symptoms of neuroleptic malignant syndrome (sweating, fever, stupor, unstable blood pressure, muscular rigidity, autonomic dysfunction) Blurred vision and /or impaired mental acuity have been reported Occasionally melanomas have been reported	*Oral:* 100 mg twice daily; may titrate up to 400 mg/day in divided doses
Bromocriptine mesylate	Dopamine receptor agonist that activates the postsynaptic dopamine receptors to inhibit prolactin secretions and it also stimulates dopamine receptors to improve motor function Therapeutic effect in the treatment of Parkinson's disease by directly stimulating the dopamine receptors in the corpus striatum		Symptomatic hypotension (orthostatic, syncope), constipation, nausea, headache, vomiting or fatigue Progressively severe headaches, hypertension or seizure activity may also be reported Possible confusion, hallucinations or unusual changes in behaviour Diabetic patients should take drug with food within 2 hours after waking in the morning Caution if used with antihypertensive medications due to orthostatic effects	*Oral:* Initial, 1.25 mg twice daily; increase by 2.5 mg daily every 14–28 days; usual maintenance dose range 2.5–40 mg/day up to 100 mg daily

(IMDs) such as tremor, hyperkinetic movements, chorea and athetosis. Table 6.6 lists the major drugs used to alleviate these symptoms.

PHYSIOTHERAPY PRACTICE POINTS: INVOLUNTARY MOVEMENTS

Since there are limited drugs available for involuntary movement disorders, physiotherapists and occupational therapists may offer suggestions regarding wrist weights, plate guards and other adaptive devices. These devices can provide considerable benefit in activities of daily living. For patients with mild tremor, minimising exposure to emotional stress, avoiding *tremorogenic foods* (e.g. caffeine) and drugs (e.g. sympathomimetics) and reassurance may be all that is required. Intermittent administration of a beta-blocker or small amounts of alcohol may be effective in special social situations.

Most patients with mild essential tremor are able to minimise functional disability, social embarrassment and personal injury by learning adaptive techniques. Examples include learning to write with the least disabled hand, placing a napkin between cup and saucer to avoid rattling, avoiding difficult foods (e.g. soup, spaghetti), using blunt-tip safety scissors, wearing clip-on neckties, having autodial on a telephone or asking the operator to place calls, learning deep breathing and other relaxation techniques, avoiding awkward or uncomfortable situations and explaining their condition to people. The number of adaptive techniques is numerous, and people can be very creative.

When tremor significantly interferes with daily activities, causes significant functional disability or if it becomes socially unacceptable long-term pharmacotherapy is indicated. Since the physiotherapist and/or occupational therapist is likely to be involved in the assessment of these patients it is imperative they are aware of the possible pharmacotherapeutic interventions and their potential side effects such as reduced cardiac output and orthostatic hypotension (see Table 6.6). These side effects may lead to an increase in the number of falls and must therefore be addressed by the treating therapist.

Spasticity

Spasticity is one of the cardinal symptoms of the upper motor neuron syndrome (UMNS). A recent review article by Pandyan et al. (2010) suggests a redefinition of spasticity as: 'disordered sensorimotor control, resulting from an upper motor neuron lesion, presenting as intermittent or sustained involuntary activation of muscles'.

Assessment of spasticity

A systematic review by Platz et al. (2005) identified a wide range of scales for spasticity. These authors argue that the definition of spasticity may have a major impact on the validity of these tests. It is beyond the scope of this handbook to enter into this discussion and the reader is directed to more comprehensive literature (Rekand 2010).

The major anti-spastic drugs are listed in Table 6.7.

TABLE 6.6 Common drugs used for involuntary movements

Medication class/ drug group	Mechanism of action	Indications for therapeutic use	Common side effects	Practice points	Common adult dosage range
Beta-blocker Propanol	Nonselective beta-blocker that reduces chronotropic, inotropic and vasodilator responses to beta-adrenergic stimulation by competing for available binding sites that stimulate the beta-adrenergic receptors	Controls tremors (including essential tremor) through incompletely understood mechanism	Oral tablet side effects may include bradyarrhythmias, cold extremities, anorexia, nausea, vomiting, insomnia, paraesthesia, dyspnoea and wheezing Possible signs of hypoglycaemia, bradycardia, exacerbation of conduction disorders or hypotension Possible bronchospasm or exacerbation of lower respiratory tract infection (i.e. difficulty breathing, wheezing)	Diabetic patients should carefully monitor blood glucose as drug may mask symptoms of hypoglycaemia Care with sudden discontinuation of drug, as this may precipitate hypertension, angina or myocardial infarction	*Oral:* 80–320 mg bds
Benzodiazepines Diazepam	Believed to be related to its capacity to enhance gamma-aminobutyric acid (GABA) activity, which is the major inhibitory neurotransmitter in the central nervous system Able to suppress the spike and wave discharges in absence seizures and decrease the frequency, duration, amplitude and spread of discharge in minor motor seizures	Controls essential tremors	Excessive salivation, ataxia, dizziness, impaired cognition, seizure, aggravation, somnolence, depression, nervousness or respiratory depression		*Oral:* 0.75–2.75 mg daily; 0.5 mg tds was most commonly used *Discontinuation of treatment:* Decrease daily dose by 0.5 mg every 3 days
Gabapentin	An anti-seizure (anti-convulsant) drug The mechanism of action is not known Gabapentin structurally resembles the neurotransmitter GABA; it is possible that this similarity is related to its mechanism of action	Restless legs syndrome	Ataxia, nystagmus Drowsiness, somnolence		

TABLE 6.7 Common drugs used for spasticity

Medication class/ drug group	Mechanism of action	Indications for therapeutic use	Common side effects	Practice points	Common adult dosage range
Baclofen	General central nervous system (CNS)-depressant actions and exerts its effects as an agonist at presynaptic gamma-aminobutyric acid (GABA)-B (bicuculline-insensitive) receptors Acts mainly at the spinal cord level to inhibit the transmission of both monosynaptic and polysynaptic reflexes, possibly by hyperpolarisation of primary afferent fibre terminals, resulting in antagonism of the release of putative excitatory transmitters (i.e. glutamic and aspartic acids) Postsynaptic effects have been demonstrated at concentrations above the therapeutic range	Generalised spasticity associated with UMNS	May cause constipation, nausea, vomiting, poor muscle tone, asthenia, headache or seizure	Intrathecal baclofen should not be discontinued abruptly; discontinuation may result in muscle rigidity, exaggerated rebound spasticity, severe high fever and altered mental status	*Oral:* Initial dose: 5 mg orally tds for 3 days, then 10 mg orally tds for 3 days, then 15 mg orally tds for 3 days, then 20 mg orally tds *Maintenance dose:* 40–80 mg/day. 80 mg/day doses should be administered in 4 divided doses Baclofen pump when in situ is adjusted by the treating doctor according to clinical response
Dantrolene sodium	Induces skeletal muscle relaxation by directly affecting the contractile response It is suggested that its interference with the release of calcium ions from the sarcoplasmic reticulum results in the dissociation of the excitation–contraction coupling in skeletal muscle	Control of spasticity associated with spinal cord injury, stroke, cerebral palsy or multiple sclerosis	Muscle weakness, general malaise, fatigue, diarrhoea	Regular liver function tests should be carried out Increased photosensitivity reactions are possible and sun protection should be used	*Oral:* Initial dose 25 mg every day; increase at 4 to 7 day intervals to 25 mg twice daily to 4 times daily, up to maximum 100 mg twice daily to 4 times daily

Benzodiazepine Diazepam	Benzodiazepine derivative is an anxiolytic Reduces neuronal depolarisation resulting in decreased action potentials Enhances the action of GABA by tightly binding to A-type GABA receptors, thus opening the membrane channels and allowing the entry of chloride ions May be effective in multiple sclerosis patients who cannot tolerate baclofen, or in combination with baclofen	Effective in the treatment of spasticity due to cerebral lesions, brain injury or stroke	Drowsiness and fatigue, weakness, confusion, light-headedness	Care in prescribing for the elderly due to increased possibility of falls	*Muscle spasm:* 2–15 mg daily in divided doses *Management of cerebral spasticity in selected cases:* 2–60 mg daily in divided doses
Botulinium toxin A	A neurotoxin produced by *Clostridium botulinum* The toxin appears to affect the presynaptic membrane of the neuromuscular junction, where it prevents calcium-dependent release of acetylcholine and produces a state of denervation Following injection of the toxin into a muscle, the degree of resultant skeletal muscle weakness or paralysis is dose dependent; muscle inactivation persists until new fibrils grow from the nerve and form junction plates on new areas of the muscle cell walls			Contraindicated in cases of: • hypersensitivity to any botulinum toxin preparation or to any other component of the product • infection at the proposed injection site Needs to be used with caution around speech or respiratory muscle since it may lead to impaired swallow or breathing	There are special tables for dosages for every muscle. Different medications have specific 'biological units'

UMNS, upper motor neurone syndrome.

PHYSIOTHERAPY PRACTICE POINTS: SPASTICITY

Since physiotherapists will often have the most regular contact with these patients who are exhibiting spasticity they must be aware of the possible pharmacological interventions of anti-spastic medications and their effects. The treating physiotherapist must also be responsible for assessing if the drug intervention is effective and if the required dosage is being administered. Through on-going assessments the physiotherapist is able to monitor the usefulness of the medications and suggest if a more general or a more selective anti-spastic medication is required (Table 6.7).

Many of the drugs used for spasticity will result in generalised weakness. It is important for the treating physiotherapist to monitor this and advise the treating doctor. The resultant weakness or reduced spasticity may increase the patient's predisposition to falls and this tendency must be taken into account when planning treatment interventions.

With regard to the intramuscular administration of botulinum toxin (BTx), physiotherapists have a very important role. Firstly, they advise the treating doctor which muscles or muscle groups are the most spastic and therefore affect the specific function. BTx acts at the neuromuscular junction to cause temporary paralysis of the muscle by inhibiting the release of acetylcholine from presynaptic motor neurons. It induces weakness of striated muscles by inhibiting transmission of alpha motor neurons at the neuromuscular junction. Following injection it may be 2–3 days before the treatment effects are observed. Adverse effects might include mild injection pain and local oedema, erythema, transient numbness, headache, malaise or mild nausea. The physiotherapist is involved in the **voluntary** strengthening of those muscles affected with post-injection weakness and must also be aware of possible adverse effects such as dysphagia following injection into spastic neck muscles. The dose units are dependent on which of the commercially produced toxins is injected.

Cognitive decline (dementia)

Dementia, defined as impairment in cognitive performance, leading to impaired functioning (DSM-5) (American Psychiatric Association 2013), is a leading cause of morbidity in the elderly population. The major causes of dementia are Alzheimer's disease, diffuse Lewy body disease and cerebrovascular disorders. Currently, there are only a few disease-specific interventions and these are reserved for Alzheimer's disease and Parkinson's disease dementia. However, behavioural and affective symptoms of the dementias can treated with the appropriate neuropsychiatric medications. Major dementia drugs are listed in Table 6.8.

PHYSIOTHERAPY PRACTICE POINTS: COGNITIVE DECLINE

A number of studies have documented the effectiveness of physiotherapy in the form of mobility and balance activities (Christofoletti et al. 2007; Kaur, Sharma & Mittal 2012; Pomeroy et al. 1999). A recent systematic review by Cabrera and colleagues (2015) suggested that sensorial therapies were amongst the most effective interventions. Some of the drugs prescribed, as outlined in Table 6.8, may cause bradykinesia that the treating physiotherapist must be aware of and take into account.

Seizures (epilepsy)

Although physiotherapists do not actually treat epilepsy as a separate condition, many of their patients with neurological disorders will have, to a greater or lesser extent, the possibility of having an epileptic fit/convulsion. Patients with epilepsy

TABLE 6.8 Common drugs used for cognitive decline

Medication class/ drug group	Mechanism of action	Indications for therapeutic use	Common side effects	Practice points	Common adult dosage range
Acetylcholine esterase inhibitors Rivastigmine Donepezil Galantamine	Increased cholinergic neurotransmission due to inhibition of acetylcholine esterase enzyme, which breaks down acetylcholine released into the synaptic cleft	Rivastigmine: Mild to moderate AD; (FDA approved for mild to moderate Parkinson's disease dementia) Donepezil: Mild, moderate to severe AD Galantamine: Mild to moderate AD	Due to increased cholinergic activity there might be cardiac side effects (bradycardia, AV block) as well as gastrointestinal discomfort (nausea, diarrhoea)	Cognitive enhancement Treats also behavioural symptoms Start with low dose due to gastrointestinal side effects	**Rivastigmine**: *Oral:* 1.5–6 mg bds *Patch:* 4.6–13.3 mg/ 24 hours **Donepezil:** 5–10 (and less common 23) mg/day **Galantamine:** IR: 4–12 mg bds ER: 8–24 mg daily
Memantine	Glutamatergic neurotransmission modulation (NMDA receptor antagonist)	Moderate to severe AD; off-label use in mild AD	Minimal side effects: fatigue, dizziness, headaches	Well tolerated	IR: 5–10 mg bds ER: 8–24 mg day

AD, Alzheimer's disease; AV, atrioventricular; ER, extended release; IR, immediate release; NMDA, N-methyl-D-aspartate.

have also been described as being non-compliant in taking their medications (Kaiser, Michael & Chanda 2009) and it may therefore fall to the treating physiotherapist to monitor this.

Common medications include: carbamazepine, phenytoin, valproate, lamotrigine, topiramate.

For common anti-epileptic drugs see Table 6.9.

CAVEAT: Table 6.9 refers only to those drugs in long-term therapeutic use for epilepsy. All drugs outlined in this table are taken orally. Prescription for acute epileptic episodes must be controlled by experts in the field and the possible combinations of medications and forms of administration are beyond the scope of this handbook.

PHYSIOTHERAPY PRACTICE POINTS: SEIZURES

Treating physiotherapists must be aware if their patients are taking anti-epileptic drugs, including the dosage and timing of their medications. Epilepsy medications may cause nausea, headache, sleep and motor disorders, effects on behaviour and mood, dizziness, drowsiness, sedation and fatigue, all of which may impact upon the patient's participation in physical activities. Patients should be advised against sudden discontinuation of drugs, as this may precipitate seizures.

It is important to note that a number of medications have been implicated as a cause of acute seizures in later life (Ding et al. 2012). Elderly individuals are most likely to be susceptible to seizures as a consequence of drugs because of a high prevalence of polypharmacy, impaired drug clearance and a heightened sensitivity to the pro-convulsant effects of medications. Seizures can also occur with alcohol, benzodiazepine or barbiturate withdrawal. Overall, drugs and drug withdrawal contribute to up to 10% of acute symptomatic seizures.

■ Specialised drugs used for specific neurological conditions

For some particular neurological conditions, in particular multiple sclerosis (MS) and motor neurone disease (MND) (amyotrophic lateral sclerosis [ALS]), specialised drugs able to reverse the condition or prevent the degenerative processes are being developed and used with some degree of success (Miller et al. 2009).

Multiple sclerosis

Multiple sclerosis (MS) is a chronic autoimmune, inflammatory neurological disease of the central nervous system (CNS). MS attacks the myelinated axons in the CNS, destroying the myelin and the axons.

Patients may be grouped into four major subgroups depending on the course of the disease:

1 relapsing–remitting MS – the most common form, in which there are relapses or exacerbations of symptoms followed by periods of remission
2 secondary progressive MS – relapsing occurs with progression of signs and symptoms, usually with permanent disability

Text continued on p. 189

TABLE 6.9 Common anti-epileptic drugs

Medication class/ drug group	Mechanism of action	Indications	Common side effects	Practice points	Common adult dosage range
Phenytoin	Sodium channel blockade	Seizures, epilepsy	Ataxia, dysarthria, motor slowing, lethargy	Long-term use may cause lethargy, peripheral neuropathy Monitor by blood level (40–79 micromol/L) Beware of suicidality and depression	*Oral:* 200–450 mg/day usually taken 1 to 4 times a day
Carbamazepine	Sodium channel blockade	Seizure disorders, bipolar disorder, trigeminal neuralgia (facial pain)	Stomach cramps, abdominal pain, diarrhoea, vomiting, ataxia, drowsiness	Anorexia Monitor blood level (25–51 micromol/L), liver function, blood count, blood urea and creatinine Beware of suicidality and depression	*Oral:* 400–1600 mg/day Available as both immediate release (IR) and extended release (ER)
Valproate	Various actions on multiple sites: increased GABA effect; inhibition of glutamate/NMDA receptor	Seizure disorder Bipolar disorder	Nausea, vomiting, tremor, headaches	Confusion, irritability, Parkinsonism, encephalopathy Monitor blood level (347–693 micromol/l mcg/mL), liver function, platelet, coagulation tests at baseline Beware of behavioural changes, suicidality and depression	*Oral:* 500–2000 mg/day Available as both immediate release (IR) and extended release (ER)

Continued

TABLE 6.9 Common anti-epileptic drugs—cont'd

Medication class/drug group	Mechanism of action	Indications	Common side effects	Practice points	Common adult dosage range
Lamotrigine	Sodium channel blockade Reduced release of glutamate	Seizure disorder Bipolar disease	Ataxia, diplopia, severe skin reaction and allergic reaction (Stevens–Johnson syndrome)	Severe skin rash and hypersensitivity syndrome Beware of behavioural changes, suicidality and depression Major interaction with valproate; care when dosing these drugs together	*Oral:* 200–600 mg/day (dose should be titrated very slowly due to the risk of severe allergic reaction)
Levetiracetam	Modulation of synaptic vesicle protein 2a	Seizure disorders	Lethargy, dizziness, headaches, vomiting	Beware of behavioural changes, suicidality and depression	*Oral:* 500–3000 mg twice daily
Topiramate	Various actions on multiple sites: sodium channel blockade; increased GABA effect; inhibition of glutamate/NMDA receptor	Seizure disorders, Migraine prevention	Ataxia, paraesthesia	Impairment of concentration, mental slowing and cognitive effects, disturbance of memory Beware of behavioural changes, suicidality and depression	*Oral:* 25–400 mg/day

GABA, gamma-aminobutyric acid; NMDA, N-methyl-D-aspartate.

3 primary progressive MS – symptoms continue to worsen gradually from the beginning; there are no relapses or remissions, but there may be occasional plateaus

4 progressive–relapsing MS – progressive from the start, with intermittent flare-ups of worsening symptoms without periods of remission.

Assessment of multiple sclerosis

Originally called 'the great pretender', MS presents great challenges in assessment. Most recently, Rudick et al. (2014) have presented a new form of assessment, the Multiple Sclerosis Performance Test (MSPT), which represents a new approach to quantifying MS related disability. The MSPT takes advantage of advances in computer technology, information technology, biomechanics and clinical measurement science. The resulting MSPT represents a computer-based platform for precise, valid measurement of MS severity. Based on, but extending the Multiple Sclerosis Functional Composite (MSFC), the MSPT provides precise, quantitative data on walking speed, balance, manual dexterity, visual function and cognitive processing speed (Rudick et al. 2014).

Specific medications used in MS have several goals; see below and Table 6.10.

1 To modify the disease course

  a The goals of using these drugs are to reduce disease activity by decreasing the timing and intensity of relapsing attacks of MS. Beta interferons, which are injected under the skin or into muscle, can reduce the frequency and severity of relapses. Beta interferons can cause side effects such as flu-like symptoms and injection-site reactions.

2 To treat during relapses (to decrease illness exacerbations)

  a The most common treatment regimen is a three-to-five-day course of high-dose, intravenous corticosteroids to reduce inflammation and end the relapse more quickly. Sometimes followed by a slow tapering dose of oral prednisone.

  b Plasma exchange (plasmapheresis) may be used if severe attack does not respond to steroid therapy. The plasma is removed and separated from the whole blood. The blood cells and albumin are placed back into the body.

3 To manage MS impairments such as spasticity (improving quality of life)

  a These medications are not specific to MS but rather are directed at the management of specific symptoms.

  b Impairments might include: bladder problems, bowel dysfunction, emotional changes (such as depression or euphoria), fatigue, itching, pain, sexual disorders, spasticity, tremors and gait difficulties.[2]

The approved Australian medications (Australian Medicines Handbook Pty Ltd 2016) listed in Table 6.10 are assumed to reduce the number of relapses and the number of new lesions. First-line treatments for MS include injectables – interferons beta-1a, beta-1b and glatiramer. Peginterferon beta 1-a has recently been approved for relapsing forms of MS. Second-line therapies include

Text continued on p. 193

---

[2]See appropriate symptoms as discussed earlier in the chapter.

TABLE 6.10 Drugs used in the treatment of multiple sclerosis

Medication class/ drug group	Mechanism of action	Indications for therapeutic use	Common side effects	Practice points	Common adult dosage range
Beta interferons Beta-1a, beta-1b	Immunomodulation possibly produced by cytokines that perform regulatory functions in the immune system via their anti-inflammatory activity	Used for reducing the incidence of relapses Recommended for patients with relapsing–remitting MS who have intolerance to glatiramer acetate	Increase risk of liver function abnormalities, leukopenia, thyroid disease and depression	It is necessary to monitor liver and white blood cell (WBC) count Flu-like symptoms (e.g. fever, chills, malaise, muscle aches and fatigue)	An example for interferon beta-1a: *Intramuscular (IM) injection:* 30 mcg once weekly
Glatiramer	Mechanism of action is distinct from that of the beta interferons Possibly glatiramer acetate-specific suppressor T cells are induced and activated in the periphery, so reducing inflammatory activity by one-third	Reducing the rate of attacks in patients with relapsing–remitting MS	Vasodilatation, rash, hypersensitivity, nausea, vomiting, asthenia and injection site reactions Localised lipoatrophy and skin necrosis	Inform patient that a transient, self-limiting post injection reaction may include flushing, palpitations, chest pain, anxiety, urticaria, dyspnoea or throat constriction	*Subcutaneous (SC) injection:* 20 mg once daily
Natalizumab	A recombinant humanised immunoglobulin (IgG4) monoclonal antibody Impairs adhesion of leukocytes to their counter receptors	Severe relapsing–remitting MS	Depression, rash, arthralgia, diarrhoea, nausea, headache, pain in extremity, abdominal discomfort and fatigue	A potential increase in the risk of progressive multifocal leukoencephalopathy (PML) An opportunistic viral infection of the brain MRI scanning is required before treatment is initiated, and an analysis of the CSF for John Cunningham virus (JCV) DNA is recommended	*IV infusion:* 300 mg 1-hour infusion every 4 weeks

Fingolimod	Blocks the migration of lymphocytes from lymph nodes, thereby reducing the number of lymphocytes in peripheral blood. Might involve the reduction of lymphocyte migration into the CNS	Reducing relapses and to delay the progression of disability in patients with relapsing forms of MS	Hypertension, headache, influenza, diarrhoea, back pain and cough; Bradycardia, especially within the first 6 hours of administration; Visual disturbances; Respiratory distress	*Oral:* 0.5 mg once daily
Teriflunomide	Selectively and reversibly inhibits dihydro-orotate dehydrogenase, a key mitochondrial enzyme in the de novo pyrimidine synthesis pathway, leading to a reduction in proliferation of activated T and B lymphocytes without causing cell death	Reducing relapses and to delay the progression of disability in patients with relapsing forms of MS	Allergic reactions; Hepatotoxicity; May cause major birth defects and therefore pregnancy must be excluded before starting the medication	*Oral:* 7 mg or 14 mg once daily; Can be taken with or without food
Dimethyl fumarate	In a class of medications called Nrf2 activators, it may work by decreasing inflammation and preventing nerve damage that may cause symptoms of multiple sclerosis	Relapsing–remitting MS	GI problems; Swallowing or breathing difficulties; Swelling of the face, throat, tongue, lips, eyes, hands, feet, ankles or lower legs; Hives, rash, itching, hoarseness; Vision problems; Weakness/clumsiness of one side of the body; Visual changes; May cause serious eye irritation	*Oral – ER capsules:* 120–240 mg bds

Continued

TABLE 6.10 Drugs used in the treatment of multiple sclerosis—cont'd

Medication class/drug group	Mechanism of action	Indications for therapeutic use	Common side effects	Practice points	Common adult dosage range
ACTH Methylprednisolone	Anti-inflammatory	For acute and relapsing attacks	May cause fluid retention, alteration in glucose tolerance, elevation in blood pressure, behavioural and mood changes, increased appetite and weight gain	Patient should be advised to avoid live vaccines during therapy due to drug-induced immunosuppression	*Intramuscular injection:* 80–120 units/day for 2 to 3 weeks After prolonged treatment, dose tapering and interval extension may be necessary to avoid adrenal insufficiency
Symptomatic treatment Dalfampridine	Contains a sustained-release formulation of 4-aminopyridine, which blocks potassium channels on the surface of nerve fibres; this blocking ability may improve the conduction of nerve signals in nerve fibres whose insulating myelin coating has been damaged by MS	Found to improve walking in patients with any type of MS Increasing walking speeds	Seizures, urinary tract infections, insomnia, dizziness, headache, nausea, weakness, back pain, balance disorders, swelling in the nose or throat, constipation, diarrhoea, indigestion, throat pain and burning, tingling or itching of the skin	The maximum recommended dosage is one 10-mg tablet twice daily, taken with or without food This dosage should not be exceeded The tablets should be taken approximately 12 hours apart, and patients should not take double or extra doses if a dose is missed	*Oral:* Maximum recommended dose is 10 mg twice daily with or without food about 12 hours apart Tablets should not be divided, crushed, chewed or dissolved

Adapted with permission from: Australian Medicines Handbook Pty Ltd, 2016. Australian Medicines Handbook (online). Australian Medicines Handbook Pty Ltd, Adelaide. *Available from: <http://amhonline.amh.net.au/>.*

natalizumab, given by IV infusion, and alemtuzumab has also recently been approved for relapsing–remitting MS. It is given in two courses of IV infusions, 12 months apart.

The interferon beta drug reduces the frequency of relapses by one-third due to its antiviral, anti-proliferative and immunomodulatory properties. One possible mechanism of action of interferon beta is to decrease permeability of the blood–brain barrier (BBB), thereby reducing damage to the brain. Glatiramer is a copolymer of four amino acids first introduced in 1996 as another first-line agent. Glatiramer has immunomodulatory properties by affecting the antigen presenting cells, such as monocytes and dendritic cells, leading to a decrease in pro-inflammatory cytokines and an increase in anti-inflammatory cytokines, thus decreasing the inflammation associated with the disease course (Schrempf & Ziemssen 2007; Ziemssen & Schrempf 2007).

Natalizumab is a recombinant humanised monoclonal antibody approved for treatment of MS. It binds to integrins on the surface of T cells thus preventing their transmigration through the BBB.

Fingolimod and teriflunomide are oral drugs for relapsing MS. Fingolimod is a competitive inhibitor of the sphingosine 1-phosphate receptor on T cells, and is assumed to reduce relapses and delays the onset of disability by affecting T cell emigration from the lymph nodes and migration into the brain, effectively reducing the number of lymphocytes in the periphery and central nervous system. The most recent drug therapy, approved in 2013, it has antioxidant and anti-inflammatory properties (Dörr & Paul 2015; Grey Née Cotte et al. 2015; Uttara et al. 2009; Wiendl & Meuth 2015). Dimethly fumerate is another oral drug that has recently been approved for relapsing–remitting MS.

PHYSIOTHERAPY PRACTICE POINTS: MULTIPLE SCLEROSIS

A recent overview of rehabilitation interventions for MS (Beer, Khan & Kesselring 2012) suggests them to be most beneficial in the early phases of the disease. Due to the variability in the presentation of the disease, regular evaluation and assessment is needed and treatment is directed to the needs of the individual. A multidisciplinary approach is recommended and all members of the team, which includes rehabilitation specialists, neurologists, physiotherapists, occupational therapists, psychologists, speech pathologists and nurses, must be aware of all possible signs and symptoms and the effects that the prescribed medications may have on the patient.

In addition to the fatigue associated with the disease itself many of the recommended drugs will also cause fatigue. The treating physiotherapists must be aware of how to gear treatments in order to maximise the benefits of treatments and minimise the effects of fatigue. Other side effects, both motor and non-motor as listed in Table 6.10, must also be taken into account and monitored by the treating physiotherapist.

As with the majority of neurological disorders that cause impairment of movement, patients with MS are also prone to multiple falls and a falls program should be implemented whenever possible.

Amyotrophic lateral sclerosis or motor neurone disease

Amyotrophic lateral sclerosis (ALS) or motor neurone disease (MND) is a degenerative disease of upper and lower motor neurones that causes rapidly progressive weakness and resultant atrophy of muscles in all parts of the body. The cause of the disease is not known, but an increased level of glutamate at the motor synapses has been demonstrated in many patients. Ten per cent of patients have a familial form of the disease, usually with autosomal dominant inheritance, while in the others the disease is apparently sporadic (Haringer & Gibson 2015).

The disease advances rapidly, leading in the late stages to patients being paralysed in the majority of the muscles of their body, but with a clear mind and preserved consciousness. The mean survival from the first symptoms to death (usually due to respiratory failure) is 5 years (Blackhall 2012). Approximately 10% of patients develop a characteristic form of dementia named frontotemporal dementia (FTD), with prominent behavioural disturbances (Lillo & Hodges 2010).

There are two approaches in ALS treatment that need to be combined: 1) treatment oriented toward slowing down the process of neurodegeneration and clinical worsening and 2) symptom-oriented treatment in order to allow patients a better quality of life (Musarò 2013) (see Table 6.11).

Assessment of ALS/MND

The ALS Functional Rating Scale (ALSFRS) is a validated rating instrument for monitoring the progression of disability in patients with ALS. The Revised ALSFRS (ALSFRS- R) retains the properties of the original scale but demonstrates strong internal consistency and construct validity. ALSFRS-R scores correlate significantly with quality of life as measured by the Sickness Impact Profile, indicating that the quality of function is strongly correlated to quality of life in ALS (Cedarbaum et al. 1999). A more recent scale based upon clinical outcomes and survival time is considered a more appropriate tool for clinical trials in ALS (Berry et al. 2013).

PHYSIOTHERAPY PRACTICE POINTS: AMYOTROPHIC LATERAL SCLEROSIS/MOTOR NEURONE DISEASE

In order to maximise function the treating physiotherapist should aim to maintain optimal muscle strength, muscle length and joint range of motion and, where necessary, manage muscle tone, which may be hypertonic or hypotonic. Advice on exercise and exercise prescription is also given as and when necessary. Recent evidence presents a strong case for the use of exercise and it has been shown that unaffected muscle fibres can respond to exercise allowing a patient to develop a small reserve of healthy usable muscle (Drory et al. 2001; Harkawik & Coyle 2012; Lewis & Rushanan 2007; Sanjak et al. 2010). Exercise can provide improvement of the neural control of muscle, leading to more effective recruitment and, therefore, stronger contractions. Short but frequent exercise sessions are recommended rather than prolonged activity in order to avoid fatigue (Berry et al. 2013). Optimal tissue length is essential for maximal muscle activation and resultant function, and it is therefore important to initiate early intervention in the form of stretching programs and/or splinting to prevent changes in tissue length. Again, falls programs are required.

The physiotherapist may also be involved in pain and fatigue management and in the treatment and monitoring of respiratory dysfunction. As the person in regular contact with the patient it is important that the physiotherapist is aware of all medications that may be required and can advise the treating doctor as to how the patient is able to cope prior to receiving specific medications or monitoring when they are receiving medications.

It is important that people with ALS/MND have enough information to help them understand their illness and plan for disability. Physiotherapists can offer advice and support and working with other team members can help to achieve the highest quality of life for this patient group.

TABLE 6.11 Drugs used in the treatment of amyotrophic lateral sclerosis/motor neurone disease

Medication class/ drug group	Mechanism of action	Indications	Common side effects	Practice points	Common adult dosage range
Riluzole	Antiglutamate agent and is the only drug approved for the treatment of ALS It appears to slow the progression of ALS and to improve survival	Disease-modifying treatment	Abdominal pain, anorexia, diarrhoea; nausea, vomiting; rarely, an elevation of liver enzymes and neutropenia that are reversible upon drug cessation	Liver function tests and blood counts should be obtained every month for the first 3 months, then every 3 months for the first year, and every 6 months thereafter while the patient is on riluzole	50 mg bid
Anticholinergics Amitryptilline Scopolamine patches		Sialorrhoea – symptom-oriented treatment to reduce excess saliva due to ineffective swallow	Drowsiness, heart rhythm disturbances, urinary retention and constipation should be taken into consideration, especially in the elderly		
Botulinum toxin into salivary glands		Sialorrhea – symptom-oriented treatment to reduce excess saliva due to ineffective swallow			
Anti-spastic medications		See Table 6.7			
Pain (see Chapter 7)		Pain is rare in ALS and is caused usually by immobility and spasticity and is of musculoskeletal origin Cannabis and opiates should be used liberally due to the poor prognosis of the disease			

■ References

AlDakheel, A., Kalia, L.V., Lang, A.E., 2014. Pathogenesis-targeted, disease-modifying therapies in Parkinson disease. Neurotherapeutics 11 (1), 6–23.

American Psychiatric Association, 2013. Diagnostic and Statistical Manual of Mental Disorders (DSM-5). American Psychiatric Publishing, Washington, DC.

Australian Medicines Handbook Pty Ltd, 2016. *Australian Medicines Handbook* (online). Adelaide: Australian Medicines Handbook Pty Ltd. [Internet] <https://amhonlineamhnetau.ezp01.library.qut.edu.au>.

Beer, S., Khan, F., Kesselring, J., 2012. Rehabilitation interventions in multiple sclerosis: an overview. Journal of Neurology 259 (9), 1994–2008.

Berry, J.D., Miller, R., Moore, D.H., et al., 2013. The Combined Assessment of Function and Survival (CAFS): a new endpoint for ALS clinical trials. Amyotrophic Lateral Sclerosis & Frontotemporal Degeneration 14 (3), 162–168.

Bickerton, W.L., Riddoch, M.J., Samson, D., et al., 2012. Systematic assessment of apraxia and functional predictions from the Birmingham Cognitive Screen. Journal of Neurology, Neurosurgery, and Psychiatry 83 (5), 513–521.

Blackhall, L.J., 2012. Amyotrophic lateral sclerosis and palliative care: where we are, and the road ahead. Muscle and Nerve 45 (3), 311–318.

Blond, S., Caparros-Lefebvre, D., Parker, F., et al., 1992. Control of tremor and involuntary movement disorders by chronic stereotactic stimulation of the ventral intermediate thalamic nucleus. Journal of Neurosurgery 77 (1), 62–68.

Burke, G., Hammans, S., 2008. Ataxia. Medicine 36 (10), 540–544.

Burke, G., Hammans, S., 2012. Ataxia. Medicine (United Kingdom) 40 (8), 435–439.

Cabrera, E., 2015. Non-pharmacological interventions as a best practice strategy in people with dementia living in nursing homes: a systematic review. European Geriatric Medicine 6 (2), 134–150.

Cedarbaum, J.M., Stambler, N., Malta, E., et al., 1999. The ALSFRS-R: a revised ALS functional rating scale that incorporates assessments of respiratory function. Journal of the Neurological Sciences 169 (1–2), 13–21.

Christofoletti, G., Oliani, M.M., Gobbi, S., et al., 2007. Effects of motor intervention in elderly patients with dementia: an analysis of randomized controlled trials. Topics in Geriatric Rehabilitation 23 (2), 149–154.

Connolly, B.S., Lang, A.E., 2014. Pharmacological treatment of Parkinson disease: a review. Journal of the American Medical Association 311 (16), 1670–1683.

Den Dunnen, W.F.A., 2013. Neuropathological diagnostic considerations in hyperkinetic movement disorders. Frontiers in Neurology 4, 7.

Ding, J.J., Zhang, Y.J., Jiao, Z., et al., 2012. The effect of poor compliance on the pharmacokinetics of carbamazepine and its epoxide metabolite using Monte Carlo simulation. Acta Pharmacologica Sinica 33 (11), 1431–1440.

Dörr, J., Paul, F., 2015. The transition from first-line to second-line therapy in multiple sclerosis. Current Treatment Options in Neurology 17 (6), 354.

Drory, V.E., Goltsman, E., Goldman Reznik, J., et al., 2001. The value of muscle exercise in patients with amyotrophic lateral sclerosis. Journal of the Neurological Sciences 191 (1–2), 133–137.

Global Burden of Disease Study 2013 Collaborators, 2015. Global, regional, and national incidence, prevalence, and years lived with disability for 301 acute and chronic diseases and injuries in 188 countries, 1990–2013: A systematic analysis for the Global Burden of Disease Study 2013. Lancet 386 (9995), 743–800.

Goldstein, L.B. (Ed.), 2011. A Primer on Stroke Prevention and Treatment: An overview based on AHA/ASA guidelines. John Wiley & Sons, New York.

Grey Née Cotte, S., Salmen Née Stroet, A., von Ahsen, N., et al., 2015. Lack of efficacy of mitoxantrone in primary progressive multiple sclerosis irrespective of pharmacogenetic factors: a multi-center, retrospective analysis. Journal of Neuroimmunology 278, 277–279.

Haringer, V.C., Gibson, S.B., 2015. Amyotrophic lateral sclerosis: clinical perspectives. Orphan Drugs: Research and Reviews 5, 19–31.

Harkawik, R., Coyle, J.L., 2012. Exercise for better ALS management? ASHA Leader 17 (11).

Heilman, K.M., Rothi, L.J.G., 1997. Limb apraxia: a look back. In: Rothi, L.J.G., Heilman, K.M. (Eds.), Apraxia: The Neuropsychology of Action. Psychology Press, Hove, UK, pp. 7–18.

Hill, K., Denisenko, S., Miller, K., et al., 2010. Clinical Outcome Measurement in Adult Neurological Physiotherapy, 4th ed. Australian Physiotherapy Association, National Neurology Group, Melbourne, Australia.

Horak, F.B., 2006. Postural orientation and equilibrium: what do we need to know about neural control of balance to prevent falls? Age and Ageing 35 (Suppl. 2), ii7–ii11.

Kaiser, M.R., Michael, S.G., Chanda, K., 2009. Preventable seizures: a prospective, cross sectional study on the influence of pharmacological factors. Journal of Clinical and Diagnostic Research: JCDR 3 (6), 1836–1840.

Kaur, J., Sharma, S., Mittal, J., 2012. Physiotherapy in dementia. Dehli Psychiatry Journal 15 (1), 200–203.

Kraus, M.F., Maki, P., 1997. Case report: the combined use of amantadine and l-dopa/carbidopa in the treatment of chronic brain injury. Brain Injury 11 (6), 455–460.

Lance, J.W., 1980. Symposium synopsis. In: Feldman, R.G., Young, R.R.Koella, W.P. (Eds.), Spasticity: Disorder of Motor Control. Year Book Medical Publishers, Chicago, pp. 485–494.

Lewis, M., Rushanan, S., 2007. The role of physical therapy and occupational therapy in the treatment of amyotrophic lateral sclerosis. Neurorehabilitation 22 (6), 451–461.

Lillo, P., Hodges, J.R., 2010. Cognition and behaviour in motor neurone disease. Current Opinion in Neurology 23 (6), 638–642.

Ling, H., Massey, L.A., Lees, A.J., et al., 2012. Hypokinesia without decrement distinguishes progressive supranuclear palsy from Parkinson's disease. Brain: A Journal of Neurology 135 (4), 1141–1153.

Louis, E.D., 2014. 'Essential tremor' or 'the essential tremors': is this one disease or a family of diseases? Neuroepidemiology 42 (2), 81–89.

Mazzoni, P., Shabbott, B., Cortés, J.C., 2012. Motor control abnormalities in Parkinson's disease. Cold Spring Harbor Perspectives in Medicine 2 (6), a009282.

McAuley, J.H., Britton, T.C., Rothwell, J.C., et al., 2000. The timing of primary orthostatic tremor bursts has a task-specific plasticity. Brain: A Journal of Neurology 123 (2), 254–266.

Miller, R.G., Jackson, C.E., Kasarskis, E.J., et al., 2009. Practice parameter update: the care of the patient with amyotrophic lateral sclerosis: multidisciplinary care, symptom management, and cognitive/behavioral impairment (an evidence-based review): report of the Quality Standards Subcommittee of the American Academy of Neurology. Neurology 73 (15), 1227–1233.

Mogyoros, I., Bostock, H., Burke, D., 2000. Mechanisms of paresthesias arising from healthy axons. Muscle and Nerve 23 (3), 310–320.

Musarò, A., 2013. Understanding ALS: new therapeutic approaches. The FEBS Journal 280 (17), 4315–4322.

National Institute for Health and Care Excellence (NICE), 2013. Diagnosis and Management of the Epilepsies in Adults, Children and Young People, NICE Commissioning Guides UK.

National Institute for Health and Care Excellence (NICE), 2014. Multiple Sclerosis: Management of Multiple Sclerosis in Primary and Secondary Care, NICE Guidelines.

NHMRC Partnership on Dealing with Dementia and Related Functional Decline in Older People (CDPC), Draft Clinical Practice Guidelines for Dementia in Australia, 2015.

Pandyan, A.D., Hermens, H., Johnson, G.R., 2010. Spasticity. In: Encyclopedia of Neuroscience. Elsevier Ltd, pp. 153–163.

Perlmutter, J.S., 2009. Assessment of Parkinson disease manifestations. Current Protocols in Neuroscience Chapter 10, Unit 10.1.

Platz, T., Eickhof, C., Nuyens, G., et al., 2005. Clinical scales for the assessment of spasticity, associated phenomena, and function: a systematic review of the literature. Disability and Rehabilitation 27 (1–2), 7–18.

Pomeroy, V.M., Warren, C.M., Honeycombe, C., et al., 1999. Mobility and dementia: is physiotherapy treatment during respite care effective? International Journal of Geriatric Psychiatry 14 (5), 389–397.

Rekand, T., 2010. Clinical assessment and management of spasticity: a review. Acta Neurologica Scandinavica. Supplementum 190, 62–66.

Rudick, R.A., Miller, D., Bethoux, F., et al., 2014. The Multiple Sclerosis Performance Test (MSPT): an iPad-based disability assessment tool. Journal of Visualized Experiments (88), e51318. doi:10.3791/51318.

Rush, A.J., Blacker, D., 2008. Handbook of Psychiatric Measures. American Psychiatric Publishing, Washington, DC.

Sanger, T.D., Chen, D., Fehlings, D.L., et al., 2010. Definition and classification of hyperkinetic movements in childhood. Movement Disorders: Official Journal of the Movement Disorder Society 25 (11), 1538–1549.

Sanjak, M., Bravver, E., Bockenek, W.L., et al., 2010. Supported treadmill ambulation for amyotrophic lateral sclerosis: a pilot study. Archives of Physical Medicine and Rehabilitation 91 (12), 1920–1929.

Schneider, W.N., Drew-Cates, J., Wong, T.M., et al., 1999. Cognitive and behavioural efficacy of amantadine in acute traumatic brain injury: an initial double-blind placebo-controlled study. Brain Injury 13 (11), 863–872.

Schrempf, W., Ziemssen, T., 2007. Glatiramer acetate: mechanisms of action in multiple sclerosis. Autoimmunity Reviews 6 (7), 469–475.

Sellbach, A., Silburn, P., 2012. Management of Parkinson's disease. Australian Prescriber 35 (6), 183–188.

Sharif-Alhoseini, M., Rahimi-Movaghar, V., Vaccaro, A.R., 2012, Underlying causes of paresthesia, Paraesthesia: InTech.

Stovner, L.J., Hoff, J.M., Svalheim, S., et al., 2014. Neurological disorders in the Global Burden of Disease 2010 study. Acta Neurologica Scandinavica. Supplementum 198, 1–6.

Trompetto, C., Marinelli, L., Mori, L., et al., 2014. Pathophysiology of spasticity: implications for neurorehabilitation. BioMed Research International 2014, 354906. doi:10.1155/2014/354906.

Uttara, B., Singh, A.V., Zamboni, P., et al., 2009. Oxidative stress and neurodegenerative diseases: a review of upstream and downstream antioxidant therapeutic options. Current Neuropharmacology 7 (1), 65–74.

Whiteford, H.A., Ferrari, A.J., Degenhardt, L., et al., 2015. The global burden of mental, neurological and substance use disorders: an analysis from the global burden of disease study 2010. PLoS ONE 10 (2), e0116820.

Wiendl, H., Meuth, S.G., 2015. Pharmacological approaches to delaying disability progression in patients with multiple sclerosis. Drugs 75 (9), 947–977.

Ziemssen, T., Schrempf, W., 2007. Glatiramer acetate: mechanisms of Action in multiple sclerosis. In: Minagar, A. (Ed.), International Review of Neurobiology. pp. 537–570.

Zwinkels, A., Geusgens, C., van de Sande, P., et al., 2004. Assessment of apraxia: inter-rater reliability of a new apraxia test, association between apraxia and other cognitive deficits and prevalence of apraxia in a rehabilitation setting. Clinical Rehabilitation 18 (7), 819–827.

Pain and analgesia

Anthony Wright, Heather AE Benson, Robert Will

■ Introduction

Pain is a common presenting problem for patients receiving physiotherapy treatment. It may be the primary reason for seeking treatment or it may be a significant concurrent problem that has the potential to impact on function. Patients may present with either acute or chronic pain (pain that persists beyond the normal time of healing, commonly 3 months [Merskey & Bogduk 1994]), and in most cases they will require some form of pharmaceutical treatment in addition to any physiotherapy interventions. There are a number of different groups of drugs available to manage pain that target different receptor systems and sites of action. There are also a number of different routes of administration for analgesic drugs. In many cases there will be some degree of trial and error in determining the appropriate medication, the best route of administration and the appropriate dosage required to manage pain in any individual, with maximum efficacy and minimal side effects.

While we commonly focus on distinctions between the management of acute and chronic pain, one of the key distinctions in the pharmaceutical field is between drugs and delivery systems that are effective in the management of inflammatory or nociceptive pain and those that are intended to reduce neuropathic pain. Inflammatory pain is pain that is initiated at the site of injury or disease and may be due to a variety of pathological insults including arthritis, fracture, muscle tear, organ trauma etc (Merskey & Bogduk 1994; Woolf 2010). Neuropathic pain is pain that originates as a result of disease or injury affecting the somatosensory system (Merskey & Bogduk 1994; Treede et al. 2008; Woolf 2010). Patients will often use different words to describe peripheral neuropathic pain and, because of the different mechanisms involved, it often requires different pharmacological management. See Treede et al. (2008) for a description of the key features of neuropathic pain. Woolf (2010) also uses the term dysfunctional pain to describe pain states in which there is no clear evidence of either an inflammatory processes or nervous system damage yet the person reports significant pain (e.g. fibromyalgia). These conditions are difficult to manage but are commonly treated using centrally acting medications in a similar manner to some forms of neuropathic pain.

The emphasis in this chapter will primarily be on the distinctions between inflammatory/nociceptive and neuropathic pain and the range of pharmaceutical agents available for the management of each type of pain. The focus will be on different classes of drugs and each category will be reviewed in terms of mechanism of action, site of action, route of administration, effects and side (adverse) effects. Examples will be provided for the different clinical situations in which particular drugs would be used. While there is a range of options available for the management of pain it is critical for all practitioners to ensure that patients are fully assessed and a correct diagnosis is determined before any treatment is implemented. It is also important to use medications with the lowest risk profile and the least invasive route of administration that is commensurate with obtaining pain relief in any particular patient. With many analgesic drugs it is also important to achieve an appropriate balance between the need to reduce and minimise pain and managing the risk of toxicity, addiction or inappropriate use of prescription medications. The primary aim of drug treatment is to reduce pain to a level where patients can function on a daily basis.

Inflammatory and neuropathic pain

A clear understanding of the neurophysiology of pain perception and pain modulation provides an important basis for understanding the actions of various classes of analgesic drugs, and there is an increasing emphasis on developing mechanism-based approaches to pain management (Woolf et al. 1998). Hence it is important to clearly differentiate the type of pain requiring treatment and the extent to which the nociceptive system has changed in response to a particular nociceptive input.

Pain is often classified as either inflammatory pain, in which peripheral nociceptors are activated by chemical mediators of inflammation or tissue damage, or neuropathic pain, where the cause of pain is injury or a disease process affecting the nervous system itself (Merskey & Bogduk 1994; Treede et al. 2008; Woolf 2010). Inflammatory pain may arise from somatic structures such as muscle, joints and bones, or from visceral organs such as the heart or liver. Neuropathic pain may arise from damage or disease affecting either the peripheral or the central nervous system (CNS). In some cases it is possible for patients to have a mixed pain presentation with features of both inflammatory and neuropathic pain. This form of mixed pain presentation is increasingly recognised in patients with chronic back pain (see Chapter 5) (Freynhagen et al. 2006, 2008).

Inflammatory pain involves activation of nociceptive afferent neurons that are normally either unmyelinated or thinly myelinated. Tissue damage or disease processes trigger a range of inflammatory mediators that activate and sensitise nociceptive neurons. This leads to changes in neuronal function and recruitment that have been termed peripheral sensitisation (Wright & Zusman 2004). One important consequence of peripheral sensitisation is that nociceptive afferents that are normally relatively insensitive begin to generate trains of action potentials that enter the dorsal horn of the spinal cord (Schmidt 1996). This afferent activity rapidly generates changes in the function and recruitment of central nervous system neurons, which has been termed central sensitisation (Woolf 2011). These processes of peripheral and central sensitisation provide important potential mechanisms for pharmaceutical interventions to control inflammatory pain. Inflammatory pain is often described using terms such as dull, throbbing and aching, and it will normally be associated with hyperalgesia (enhanced response to a stimulus that is normally painful) (Merskey 2007) in the affected area and also potentially with the development of somatic referred pain related to the degree of central sensitisation (Graven-Nielsen 2006). Somatic referred pain often occurs in specific anatomical locations but it does not follow a dermatomal pattern (Graven-Nielsen 2006). Importantly, there are significant numbers of 'silent' nociceptors in visceral organs (Cervero & Janig 1992) so the presence of disease and inflammatory processes may substantially increase nociceptive inputs from the viscera and visceral organs may also trigger referred pain (Sikandar & Dickenson 2012).

Importantly, when damage to the nervous system occurs nociceptive activity is generated from the site of damage within the nervous system rather than at the peripheral nociceptive ending. Damage and disease of the nerve tissue also often affects larger myelinated afferent neurons as well as the thinly myelinated and unmyelinated nociceptive afferents. Ectopic neuronal activity arising at some point along the axon rather than at the peripheral receptor seems to be one of the key mechanisms for triggering neuropathic pain (Devor 1991). This tends to result in a very distinctive pattern of pain and dysaesthesia that is not easily modulated. This aberrant neuronal activity may also initiate central sensitisation but, importantly, damage to the nervous system will also often trigger some degree of neuroanatomical reorganisation within the nervous system (Woolf & Mannion 1999) and may also initiate apoptosis (programmed cell death) in some neurons that have lost their normal neuronal inputs (Scholz et al. 2005). These changes often mean that the capacity for the nervous system to modulate neuropathic pain is significantly impaired. As a consequence, some common analgesic medications are known to be less effective in managing neuropathic pain (Gilron, Baron & Jensen 2015). Stabilisation of neuronal membranes, minimisation of impulse activity and enhancement of CNS pain modulatory systems provide important potential mechanisms for pharmaceutical interventions to control neuropathic pain. Peripheral neuropathic pain is often described using terms such as tingling/prickling, hot/burning and shooting/ electric shocks (Gilron, Baron & Jensen 2015), and may be accompanied by sensations such as numbness or paraesthesia. It will commonly be associated with hyperalgesia but also, importantly, in some cases it will be associated with allodynia (pain due to a stimulus that does not usually provoke pain) (Merskey 2007) in which normally innocuous stimuli (e.g. light touch) begin to trigger pain, potentially as a reflection of neuroanatomical reorganisation (Woolf & Mannion 1999). Injury or inflammation of peripheral nerve structures may produce referred pain that will normally follow a dermatomal or peripheral nerve distribution pattern (Graven-Nielsen 2006).

There are a number of questionnaires that can be used in the clinical setting to identify patients with features of neuropathic pain (Bennett 2001; Bouhassira et al. 2004; Freynhagen et al. 2006), although a definitive diagnosis of neuropathic pain also requires the presence of clear evidence of damage or impairment affecting the nervous system (Treede et al. 2008).

Some pain presentations are not easily classified as either inflammatory or neuropathic pain. These include disorders such as complex regional pain syndrome (CRPS) and phantom limb pain (Merskey & Bogduk 1994). CRPS is a condition in which people experience excessive pain that is often associated with swelling and trophic changes in the skin. A distinction can be made between CRPS type I and CRPS type II. In CRPS type I the problem may be caused by a relatively minor injury (e.g. Colles fracture), and the degree of pain experienced is disproportionate to the severity of the injury. In CRPS type II the causative injury involves damage to the nervous system. Patients may have high levels of circulating cytokines suggesting an inflammatory basis for the pain, but they also exhibit features such as allodynia that are often associated with neuropathic pain problems and there is evidence of significant neuroanatomical reorganisation within their somatosensory systems (Marinus et al. 2011). The problem can persist for a prolonged period of time and patients will often require detailed assessment and specialist pain clinic management to develop an optimal treatment protocol.

Phantom limb pain is another chronic pain disorder that might generally be classified as neuropathic but it can also be influenced by nociceptive inputs from the residual limb. Amputation of a limb triggers very significant neuroanatomical reorganisation that often leaves individuals with the perception of a phantom limb that may or may not be painful (Ramachandran & Hirstein 1998). Neurons associated with the affected limb in the somatosensory cortex will acquire synaptic connections with adjacent cortical neurons and paradoxical situations may arise where, for example, stimulation of the face may induce pain and other sensations in a phantom hand (Ramachandran & Hirstein 1998). This may also be exacerbated by nociceptive stimuli affecting the residual stump or nociceptive inputs from the face. Phantom limb pain will often require specialist pain management and it may be important to time rehabilitation activities to coincide with the optimal effects of pain medications.

Pharmaceutical management of inflammatory pain

Inflammatory pain involves the activation of peripheral nociceptors by chemical mediators released during inflammation. Nociceptive signals are then transmitted to the brain via peripheral afferent neurons and spinal cord neurons. There are four key sites at which drugs can potentially modulate this nociceptive input: the peripheral tissues, the peripheral nerve fibres, the dorsal horn of the spinal cord and key brain sites.

Medications acting on the peripheral tissues and nociceptors

Orally administered non-steroidal anti-inflammatory drugs

Non-steroidal anti-inflammatory drugs (NSAIDs) are well recognised for their anti-inflammatory actions but they also have demonstrable analgesic and antipyretic effects, which are independent of their anti-inflammatory action (Insel 1996). There is variation in the degree to which different drugs in this class exert each of these actions. For example, paracetamol has a weak anti-inflammatory action but is well recognised for its analgesic and antipyretic effects (Insel 1996). The actions of NSAIDs have been primarily attributed to inhibition of cyclooxygenase (COX1 and COX2) enzymes but there are a number of other mechanisms that may contribute to the actions of drugs in this category. These include: inhibition of leucocyte function, inhibition of cytokine release, inhibition of platelet aggregation, inhibition of free radical formation, amelioration of complement-mediated cell lysis and inhibition of central sensitisation (Insel 1996). They have both peripheral and central nervous system effects. Table 7.1 describes a number of different drugs within this class. In terms of pain management they are commonly used to treat pain related to soft tissue injuries, inflammatory arthritic conditions, inflammatory conditions of internal organs and postoperative pain (Atkinson et al. 2013). Many patients who receive treatment from physiotherapists will also be taking NSAIDs. In relation to the arthritides, there are also other classes of disease-modifying anti-rheumatic drugs (DMARDs) that may produce pain relief as a result of modifying the immune process or the inflammatory process. This category of drugs is dealt with in Chapter 5.

Text continued on p. 206

TABLE 7.1 Non-steroidal anti-inflammatory drugs

Medication class/drug name	Mechanism of action	Common side effects	Practice points	Common adult dosage range	Availability
Paracetamol	Analgesic and antipyretic	Generally well tolerated Potentially fatal hepatotoxicity in overdose	Available in many brands and in cough and cold products Avoid using multiple products containing paracetamol	0.5–1 g every 4–6 hours (maximum 4 g daily); also available as SR tablets and capsules	Over the counter (OTC)
Aspirin	Analgesic with poor anti-inflammatory activity	Gastrointestinal irritation, gastrointestinal bleeding; indigestion or heartburn; allergic reactions such as swelling, rash, difficulty in breathing	Paracetamol may be taken with this medicine	300–900 mg every 4–6 hours (maximum 4 g daily)	OTC
Diclofenac	Reduces the production of prostaglandins by inhibiting the enzyme cyclooxygenase (COX)	Gastrointestinal discomfort, nausea, diarrhoea Patients at risk of duodenal or gastric ulceration (including the elderly) should receive COX-2 or NSAID with gastro-protective treatment	Do not combine with other anti-inflammatory medicines	75–150 mg daily in 2–3 divided doses (also available as modified release oral tablets/capsules, suppositories, injections)	OTC
Ibuprofen				200–400 mg 3–4 times daily (maximum 2400 mg)	OTC
Indomethacin				50–200 mg daily in 2–4 divided doses	Prescription only

Ketoprofen		25–50 mg orally every 6–8 hours; dose may be increased up to a maximum of 75 mg	Prescription only
Mefenamic acid		500 mg orally followed by 250 mg every 6 hours as needed, not to exceed 7 days use	Pack of 20 available OTC
Naproxen, Naproxen sodium		250–1250 mg daily in 2–4 doses; controlled release formulations 750–1000 mg once daily	OTC
Piroxicam		10–20 mg once daily	Prescription only
Sulindac		200–400 mg daily in 1 or 2 doses	Prescription only
Celecoxib	Selective COX-2 inhibitor	200 mg daily in 1–2 divided doses	Prescription only
Etoricoxib		30–90 mg once daily	Prescription only
Meloxicam		7.5–15 mg daily	Prescription only

SR, slow release.

There are two different forms of the cyclooxygenase enzyme, cyclooxygenase-1 (COX-1) and cyclooxygenase-2 (COX-2) (Abate & Buttaro 2015). The enzyme catalyses the conversion of arachidonic acid to prostaglandin H2 (PGH2), which is the precursor for a number of other molecules that have significant roles in relation to inflammation and pain (O'Banion 1999). COX-1 is present in many tissues and is constitutively expressed whereas expression of COX-2 is more selective and occurs in response to specific stimuli such as tissue damage and inflammation. Inhibition of COX-1 has been linked to many of the adverse effects of NSAIDs, which encouraged the development of COX-2 selective NSAIDs (see Table 7.1), but increasing experience with COX-2 NSAIDs has shown that they also have a significant adverse effect profile and that in relation to cardiovascular adverse effects they may carry greater risk than the traditional COX-1 grouping (Abate & Buttaro 2015). Adverse effects include gastrointestinal bleeds, ulcers and gastritis or esophagitis, hypertension, fluid retention, kidney problems, heart problems and cutaneous rashes (Table 7.1). There is considerable interindividual variation in response and adverse effect profiles so patients may be switched between NSAIDS to determine the drug with the best efficacy and adverse effect profile for their condition.

Topically applied NSAIDs

NSAID gels and sprays applied to the skin at the site of pain can provide local anti-inflammatory and pain relieving effects. A number of topical preparations containing NSAIDs are available over the counter at pharmacies (Table 7.2). The intent of administering NSAIDs via the skin is to achieve local tissue levels of the drug at the target tissue with minimal systemic absorption. The concept is that, if drug delivery can be targeted to the injured/inflamed tissues in this way, the dosage required can be reduced. This will reduce adverse effects, particularly gastrointestinal adverse effects, while at the same time achieving a therapeutic outcome. In order to achieve a therapeutic outcome the topical NSAID must be formulated to effectively penetrate the stratum corneum and diffuse through the viable epidermis and dermis. Various approaches have been used to formulate NSAIDs to ensure effective penetration. These can involve modifying the drug (e.g. diclofenac diethyl ammonium salt) or modifying the formulation (e.g. solvent enhancers such as alcohols, liposomes or microemulsions). Penetration may then occur into the deeper soft tissues directly or via the local circulation. Direct penetration of NSAIDs to the underlying soft tissues has been demonstrated although there is less evidence of penetration into synovial fluid in underlying joints (Vaile & Davis 1998). Topical application can result in local adverse effects such as erythema, irritation and itch. While the incidence of adverse effects is relatively low it tends to increase with repeated application (Vaile & Davis 1998). Topical NSAIDs are regularly used to reduce pain and inflammation associated with a range of localised soft tissue injuries. There is also evidence to support their use in conditions such as osteoarthritis (Baraf et al. 2011) although caution is required with regular daily use.

Corticosteroids

Corticosteroids (Table 7.3) are potent anti-inflammatory agents and a short course of high-dose oral steroids is sometimes indicated for painful conditions

TABLE 7.2 Topical creams, ointments, gels, sprays and rubs/liniments

Medication class/drug name	Mechanism of action	Common side effects	Practice points	Common adult dosage range	Availability
Salicylate esters	Rubefacient: stimulates blood flow and creates a sense of warmth, which may contribute to pain relief by masking the sensation of pain	Infrequent skin irritation, erythema, itching, rash	Should not be applied over broken skin Contact with eyes and other mucous membranes to be avoided	Apply 2–4 times daily for up to 14 days; review treatment after 14 days	OTC
Capsaicin	Depletes substance P to reduce nerve conduction	Stinging or burning sensation	As above Transient burning sensation may occur with initial treatment Hot shower or bath should be avoided before or immediately after application	Apply 3–4 times daily for 3–4 weeks then review treatment outcome	OTC
Benzydamine hydrochloride	Non-steroidal anti-inflammatory drug (NSAID)	Infrequent skin irritation, erythema, itching, rash		Apply 2–4 times daily for up to 14 days; review treatment after 14 days	OTC
Diclofenac diethylammonium					OTC
Ibuprofen					OTC
Ketoprofen					OTC
Piroxicam					OTC

such as polymyalgia rheumatica or rheumatoid arthritis (Chapter 5). They act to limit inflammation by suppressing neutrophil and macrophage function, including the release of inflammatory mediators from these cells. While they have potent effects they are also associated with a significant number of adverse effects (Table 7.3), which limit their long-term use (Frauman 1996).

Patients who have symptoms related to one or two joints may benefit from intra-articular injection of active steroid formulations to relieve pain and improve mobility. Triamcinolone acetonide is often used for intra-articular injection because it is relatively insoluble and therefore provides a long-acting effect (Bodick et al. 2015). Local steroid injections into soft tissues may be used to treat tendonitis in various locations (e.g. Achilles tendon, supraspinatus tendon).

PHYSIOTHERAPY PRACTICE POINTS: INFLAMMATORY PAIN

In patients with complex regional pain syndrome, physiotherapy rehabilitation of the affected limb is an important component of treatment and may include strategies such as graded motor imagery (Walz et al. 2013). It is important that rehabilitation is timed to coincide with periods of optimum analgesia in order to minimise any increase in pain.

Patients on corticosteroids are normally advised to rest the injected area for 24–48 hours and then to gradually restore range of motion and muscle function in the affected area. Some physiotherapists have begun to use steroid injections as a component of their management of musculoskeletal disorders.

Text continued on p. 211

TABLE 7.3 Corticosteroids administered orally or by injection

Medication class/ drug name	Mechanism of action	Common side effects	Practice points	Common adult dosage range
Prednisolone	Reduces inflammation and suppresses the immune system	Long-term therapy: weight gain, hypertension, osteoporosis Can worsen conditions such as peptic ulcer disease, diabetes, hypertension and heart failure, osteoporosis particularly in long-term use	Medication taken only once a day should be taken in the morning (to prevent possible sleep disturbance) Medication should also be taken with food Medication dosages should not be ceased or altered without consultation with the treating doctor	*Oral:* 5–10 mg once daily (may be twice daily initially); maintenance 2.5–15 mg daily
Prednisone				*Oral:* 5–10 mg once daily (may be twice daily initially); maintenance 2.5–15 mg daily
Betamethasone Dexamethasone Methylprednisolone Triamcinolone	As above: direct injection into joint or soft tissue reduces heat, swelling, erythema, tenderness	Side effects are rare but may include infection, intraarticular pain, flare, hypopigmentation	Relief of symptoms usually occurs within 2–4 hours and lasts at least 4 weeks	*Intraarticular or soft tissue injection:* dose depends on site of injection

	TABLE 7.4 Cytokine modulators				
Medication class/ drug name	Mechanism of action	Indication	Common side effects	Practice points	Common adult dosage range
Adalimumab	TNF-α inhibitor; monoclonal antibody	Moderate to severe active RA, often in combination with methotrexate; active and progressive psoriatic arthritis; severe active ankylosing spondylitis	Mild pain, swelling or itching; headaches, cough, stomach and bowel discomfort; upper respiratory tract infections (colds, sinusitis)	*All medicines in this group can reduce the immune response; therefore any sign of infection should be reported and live vaccines should be avoided*	*SC injection:* 40 mg every 2 weeks
Etanercept			Less common side effects: blood disorders; severe infections	These medications may be given subcutaneously or intravenously (see next column)	*SC injection:* 50 mg once weekly or 25 mg twice weekly
Infliximab					*IV infusion:* 3 mg/kg, repeated 2 and 6 weeks, then every 8 weeks
Golimumab				When applied subcutaneously the medicine is administered by injection into a skin fold on the thigh or abdomen; injections should be rotated between the thigh and abdomen	*SC injection:* 50 mg once per month
Certolizumab pegol					*SC injection:* 400 mg every 2 weeks for 3 doses, then 200 mg every 2 weeks
Rituximab	Prevents full activation of B lymphocytes	Severe active arthritis			*IV infusion:* 1 g repeated after 2 weeks; may repeat every 16–24 weeks (see institutional protocols)

Continued

TABLE 7.4 Cytokine modulators—cont'd

Medication class/ drug name	Mechanism of action	Indication	Common side effects	Practice points	Common adult dosage range
Anakinra	Interleukin-1 inhibitor	In combination with methotrexate for RA that has not responded to methotrexate alone			*SC injection:* 100 mg every 24 hours
Abatacept	Prevents full activation of T lymphocytes	Moderate to severe RA in combination with methotrexate			*SC injection:* Every week (or by IV infusion); Adjust for weight: 60–100 kg: 125 mg SC every week
Tocilizumab	Blocks interleukin-6		Mild pain, swelling or itching; headaches/dizziness, stomach and bowel discomfort; upper respiratory tract infections (colds, sinusitis); skin irritation/ rashes; high blood pressure; weight gain		*IV infusion:* 8 mg/kg (maximum 800 mg) every 4 weeks (also SC formulations)
Tofacitinib	Inhibits cytokine production		Upper respiratory tract infections, headache, diarrhoea and nasopharyngitis		*Oral:* 5 mg twice a day

IV, intravenous; RA, rheumatoid arthritis; SC, subcutaneous; TNF, tumour necrosis factor.

Cytokine modulators

Cytokine modulators (Table 7.4) are a relatively new category of medication that have a major anti-inflammatory but also a pain relieving action. The main group of such agents is the tumour necrosis factor alpha (TNF-α) blockers, which are monoclonal antibodies that bind to TNF-α and prevent it from triggering a cascade of inflammatory processes. They are normally administered as an injection or an infusion and can have a relatively rapid and potent effect on pain and inflammation. They are used to treat a range of painful arthritic conditions such as rheumatoid arthritis (RA), ankylosing spondylitis, psoriatic arthritis and juvenile idiopathic arthritis (JIA) (Breedveld 2014; Lomholt, Thastum & Herlin 2013; Machado et al. 2013). Commonly used TNF inhibitors in Australia include adalimumab, etanercept, infliximab, golimumab and certolizumab pegol. Other drugs in this category include: rituximab, which blocks the production and activity of B lymphocytes; abatacept, which blocks T lymphocytes; and tociliziumab, which blocks interleukin-6. These monoclonal antibodies have been approved to treat RA and JIA (tocilizumab). Tofacitinib, a Janus kinase (JAK) inhibitor, which inhibits cytokine production, has recently been approved in Australia to treat RA.

Topical local anaesthetics

Local anaesthetic drugs act by producing a reversible conduction block in sensory afferents. There are a number of different local anaesthetic drugs that vary in their potency, duration of action and potential for adverse effects. Local anaesthetic preparations for topical application (Table 7.5) include lignocaine creams/gels and they are primarily used to reduce or eliminate pain related to venepuncture and minor surgical procedures such as tattoo removal. This may include vaccinations and they are often used in younger patients who may require multiple venepunctures for monitoring or treatment. It does require some time (30–60 minutes) for the anaesthetic to penetrate the stratum corneum and the product may need to be applied under an occlusive dressing to enhance penetration. These products provide effective short-term pain relief but are of limited value for ongoing painful conditions. Adverse effects are normally mild but may include erythema, burning and itch (Russell & Doyle 1997).

Oral opioid analgesics

The term opium is derived from the ancient Greek word for juice and the drug is derived from the juice of the poppy. It is a form of pain relief that has been utilised for millennia. Opioid drugs mimic the effects of endogenous opioids and act on receptors within the central nervous system, but they can also act on opioid receptors in peripheral tissues that are induced in response to inflammation (Stein, Schafer & Hassan 1995). There are three main groups of opioid receptors, which are classified as mu (μ), kappa (κ) and delta (δ) (Pleuvry 1983). Binding of opioids to these receptors on neurons within the nociceptive system elicits analgesia.

Drugs in this class (Table 7.6) are divided into weak and strong opioids. Weak opioids include codeine, dihydrocodeine and dextropropoxyphene, which are available as single agent formulations or in combination with paracetamol. Strong opioid analgesics include morphine, hydromorphone, oxycodone,

TABLE 7.5 Local anaesthetics: topical

Medication class/ drug name	Mechanism of action	Common side effects	Practice points	Common adult dosage range
Amethocaine (tetracaine)	Interrupts impulse conduction in peripheral nerves and stabilises cell membranes by blocking sodium channels	Transient, localised erythema	Supplied in various forms: topical spray, cream, gel, ointment, medicated plaster	Apply approx. 0.5 g gel and cover with occlusive dressing
Lidocaine (lignocaine)		As above		Example of lignocaine/ prilocaine topical: Apply 1–2 g cream and cover with occlusive dressing; apply patch 1 hour before procedure
Prilocaine				

methadone, buprenorphine, fentanyl and pethidine. Several of the medications such as oxycodone are available as sustained release formulations that extend their duration of action making them more effective for the management of chronic pain (Richarz et al. 2013). Oxycodone, fentanyl and buprenorphine are commonly used to treat conditions of chronic non-malignant pain such as lumbar spondylosis and osteoporotic fracture where other treatments have been ineffective or not tolerated. These medications are prescribed predominantly in the elderly population and side effects are common and include constipation, nausea, sedation and addiction (see Chapter 11). Particular care is required in using these medications where patients are using other sedating drugs such as anti-anxiolytics, antidepressants, hypnotics and gabinoids. Methadone and buprenorphine are primarily used to manage opioid addiction (Bonhomme et al. 2012). Pethidine is a powerful analgesic that is commonly used as a postoperative medication or for obstetric analgesia. In relation to inflammatory pain these drugs are likely to have analgesic actions in the peripheral tissues and via spinal cord and brain receptors.

Morphine and pethidine may be administered by continuous infusion or by intermittent intravenous dosing as well as intramuscular and subcutaneous injection. Patient controlled analgesia (PCA) is a specific drug administration system that allows patients to control their intravenous dosage (Walder et al. 2001). PCA is often used for postoperative or obstetric analgesia. It can also be used to manage ongoing pain associated with cancer.

Fentanyl is available in a number of formulations including a sustained release transdermal patch, IV infusion, subcutaneous injection and a lollipop or lozenge for buccal delivery in cases of breakthrough pain[1] (Stanley et al. 1989). The fentanyl patch provides sustained drug administration for 72 hours to induce analgesia in chronic cancer pain and chronic pain of non-malignant origin (Park et al. 2011).

Common adverse effects of opioid drugs include nausea, vomiting, constipation and drowsiness (Table 7.6). They may also produce potentially fatal

---

[1]Breakthrough pain (BTP) is a sudden flare of pain that 'breaks through' the long-acting medication prescribed to treat moderate to severe persistent pain.

TABLE 7.6 Opioid analgesics

Medication class/drug name	Mechanism of action	Common side effects	Practice points	Common adult dosage range
Buprenorphine	Partial agonist at μ opioid receptors and an antagonist at δ and κ receptors	Nausea, vomiting and dry mouth on initiation of therapy (should settle with continued use), constipation (take laxative), drowsiness and dizziness Dependence, tolerance, withdrawal symptoms	Patch: apply to dry, hairless skin on upper arm, chest or back; rotate site to avoid irritation SL tab: allow to dissolve under the tongue; do not swallow for about 10 minutes	Patch: Initially 5 mcg/hour (maximum 20 mcg/hour) (apply new patch every 7 days) SL tablet: 0.2–0.4 mg every 6–8 hours
Fentanyl	μ opioid receptor agonist	As above	Patch: apply to dry, hairless skin on upper arm, chest or back; rotate site to avoid irritation	Patch: Individualised treatment
Hydromorphone	μ opioid receptor agonist	As above		Initially 4–8 mg once daily (modified release) or 2–4 mg every 4 hours (immediate release), increasing as required
Methadone	μ opioid receptor agonist with additional ketamine-like antagonism at the NMDA receptor	As above		2.5 mg every 8–12 hours
Morphine	μ opioid receptor agonist	As above		Initially 5–20 mg every 4 hours (immediate release) or 5–60 mg daily (SR)

Continued

TABLE 7.6 Opioid analgesics—cont'd

Medication class/drug name	Mechanism of action	Common side effects	Practice points	Common adult dosage range
Oxycodone	κ opioid receptor agonist with less activity at μ and δ receptors	As above		Initially 5–15 mg every 4–6 hours (immediate release) or 10 mg every 12 hours (modified release)
Tapendatol	μ opioid receptor agonist and noradrenaline uptake inhibitor	As above; headaches		*Oral:* 50–100 mg every 4–6 hour (maximum 600 mg/day)
Tramadol	μ opioid receptor agonist and reuptake inhibitor of serotonin and noradrenalin	As above; headaches		Initially 50–100 mg every 4–6 hours (immediate release) or 100–200 mg every 12 hours (modified release) (maximum daily dose 400 mg)

SL, sublingual; SR, sustained release.

respiratory depression. Opioid medications are associated with the development of physical dependence and also with the development of tolerance (Reisine & Pastarnak 1996). This means that addiction and diminished effect leading to increased dosage with the likelihood of greater adverse effects are significant clinical problems with sustained use.

Medications acting on peripheral nerve fibres

Local anaesthetics

Local anaesthetic blockade involves blockade of specific sodium channels in peripheral neurons to limit the generation of action potentials (French, Zamponi & Sierralta 1998). Anaesthetic blockade can be used to treat localised inflammatory conditions and pain associated with tissue injury as well as providing intraoperative and postoperative regional analgesia. A wide range of techniques are available to produce regional analgesia and a number of different drugs are used depending on the extent and duration of analgesia required (Liu, Ngeow & Yadeau 2009). Some of the most commonly used local anaesthetics (Table 7.5) include lignocaine, mepivacaine, bupivacaine and ropivicaine. Lidocaine is the most commonly used local anaesthetic with good effect, rapid onset and moderate duration of action. Bupivicaine has a relatively long duration of action and it can be used effectively to produce a differential block of sensory and motor fibres. This makes it useful for procedural applications in outpatient pain management.

The more commonly used techniques for pain management include greater occipital, brachial plexus, intercostal, ilioinguinal, sciatic and tibial nerve blocks (Lubenow 1996). These procedures are relatively safe but complications can include cardiovascular and CNS effects and peripheral nerve injury. These effects are of particular concern where long acting local anaesthetic agents are used.

Analgesia provided by a regional block may be beneficial in promoting restoration of movement through physiotherapy treatment or the utilisation of continuous passive motion. Thoracic nerve blocks provide pain relief and facilitate respiratory therapy in patients with painful rib fractures.

Medications acting on the dorsal horn of the spinal cord

Opioid analgesics

Opioid analgesics have an analgesic action via receptors located in the dorsal horn of the spinal cord (Pleuvry 1983). In addition to the potential action of oral opioids at these sites, opioids (Table 7.6) can be administered epidurally or intrathecally to achieve analgesia (Bujedo, Santos & Azpiazu 2012). Morphine and fentanyl are commonly administered by the epidural or intrathecal routes for obstetrics and for surgical procedures. These short-term uses are normally unproblematic but more sustained administration tends to increase the risk of problems related to addiction, diminished effect and accidental overdose.

Local anaesthetics

Opioids may be administered in combination with local anaesthetics. Effective postoperative analgesia with minimal motor block facilitates early mobilisation and return to function, particularly after major surgery. This approach is commonly used after major abdominal surgery.

Epidural or intrathecal opioid administration can also be used for the management of cancer pain or for chronic inflammatory pain. In most cases this will involve the implantation of an infusion pump with a subcutaneous reservoir that allows for repeated replenishment (Carr & Cousins 1998).

The α-2 agonist clonidine is also frequently used for spinal analgesia in combination with local opioids and local anaesthetics (Carr & Cousins 1998). The action of clonidine is thought to involve activation of the descending noradrenergic pain modulation system.

NSAIDs

Sensitisation of the nociceptive system results in increased levels of intracellular calcium ions, which leads to activation of phospholipase C and increased production of arachidonic acid. The COX enzymes can then convert this substrate to the various elements of the prostaglandin cascade. These prostaglandins then diffuse through the spinal cord to sensitise adjacent neurons. NSAIDs have an important action within the CNS to block or reverse this sensitisation process (Malmberg & Yaksh 1992). They may also contribute to this process by blocking the release of nitric oxide, which also diffuses through the dorsal horn to promote sensitisation (Gordh, Karlsten & Kristensen 1995). While paracetamol has only a weak anti-inflammatory effect it is likely that a significant component of its analgesic effect involves inhibition of COX within the CNS rather than in the peripheral tissues. It is also thought to have a significant inhibitory effect on nitric oxide synthase (NOS) (Bjorkman 1995). These central nervous system effects provide an important contribution to the analgesic effect of NSAIDs.

Medications acting on supraspinal sites

Opioid analgesics

The analgesic actions of opioids in the peripheral tissues and the dorsal horn of the spinal cord have been described. Their most potent analgesic effect occurs upon binding to receptors in the periaquaductal gray (PAG) region and adjacent brainstem nuclei. All routes of administration have the capacity to activate opioid receptors in the brain but the most effective route of administration is direct intraventricular administration. This results in high concentrations of drug in supraspinal sites such as the PAG. This method of treatment is sometimes used for patients with severe pain due to a terminal illness who have become relatively tolerant to morphine administered via other routes (Karavelis et al. 1996).

Tricyclic antidepressants

The tricyclic antidepressants (see Table 7.8 later) are a class of drugs originally developed to treat depression (see Chapter 10) but they are now increasingly used to treat chronic pain states. They are often effective in providing analgesia at doses lower than the dose required to alleviate depression. Noradrenaline and serotonin (5-hydroxytryptamine, 5-HT) are two neurotransmitters released by descending pain inhibitory neurons projecting from the brain to the spinal cord. The tricyclic antidepressants inhibit the reuptake of these neurotransmitters increasing their capacity to inhibit nociceptive transmission through the spinal

Medication class/ drug name	Mechanism of action	Common side effects	Practice points	Common adult dosage range
Amitriptyline Clomipramine Dothiepin Doxepin Imipramine	Inhibits reuptake of noradrenaline and serotonin	Drowsiness and blurred vision on initiation of therapy (should settle with continued use), dry mouth, dizziness on standing up (postural hypotension), urinary retention, constipation	The medicine can take time (2–4 weeks) before any improvement is perceived Most effective as single dose at night Alcohol to be avoided when taking this drug	25–100 mg/day Imipramine: 25–300 mg/day

TABLE 7.7 Tricyclic antidepressants

cord (Godfrey 1996). There are a number of drugs in this category (Table 7.7) although amitriptyline is the main tricyclic antidepressant used in the management of chronic pain (Kajdasz et al. 2007).

The normal approach is to give amitriptyline 10–25 mg 2 hours before bedtime (Karavelis et al. 1996). This helps to promote sleep and improve sleep quality as well as alleviating pain, although this effect tends to diminish over time. It may take 2–3 months before noticeable improvements in pain occur. The dose is then titrated to achieve optimal pain relief while minimising adverse effects.

The main limitation of these drugs is their adverse effect profile. Common adverse effects include drowsiness, dry mouth, blurred vision, constipation, urinary retention and sweating (Table 7.7). More severe adverse effects include hypertension, arrhythmias and myocardial infarction. Nevertheless, there is evidence that the tricyclic antidepressants are valuable in the management of pain associated with conditions such as fibromyalgia and chronic low back pain (Godfrey 1996; Ward 1986).

Pharmacological management of neuropathic pain

Neuropathic pain is pain that arises as a result of disease or injury affecting the nervous system. Common neuropathic pain syndromes include post-herpetic neuralgia, pain related to peripheral neuropathies secondary to various disease processes (e.g. diabetes mellitus), phantom limb pain and trigeminal neuralgia. There is considerable individual variation in the presentation of neuropathic pain syndromes, and consequently there may be variation in the efficacy of different pain treatments. There are a range of approaches that can be taken to the management of neuropathic pain states. These include treatments for the underlying disease process, topical agents, local anaesthetic blocks and various systemic drugs addressing different components of the pathophysiological process (Belgrade 1999). There is an increased focus on medications that specifically address the pathophysiological processes associated with neuropathic pain and an understanding that some of the drugs that are commonly used to address inflammatory pain are not effective for neuropathic pain disorders (Eisenberg & Suzan 2014).

Disease management

Treatment of the underlying disease may be an important factor in the management of some forms of neuropathic pain. Examples include improved blood glucose control in patients with diabetes, which may limit the development of complications such as diabetic neuropathy, or the use of surgery and chemotherapy in managing tumours that impact on nerve structures.

As with inflammatory pain, drug therapy for neuropathic pain targets four major sites: the peripheral tissues, the peripheral nerve fibres, the dorsal horn of the spinal cord and key brain sites.

Medications acting on the peripheral tissues and nociceptors

Capsaicin cream

Capsaicin derived from capsicum has the ability to deplete peripheral C fibres of a number of neurotransmitters including substance P. If the cream (Table 7.2) is applied regularly (4 times per day) it can be effective in reducing some forms of neuropathic pain (Rains & Bryson 1995). This is particularly the case for small areas of allodynia in conditions such as post-herpetic neuralgia or stump pain. There is also evidence to support the efficacy of high-dose capsaicin in the management of pain associated with post-herpetic neuralgia (Baranidharan, Das & Bhaskar 2013).

Local anaesthetics

Local anaesthetics can be administered topically to areas of allodynia and may be of some value in the management of conditions such as post-herpetic neuralgia, although there is considerable individual variation in skin penetration (Rowbotham et al. 1996).

Medications acting on peripheral nerve fibres

Local anaesthetics

A range of local anaesthetics (Table 7.5) can be used to provide regional blocks for injured or disease affected peripheral nerves. Local anaesthetics have a stabilising effect on the nerve membrane and can act to reduce spontaneous activity from neuromas that are important for some neuropathic pain states (e.g. Morton's (or intermetatarsal) neuroma). It may be necessary to provide a series of anaesthetic blocks or a continuous infusion of anaesthetic over a longer period of time in order to diminish spontaneous activity and reduce nociceptive input. The most commonly used local anaesthetics are lignocaine, bupivicaine and ropivicaine. There is evidence to support the use of lignocaine in the management of painful diabetic neuropathy, post-herpetic neuralgia and peripheral nerve injury (Kingery 1997; Challapalli et al. 2005). Anaesthetic blocks may also be used as a means of promoting rehabilitation and restoration of function in some patients, particularly those with nerve injury or stump and phantom pain post amputation.

Medications acting on the dorsal horn of the spinal cord

Anticonvulsants and calcium channel blockers

Anticonvulsants (also discussed in Chapter 5) and calcium channel blockers (Table 7.8) are regarded as some of the most effective forms of treatment for

TABLE 7.8 Anticonvulsants and calcium channel blockers

Medication class/ drug name	Mechanism of action	Common side effects	Practice points	Common adult dosage range
Gabapentin	Structurally related to the neurotransmitter GABA	Dizziness, drowsiness, dry mouth, peripheral oedema, gait disturbance, weight gain	Medication should be initially taken at night	900–3600 mg daily in 3 doses, starting with 300 mg daily
Pregabalin	Antiepileptic indicated for neuropathic pain		Medication may take 2–4 weeks before the pain improves	75–300 mg twice daily

neuropathic pain (MacFarlane et al. 1997). This is particularly the case in terms of managing lancinating pain in conditions such as trigeminal neuralgia and in other conditions where ectopic discharge arising at a site of nerve inflammation or injury is a key pathophysiological process contributing to pain (MacFarlane et al. 1997).

This category of drugs is primarily used in conditions such as epilepsy (see Chapter 6) where they stabilise the neuronal membrane, limit ectopic discharge and reduce the risk of seizures. Drugs commonly used in the management of neuropathic pain include pregabalin, gabapentin and carbamazepine (Morello et al. 1999). Gabapentin is used in the treatment of a variety of neuropathic pain states because, in addition to its membrane stabilisation properties, it is an analogue of gamma-aminobutyric acid (GABA) and therefore has a direct pain inhibitory action (Rosenberg et al. 1997). There is evidence to support its use in post-herpetic neuralgia and painful diabetic neuralgia (Morello et al. 1999; Rosenberg et al. 1997). Adverse effects include sleepiness, dizziness and ataxia (Table 7.8). Carbamazepine is considered to be particularly useful in the management of trigeminal neuralgia and there is good evidence to support its efficacy for this condition (MacFarlane et al. 1997; Sindrup & Jensen 1999). Trigeminal neuralgia is a particular form of neuropathic pain that may also benefit from antispasmodic agents or muscle-relaxing agents such as baclofen.

Over the past decade pregabalin (Table 7.8), which is also structurally similar to GABA, has become one of the most commonly used drugs to manage neuropathic pain (Zhang et al. 2015). It acts on pre-synaptic alpha-2/delta-1 calcium channels to modulate neurotransmitter release and thereby reduce nociceptive input (Zhang et al. 2015). It shares similarities of action with gabapentin. It may also have an effect in limiting synaptogenesis, which is potentially important in controlling the development of widespread hyperalgesia and allodynia. Patients are treated initially with relatively low doses of 25–50 mg daily, particularly in the elderly, but if the drug is well tolerated doses can be increased to 300–600 mg per day. It is normally given twice a day with most of the medication taken at night because of its sedative properties. There is evidence to support the effectiveness of pregabalin in the management of painful diabetic neuropathy, post-herpetic neuropathy and neuropathic pain associated with low back pain conditions (Moore et al. 2009; Zhang et al. 2015). It has also demonstrated effectiveness in the management of fibromyalgia (which can be considered as an example of dysfunctional pain) and is frequently used to limit the development of neuropathic pain during surgery (Dauri et al. 2009; Moore et al. 2009). Adverse effects include dizziness, sedation, dry mouth and peripheral oedema (Table 7.8). In many cases these adverse effects may limit the maximum tolerable dose and the effectiveness of the drug. It is frequently combined with other analgesics such as opiates. If tapentadol[2] is introduced, the dose of pregabalin can be reduced because in combination the drugs act synergistically due to their combined mechanisms of action (Christoph et al. 2011).

Local anaesthetics

Local anaesthetics can also be administered via the epidural route in patients with neuropathic pain. In many cases this will be in combination with clonidine as outlined above. Mexiletine is an antiarrhythmic agent and oral analogue of lignocaine that is effective in the management of some neuropathic pain states (Challapalli et al. 2005). It does, however, have a range of adverse effects including dizziness, ataxia, nausea and vomiting.

Medications acting on supraspinal sites

Tricyclic antidepressants

The tricyclic antidepressants (see Chapter 10 and Table 7.7) are frequently used in the management of neuropathic pain (Gilron, Baron & Jensen 2015). In many neuropathic pain disorders there appears to be reduced effectiveness of descending pain modulatory systems and so the tricyclic antidepressants can be used to increase the capacity of these systems to modulate pain. There is evidence to support their effectiveness in the management of a number of neuropathic pain conditions including post-herpetic neuralgia and painful diabetic neuropathy (Sindrup et al. 2005). The main limitation associated with these drugs is their adverse effect profile and it is clear that in practice the need to reduce dosage in order to limit adverse effects may result in less than optimal pain management for some patients.

Serotonin–noradrenaline reuptake inhibitor

Duloxetine is a newer serotonin and noradrenaline reuptake inhibitor (SNRI), which is used extensively to treat neuropathic pain (Ormseth, Scholz & Boomershine 2011). There is evidence to support its effectiveness in the management of painful diabetic neuropathy (Ormseth, Scholz & Boomershine 2011). It is associated with a range of adverse effects including nausea, dry mouth, constipation, sweating, tiredness and insomnia (Table 7.7).

Opioid analgesics

There has been considerable controversy about the value of opioid analgesics in the management of neuropathic pain (Sindrup & Jensen 1999). It has been suggested that neuropathic pains states are unresponsive to opioids, and it does seem that in many cases there is a reduced responsiveness to opioids, which means that higher dosages are required (Gilron, Baron & Jensen 2015; Sindrup & Jensen 1999). It is not appropriate, however, to suggest that opioids are of no

---

[2]For further explanation on this drug see 'Tapentadol' below.

value in managing neuropathic pain. Evidence suggests that morphine and oxycodone are effective in post-herpetic neuralgia (Rowbotham 1994) and fentanyl has demonstrated efficacy for a number of neuropathic pain states (Dellemijn & Vanneste 1997). It is likely that there will be individual variation in the effectiveness of opioids for patients with a range of neuropathic pain states depending on the nature of the pathophysiological mechanisms involved.

Tapentadol

Tapentadol is a sustained release preparation that in one molecule combines mu agonist and noradrenaline reuptake inhibition actions, similar to tramadol (Vadivelu et al. 2011). It has been shown to be beneficial in chronic neuropathic pain states such as diabetic peripheral neuropathy and low back pain (Vadivelu et al. 2011). The dose varies between 50 mg twice daily up to 250 mg twice daily. It is classed as an opioid but has weak opioid action. It has a lower adverse effect profile than opioids (Riemsma et al. 2011) and GABA agonists and can replace these drugs for some patients. Nausea, dizziness and somnolence may occur with its use.

PHYSIOTHERAPY PRACTICE POINTS: PAIN

The pharmacological management of pain is a complex area. No one drug provides effective relief for all pain states in every patient. It is often necessary to trial different pain medications or different routes of administration and, in some cases, it may be necessary to use drug combinations in order to provide effective pain relief. Dosage is often limited by adverse effects and the efficacy of some drugs may decline over time. It is important for physiotherapists to be aware of the actions and adverse effects of the main groups of analgesic drugs and the requirements to monitor drug response over time in order to ensure efficacy and minimise adverse events. It is also important to be aware of the onset of action and the duration of action of drugs, particularly local anaesthetics, in order to use them effectively as an aid to improving function.

CAVEAT: Physiotherapists must be aware that many of the drugs used for pain relief have multiple usages with varying dosages according to specific indications.

■ References

Abate, K.S., Buttaro, T.M., 2015. Safe and effective NSAID use. The Nurse Practitioner 40 (6), 18–22.

Atkinson, T.J., Fudin, J., Jahn, H.L., et al., 2013. What's new in NSAID pharmacotherapy: oral agents to injectables. Pain Medicine: The Official Journal Of the American Academy of Pain Medicine 14 (Suppl. 1), S11–S17.

Baraf, H.S., Gloth, F.M., Barthel, H.R., et al., 2011. Safety and efficacy of topical diclofenac sodium gel for knee osteoarthritis in elderly and younger patients: pooled data from three randomized, double-blind, parallel-group, placebo-controlled, multicentre trials. Drugs and Aging 28 (1), 27–40.

Baranidharan, G., Das, S., Bhaskar, A., 2013. A review of the high-concentration capsaicin patch and experience in its use in the management of neuropathic pain. Therapeutic Advances in Neurological Disorders 6 (5), 287–297.

Belgrade, M.J., 1999. Following the clues to neuropathic pain: distribution and other leads reveal the cause and the treatment approach. Postgraduate Medicine 106 (6), 127–132, 135–140.

Bennett, M., 2001. The LANSS Pain Scale: the Leeds assessment of neuropathic symptoms and signs. Pain 92 (1–2), 147–157.

Bjorkman, R., 1995. Central antinociceptive effects of non-steroidal anti-inflammatory drugs and paracetamol: experimental studies in the rat. Acta Anaesthesiologica Scandinavica Supplementum 103, 1–44.

Bodick, N., Lufkin, J., Willwerth, C., et al., 2015. An intra-articular, extended-release formulation of triamcinolone acetonide prolongs and amplifies analgesic effect in patients with osteoarthritis of the knee: a randomized clinical trial. The Journal of Bone and Joint Surgery (American) 97 (11), 877–888.

Bonhomme, J., Shim, R.S., Gooden, R., et al., 2012. Opioid addiction and abuse in primary care practice: a comparison of methadone and buprenorphine as treatment options. Journal of the National Medical Association 104 (7–8), 342–350.

Bouhassira, D., Attal, N., Fermanian, J., et al., 2004. Development and validation of the Neuropathic Pain Symptom Inventory. Pain 108 (3), 248–257.

Breedveld, F., 2014. TNF antagonists opened the way to personalized medicine in rheumatoid arthritis. Molecular Medicine 20 (Suppl. 1), S7–S9.

Bujedo, B.M., Santos, S.G., Azpiazu, A.U., 2012. A review of epidural and intrathecal opioids used in the management of postoperative pain. Journal of Opioid Management 8 (3), 177–192.

Carr, D.B., Cousins, M.J., 1998. Spinal route of analgesia – opioids and future options. In: Cousins, M.J., Bridenbaugh, P.O. (Eds.), Neural Blockade in Clinical Anaesthesia. Lippincott-Raven Publishers, Philadelphia., pp. 915–983.

Cervero, F., Janig, W., 1992. Visceral nociceptors: a new world order? Trends in Neuroscience 15 (10), 374–378.

Challapalli, V., Tremont-Lukats, I.W., McNicol, E.D., et al., 2005. Systemic administration of local anesthetic agents to relieve neuropathic pain. The Cochrane Database of Systematic Reviews (4), CD003345.

Christoph, T., De Vry, J., Schiene, K., et al., 2011. Synergistic antihypersensitive effects of pregabalin and tapentadol in a rat model of neuropathic pain. European Journal of Pharmacology 666 (1–3), 72–79.

Dauri, M., Faria, S., Gatti, A., et al., 2009. Gabapentin and pregabalin for the acute post-operative pain management: a systematic-narrative review of the recent clinical evidences. Current Drug Targets 10 (8), 716–733.

Dellemijn, P.L., Vanneste, J.A., 1997. Randomised double-blind active-placebo-controlled crossover trial of intravenous fentanyl in neuropathic pain. Lancet 349 (9054), 753–758.

Devor, M., 1991. Neuropathic pain and injured nerve: peripheral mechanisms. British Medical Bulletin 47 (3), 619–630.

Eisenberg, E., Suzan, E., 2014. Drug combinations in the treatment of neuropathic pain. Current Pain and Headache Reports 18 (12), 463.

Frauman, A.G., 1996. An overview of the adverse reactions to adrenal corticosteroids. Adverse Drug Reactions and Toxicological Reviews 15 (4), 203–206.

French, R.J., Zamponi, G.W., Sierralta, I.E., 1998. Molecular and kinetic determinants of local anaesthetic action on sodium channels. Toxicology Letters 100–101, 247–254.

Freynhagen, R., Baron, R., Gockel, U., et al., 2006. painDETECT: a new screening questionnaire to identify neuropathic components in patients with back pain. Current Medical Research and Opinion 22 (10), 1911–1920.

Freynhagen, R., Rolke, R., Baron, R., et al., 2008. Pseudoradicular and radicular low-back pain – a disease continuum rather than different entities? Answers from quantitative sensory testing. Pain 135 (1–2), 65–74.

Gilron, I., Baron, R., Jensen, T., 2015. Neuropathic pain: principles of diagnosis and treatment. Mayo Clinic Proceedings 90 (4), 532–545.

Godfrey, R.G., 1996. A guide to the understanding and use of tricyclic antidepressants in the overall management of fibromyalgia and other chronic pain syndromes. Archives of Internal Medicine 156 (10), 1047–1052.

Gordh, T., Karlsten, R., Kristensen, J., 1995. Intervention with spinal NMDA, adenosine, and NO systems for pain modulation. Annals of Medicine 27 (2), 229–234.

Graven-Nielsen, T., 2006. Fundamentals of muscle pain, referred pain, and deep tissue hyperalgesia. Scandinavian Journal of Rheumatology. Supplement 122, 1–43.

Insel, P.A., 1996. Analgesic–antipyretic and aniinflammatory agents and drugs employed in the treatment of gout. In: Hardman, J.G., et al. (Eds.), Goodman and Gilman's Pharmacological Basis of Therapeutics. McGraw-Hill, New York, pp. 617–657.

Kajdasz, D.K., Iyengar, S., Desaiah, D., et al., 2007. Duloxetine for the management of diabetic peripheral neuropathic pain: evidence-based findings from post hoc analysis of three multicenter, randomized, double-blind, placebo-controlled, parallel-group studies. Clinical Therapeutics 29 (Suppl.), 2536–2546.

Karavelis, A., Foroglou, G., Selviaridis, P., et al., 1996. Intraventricular administration of morphine for control of intractable cancer pain in 90 patients. Neurosurgery 39 (1), 57–61, discussion 61-2.

Kingery, W.S., 1997. A critical review of controlled clinical trials for peripheral neuropathic pain and complex regional pain syndromes. Pain 73 (2), 123–139.

Liu, S.S., Ngeow, J.E., Yadeau, J.T., 2009. Ultrasound-guided regional anesthesia and analgesia: a qualitative systematic review. Regional Anesthesia and Pain Medicine 34 (1), 47–59.

Lomholt, J.J., Thastum, M., Herlin, T., 2013. Pain experience in children with juvenile idiopathic arthritis treated with anti-TNF agents compared to non-biologic standard treatment. Pediatric Rheumatology Online Journal 11 (1), 21.

Lubenow, T., 1996. Analgesic techniques. In: Brown, D.L. (Ed.), Regional Anesthesia and Analgesia. WB Saunders Company, Philadelphia., pp. 644–657.

MacFarlane, B.V., Wright, A., O'Callaghan, J., et al., 1997. Chronic neuropathic pain and its control by drugs. Pharmacology and Therapeutics 75 (1), 1–19.

Machado, M.A., Barbosa, M.M., Almeida, A.M., et al., 2013. Treatment of ankylosing spondylitis with TNF blockers: a meta-analysis. Rheumatology International 33 (9), 2199–2213.

Malmberg, A.B., Yaksh, T.L., 1992. Hyperalgesia mediated by spinal glutamate or substance P receptor blocked by spinal cyclooxygenase inhibition. Science 257 (5074), 1276–1279.

Marinus, J., Moseley, G.L., Birklein, F., et al., 2011. Clinical features and pathophysiology of complex regional pain syndrome. The Lancet. Neurology 10 (7), 637–648.

Merskey, H., 2007. The taxonomy of pain. Medical Clinics of North America 91 (1), 13–20, vii.

Merskey, H., Bogduk, N., 1994. Classification of Chronic Pain: Descriptions of chronic pain syndromes and definitions of pain terms. IASP Press, Seattle, p. 222.

Moore, R.A., Straube, S., Wiffen, P.J., et al., 2009. Pregabalin for acute and chronic pain in adults. The Cochrane Database of Systematic Reviews (3), CD007076.

Morello, C.M., Leckband, S.G., Stoner, C.P., et al., 1999. Randomized double-blind study comparing the efficacy of gabapentin with amitriptyline on diabetic peripheral neuropathy pain. Archives of Internal Medicine 159 (16), 1931–1937.

O'Banion, M.K., 1999. Cyclooxygenase-2: molecular biology, pharmacology, and neurobiology. Critical Reviews in Neurobiology 13 (1), 45–82.

Ormseth, M.J., Scholz, B.A., Boomershine, C.S., 2011. Duloxetine in the management of diabetic peripheral neuropathic pain. Patient Preference and Adherence 5, 343–356.

Park, J.H., Kim, J.H., Yun, S.C., et al., 2011. Evaluation of efficacy and safety of fentanyl transdermal patch (Durogesic D-TRANS) in chronic pain. Acta Neurochirurgica 153 (1), 181–190.

Pleuvry, B.J., 1983. An update on opioid receptors. British Journal of Anaesthesia 55 (Suppl. 2), 143S–146S.

Rains, C., Bryson, H.M., 1995. Topical capsaicin: a review of its pharmacological properties and therapeutic potential in post-herpetic neuralgia, diabetic neuropathy and osteoarthritis. Drugs and Aging 7 (4), 317–328.

Ramachandran, V.S., Hirstein, W., 1998. The perception of phantom limbs. The D. O. Hebb lecture. Brain: A Journal of Neurology 121 (9), 1603–1630.

Reisine, T., Pastarnak, G., 1996. Opioid analgesic and antagonists. In: Hardman, J.G., et al. (Eds.), Goodman and Gilman's Pharmacological Basis of Therapeutics. McGraw-Hill, New York, pp. 521–555.

Richarz, U., Waechter, S., Sabatowski, R., et al., 2013. Sustained safety and efficacy of once-daily hydromorphone extended-release (OROS(R) hydromorphone ER) compared with twice-daily oxycodone controlled-release over 52 weeks in patients with moderate to severe chronic noncancer pain. Pain Practice 13 (1), 30–40.

Riemsma, R., Forbes, C., Harker, J., et al., 2011. Systematic review of tapentadol in chronic severe pain. Current Medical Research and Opinion 27 (10), 1907–1930.

Rosenberg, J.M., Harrell, C., Ristic, H., et al., 1997. The effect of gabapentin on neuropathic pain. The Clinical Journal of Pain 13 (3), 251–255.

Rowbotham, M.C., 1994. Managing post-herpetic neuralgia with opioids and local anesthetics. Annals of Neurology 35 (Suppl.), S46–S49.

Rowbotham, M.C., Davies, P.S., Verkempinck, C., et al., 1996. Lidocaine patch: double-blind controlled study of a new treatment method for post-herpetic neuralgia. Pain 65 (1), 39–44.

Russell, S.C., Doyle, E., 1997. A risk–benefit assessment of topical percutaneous local anaesthetics in children. Drug Safety 16 (4), 279–287.

Schmidt, R.F., 1996. The articular polymodal nociceptor in health and disease. Progress in Brain Research 113, 53–81.

Scholz, J., Broom, D.C., Youn, D.H., et al., 2005. Blocking caspase activity prevents transsynaptic neuronal apoptosis and the loss of inhibition in lamina II of the dorsal horn after peripheral nerve injury. The Journal of Neuroscience : The Official Journal of the Society for Neuroscience 25 (32), 7317–7323.

Sikandar, S., Dickenson, A.H., 2012. Visceral pain: the ins and outs, the ups and downs. Current Opinion in Supportive and Palliative Care 6 (1), 17–26.

Sindrup, S.H., Jensen, T.S., 1999. Efficacy of pharmacological treatments of neuropathic pain: an update and effect related to mechanism of drug action. Pain 83 (3), 389–400.

Sindrup, S.H., Otto, M., Finnerup, N.B., et al., 2005. Antidepressants in the treatment of neuropathic pain. Basic and Clinical Pharmacology and Toxicology 96 (6), 399–409.

Stanley, T.H., Hague, B., Mock, D.L., et al., 1989. Oral transmucosal fentanyl citrate (lollipop) premedication in human volunteers. Anesthesia and Analgesia 69 (1), 21–27.

Stein, C., Schafer, M., Hassan, A.H., 1995. Peripheral opioid receptors. Annals of Medicine 27 (2), 219–221.

Treede, R.D., Jensen, T.S., Campbell, J.N., et al., 2008. Neuropathic pain: redefinition and a grading system for clinical and research purposes. Neurology 70 (18), 1630–1635.

Vadivelu, N., Timchenko, A., Huang, Y., et al., 2011. Tapentadol extended-release for treatment of chronic pain: a review. Journal of Pain Research 4, 211–218.

Vaile, J.H., Davis, P., 1998. Topical NSAIDs for musculoskeletal conditions: a review of the literature. Drugs 56 (5), 783–799.

Vargas-Espinosa, M.L., Sanmartí-García, G., Vázquez-Delgado, E., et al., 2012. Antiepileptic drugs for the treatment of neuropathic pain: a systematic review. Medicina Oral, Patología Oral y Cirugía Bucal 17 (5), e786–e793.

Walder, B., Schafer, M., Henzi, I., et al., 2001. Efficacy and safety of patient-controlled opioid analgesia for acute postoperative pain: a quantitative systematic review. Acta Anaesthesiologica Scandinavica 45 (7), 795–804.

Walz, A.D., Usichenko, T., Moseley, G.L., et al., 2013. Graded motor imagery and the impact on pain processing in a case of CRPS. The Clinical Journal of Pain 29 (3), 276–279.

Ward, N.G., 1986. Tricyclic antidepressants for chronic low-back pain: mechanisms of action and predictors of response. Spine 11 (7), 661–665.

Woolf, C.J., 2010. What is this thing called pain? Journal of Clinical Investigation 120 (11), 3742–3744.

Woolf, C.J., 2011. Central sensitization: implications for the diagnosis and treatment of pain. Pain 152 (Suppl. 3), S2–S15.

Woolf, C.J., Bennett, G.J., Doherty, M., et al., 1998. Towards a mechanism-based classification of pain? Pain 77 (3), 227–229.

Woolf, C.J., Mannion, R.J., 1999. Neuropathic pain: aetiology, symptoms, mechanisms, and management. Lancet 353 (9168), 1959–1964.

Wright, A., Zusman, M., 2004. Neurophysiology of pain and pain modulation. In: Boyling, J.D., Jull, G.A. (Eds.), Grieve's Modern Manual Therapy: the Vertebral Column. Churchill Livingstone, Edinburgh, pp. 155–171.

Zhang, S.S., Wu, Z., Zhang, L.C., et al., 2015. Efficacy and safety of pregabalin for treating painful diabetic peripheral neuropathy: a meta-analysis. Acta Anaesthesiologica Scandinavica 59 (2), 147–159.

Endocrine system

Joanne Morris, Chandima Perera, Jacqueline Reznik,
Ofer Keren, Iftah Biran

OBJECTIVES

This chapter will discuss the major endocrine systems and endocrine
disorders that physiotherapists may be involved with and examine the
roles that the most commonly used medications have in the management
of these conditions. By the end of this chapter the reader should gain an
understanding of the following:

* the major classification of endocrine disorders according to structure,
  location, signs and symptoms
* pharmacotherapy options commonly used in the management of the
  major endocrine disorders
* usual dosages, routes of administration and major contraindications and
  precautions associated with these medications
* any potential impact of medication on physiotherapeutic management.

OVERVIEW

Glucose metabolism
Diabetes mellitus
Type 1 diabetes mellitus
Type 2 diabetes mellitus
Gestational diabetes
Bone metabolism and calcium
balance
Osteoporosis
Osteogenesis imperfecta
Parathyroid disease
Metabolic syndrome
Thyroid disorders
Hashimoto's disease
Graves' disease
Goitre
Thyroid nodules

Pharmacological management for
thyroid disorders
Adrenal disorders
Primary adrenal insufficiency
(Addison's disease)
Secondary adrenal insufficiency
Adrenal hyperfunction (Cushing's
syndrome)
Pharmacological management for
adrenal diseases
Pituitary gland syndromes
Pineal gland disorders
Pharmacological management for
pineal gland disorders

Introduction

The endocrine system is made up of a group of organs that control metabolic equilibrium or homeostasis; the mediators of this system are the hormones. By definition an endocrine gland is one that secretes its hormones directly into the bloodstream from where they are transported to the target (cells, tissues or organs). In contrast, an exocrine gland, namely sweat, salivary or mammary glands, secretes its products into a system of ducts that lead to the external environment.

The major glands of the endocrine system are the hypothalamus, pituitary (hypophysis), thyroid, parathyroid, adrenals, pineal body and the reproductive organs (ovaries and testes). The pancreas is also a part of this system due to its role in hormone production; however, the pancreas (and the liver) are both endocrine and exocrine glands as they secrete externally through the pancreatic and hepatic ducts, respectively (see Figure 8.1 and Table 8.1) (Greenstein & Wood 2011).

Endocrine hormones circulate in the bloodstream and have a very specific action on specific tissues/organs and, upon reaching a target site, bind to a receptor. Hormones regulate the body's growth and development, metabolism, tissue function, sexual development and function, reproduction, sleep, use of foods in energy production and mood. Very small amounts of hormones can trigger very large responses in the body. Hormones are classified into three groups: amines, proteins and steroids. They are secreted in response to changes in the blood (such as glucose levels) and/or other hormones within the blood (Scanlon & Sanders 2010).

Hypothalamic–pituitary axes

The *hypothalamic–pituitary–adrenal axis* (HPA) is a complex feedback system between the hypothalamus, the pituitary gland and the adrenals (Figure 8.2).

The HPA axis is a highly sensitive negative feedback system that acts on signals from upper cortical inputs, autonomic function, environmental cues such as light and temperature and peripheral endocrine feedback. The hypothalamus then delivers specific signals to the pituitary glands, which release hormones that influence most endocrine systems in the body in response to alterations in homeostasis. Specifically, the hypothalamic–pituitary axis directly affects the functions of the thyroid gland, the adrenal gland and the gonads, as well as influencing growth, energy expenditure, milk production and water balance.

The *hypothalamic–pituitary–thyroid axis* (HPT axis or the thyroid homeostasis or thyrotropic feedback control) is part of the neuroendocrine system responsible for the regulation of metabolism (Figure 8.3).

The hypothalamus senses low circulating levels of thyroid hormone (triiodothyronine [T_3] and thyroxine [T_4]) and responds by releasing thyrotropin-releasing hormone (TRH). TRH stimulates the pituitary to produce thyroid-stimulating hormone (TSH). TSH, in turn, stimulates the thyroid to produce thyroid hormone until levels in the blood return to normal. Thyroid hormone exerts negative feedback control over the hypothalamus as well as the anterior pituitary, thus controlling the release of both TRH from the hypothalamus and TSH from the anterior pituitary gland (Dietrich, Landgrafe & Fotiadou 2012; Fekete & Lechan 2014).

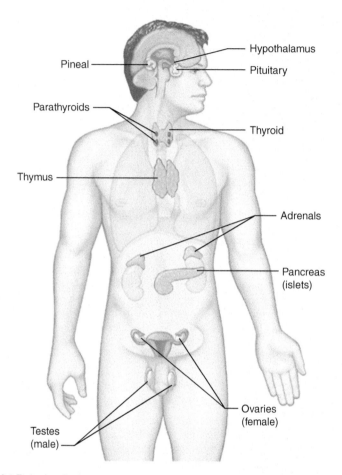

Figure 8.1 Endocrine glands.
Reproduced with permission from: Patton KT, Thibodeau GA, 2013. Anatomy and Physiology, eighth ed. St Louis, Mosby.

Disorders of the endocrine system

Allostasis, the process of achieving stability or homeostasis, through physiological or behavioural change, is normally carried out by means of alteration in HPA axis hormones, the autonomic nervous system, cytokines or a number of other systems, and is generally adaptive in the short term (McEwen & Wingfield 2010). Impairment of endocrine function may be due to a gland producing too much or too little of a hormone (or a functional decrease due to an autoimmune disease, such as Hashimoto disease), leading to a hormonal imbalance. Endocrine disease may also be due to the development of lesions (such as nodules or tumours) within the endocrine system, which may or may not affect hormone levels.

Text continued on p. 232

TABLE 8.1 Glands of the endocrine system

Gland	Anatomical position	Hormones secreted	Function/Effect
Hypothalamus	Located in the lower forebrain	Thyrotropin-releasing hormone (TRH) Corticotropin-releasing factor (CRF) Luteinising hormone-releasing hormone (LHRH) and gonadotropin-releasing hormone (GnRH) Growth hormone-releasing hormone (GHRH) Vasopressin (ADH) Oxytocin	All of these are released into the blood in the capillaries and travel immediately – in the portal veins – to a second capillary bed in the anterior lobe of the pituitary, where they exert their effects ADH and oxytocin travel in the neurons themselves to the posterior lobe of the pituitary where they are released into the circulation All are important in regulation of satiety, metabolism and body temperature

Pituitary	Located at the base of the brain beneath the hypothalamus, it is often considered the most important part of the endocrine system because it produces hormones that control many functions of other endocrine glands
	The pituitary gland is divided into two parts: the anterior lobe and the posterior lobe
		Anterior lobe:
		Thyroid-stimulating hormone (TSH)
		Gonadotropins
		• follicle-stimulating hormone (FSH)
		  • FSH in females
		  • FSH in males
		• luteinising hormone (LH)
		  • LH in females
		  • LH in males
		Prolactin (PRL)
		Growth hormone (GH)
		Adrenocorticotropin hormone (ACTH)
		Alpha-melanocyte-stimulating hormone (α-MSH)
		[intermediate lobe]
		Posterior lobe:
		Vasopressin (ADH)
		Oxytocin
			The anterior lobe contains 6 types of secretory cells, all but one of which are specialised to secrete only one of the anterior lobe hormones
			All of them secrete their hormone in response to hormones reaching them from the hypothalamus of the brain
			
			The posterior lobe of the pituitary releases two hormones – both synthesised in the hypothalamus – into the circulation

Continued

TABLE 8.1 Glands of the endocrine system—cont'd

Gland	Anatomical position	Hormones secreted	Function/Effect
Thyroid	Located in the lower part of the neck, wrapped around the trachea It has the shape of a butterfly: two lobes attached to one another by the isthmus	Thyroxine (T_4) Triiodothyronine (T_3)	The thyroid produces hormones that regulate the body's metabolism; it also plays a role in bone growth and development of the brain and nervous system in children Thyroid hormones also help maintain normal blood pressure, heart rate, digestion, muscle tone and reproductive functions
		Calcitonin	Involved in calcium metabolism and stimulating bone cells to add calcium to bone The pituitary gland controls the release of thyroid hormones
Parathyroid	Two pairs of small glands embedded in the surface of the thyroid gland	Parathyroid hormone	Regulates calcium levels in the blood and bone metabolism
Adrenal	The two adrenal glands are triangular-shaped glands located on top of each kidney Adrenal medulla	Corticosteroids Catecholamines (e.g. adrenaline)	Regulates the body's metabolism, the balance of salt and water in the body, the immune system and sexual function
Pineal body	Located in the middle of the brain	Melatonin	Regulates the sleep–wake cycle
Reproductive organs		Main source of sex hormones during the reproductive years	
Pancreas		The exocrine pancreas secretes digestive enzymes, while the endocrine pancreas secretes insulin and glucagon; these hormones regulate the level of glucose in the blood	Digestive and hormonal functions

ADH, antidiurectic hormone.

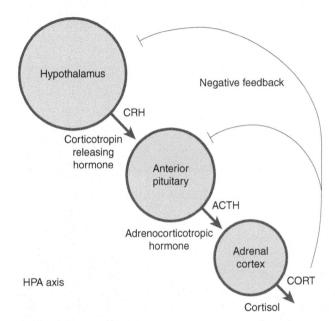

Figure 8.2 Hypothalamus–pituitary–adrenal axis.
Adapted with permission from: Neuroscientifically Challenged, *What is the HPA axis?* <http://
www.neuroscientificallychallenged.com/blog/2014/5/31/what-is-the-hpa-axis> (image courtesy of
BrianMSweis, CC BY SA 3.0).

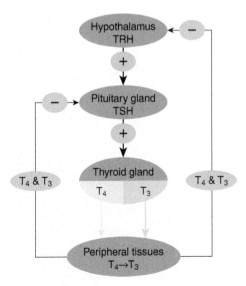

Figure 8.3 Hypothalamic–pituitary–thyroid axis.
Adapted from *Orlander P.R. et al, Hypothyroidism: Practice Essentials. Medscape, 19 February 2015,*
<http://emedicine.medscape.com/article/122393-overview>.

The body's metabolism (allostasis) is controlled by hormones; hence diseases/disorders of the endocrine system will affect this body metabolism. For example, obesity might develop due to specific endocrine disease (McEwen 2000). Table 8.2 summarises the conditions, hormones released and glands associated with disorders of the endocrine system.

TABLE 8.2 Disorders of the endocrine system

	Condition	Hormone released	Gland	Relevance for physiotherapists
Glucose metabolism disorders	Type 1 diabetes Type 2 diabetes Gestational diabetes Pre-diabetes Hyperglycaemia Hypoglycaemia	Insulin	Pancreas	+++
Calcium metabolism disorders	Osteopenia/porosis Hyperparathyroidism Hypoparathyroidism	Parathyroid hormone (PTH) Calcitonin	Parathyroid glands C cells in the thyroid gland	+++ +++
Thyroid disorders	Hashimoto's disease Thyroiditis Hyperthyroidism Hypothyroidism Graves' disease Thyroid nodules Thyroid storm	Triiodothyronine (T$_3$) Thyroxine (T$_4$)	Thyroid gland	+
Adrenal disorders	Addison's disease Cushing's syndrome Phaeochromocytoma	*Adrenal cortex*: Cortisol Aldosterone Androgen hormones *Adrenal medulla*: Adrenaline Noradrenaline	Adrenal glands	+
Pituitary disorders	Acromegaly Growth hormone deficiency (Inappropriate ADH secretion – diabetes insipidus)	Human growth hormone (HGH) Thyroid-stimulating hormone (TSH) Adrenocorticotropin hormone (ACTH) Luteinising hormone (LH) and follicle-stimulating hormone (FSH) Vasopressin (ADH) Oxytocin	Pituitary gland	+
Sex hormones disorders	Low testosterone Menopause	Testosterone Oestrogen ± progesterone	Reproductive glands	+

ADH, antidiurectic hormone; MS, multiple sclerosis.

■ Glucose metabolism

Diabetes mellitus

Diabetes mellitus (DM) is a chronic, lifetime condition affecting the body's ability to use the energy found in food. Diabetes is due to either the pancreas not producing enough insulin or the cells of the body not responding properly to the insulin produced. Symptoms of high blood glucose include frequent urination, increased thirst and increased hunger (see Table 8.3). There are three major types of diabetes: type 1 diabetes, type 2 diabetes and gestational diabetes.

1 Type 1 diabetes (formerly known as insulin-dependent diabetes mellitus or IDDM) is an autoimmune disease characterised by an inability to metabolise fuels, carbohydrates, proteins and fats because of absolute insulin deficiency. Type 1 diabetes can occur at any age, but it is more common in children.

2 Type 2 diabetes (formerly known as non-insulin dependent diabetes mellitus or NIDDM) is a chronic metabolic disorder. Onset is usually after 40 years of age but can occur at any age, including during childhood and adolescence. Often, environmental factors such as obesity and a sedentary lifestyle, superimposed on genetic susceptibility, are involved in the onset on type 2 DM (Alberti, Zimmet & Shaw 2007).

TABLE 8.3 Common signs and symptoms in diabetes mellitus (DM) types I and 2

Signs and symptoms	DM type 1 (acute onset)	DM type 2 (slower onset – milder signs and symptoms)	Gestational diabetes
Excessive thirst (polydipsia)	√	√	Often no noticeable signs and symptoms
Frequent urination (polyuria)	√	√	
Rapid weight loss	√	√	
Increased hunger	√	√	
Tiredness	√	√	
Nausea, vomiting, irritability	√	√	
Blurred vision		√	
Excessive itching		√	
Skin infections		√	
Sores that heal slowly		√	
Dry, itchy skin		√	
Pins and needles or numbness in feet		√	
Peripheral neuropathy (chronic)	√		

3 Gestational diabetes occurs when pregnant women without a previous history of diabetes develop a high blood sugar level (Barr et al. 2007).

Complications occurring with diabetes

As key members of the treating team physiotherapists need to be aware of the complications associated with DM and how affected patients will present.

Acute: Diabetic ketoacidosis and non-ketotic hyperosmolar coma

Diabetic ketoacidosis (DKA) is characterised by hyperglycaemia, metabolic acidosis and increased circulating total body ketone concentration. Ketoacidosis results from the lack (or ineffectiveness) of insulin with concomitant elevation of counter-regulatory hormones (glucagon, catecholamines, cortisol and growth hormone). Hyperglycaemia results from increased hepatic and renal glucose production (gluconeogenesis and glycogenolysis) and impaired glucose utilisation in peripheral tissues. Most patients in a hyperosmolar hyperglycaemic state (HHS) have type 2 diabetes. DKA usually develops rapidly, over a period of less than 24 hours. The clinical presentation of DKA includes polyuria, polydipsia, vomiting and abdominal pain. There will also be signs of dehydration including loss of skin turgor, dry mucous membranes, tachycardia and hypotension, reduction of mental status, lethargy and, in severe cases, dehydration may result in loss of consciousness (Houshyar, Bahrami & Aliasgarzadeh 2015). Acetone can be smelled on the breath of these patients (Li et al. 2015).

Long-term: Vascular damage and neuritis

Long-term complications of DM may include cardiovascular disease, stroke, peripheral neuropathy and chronic kidney failure. Other morbidities such as foot ulcers (a malfunction of the immune system and/or poor wound recovery) and impact on eye function are mostly due to vascular impairments.

PHYSIOTHERAPY PRACTICE POINTS: DIABETES MELLITUS

It is well recognised that cardiovascular exercise can assist with the management of DM, particularly type 2 (Taylor et al. 2014; Taylor, Fletcher & Tiarks 2009). Evidence suggests that cardiovascular exercise will:

- help insulin work better to improve diabetes control
- assist with weight control
- reduce blood pressure
- reduce the risk of heart disease
- reduce stress.

As an important member of the multidisciplinary team (MDT) the treating physiotherapist must be aware of when to refer the patient to another member of the team (i.e. due to ophthalmic impairments such as diabetic retinopathy, diabetic macular oedema [DME], cataract and glaucoma) since these secondary impairments may lead to severe vision loss and blindness. Physiotherapists need to be aware of which medications their patients are currently taking and the potential side effects of these medications, as they may impact on the patient's ability to undertake an exercise program (see Table 8.4 later).

TABLE 8.4 Common drugs used for diabetes mellitus

Drug group/name	Mechanism of action	Indications	Common side effects	Practice points	Common adult dosage range
Insulin U-100 insulin pen device containing U-300 insulin glargine	Mimics the natural activity Insulin is not orally absorbed, but is digested to its component amino acids and cannot be reconstructed to insulin due to beta-islet cell dysfunction. Therefore, insulin must currently be injected subcutaneously, although inhaled insulin dose forms are currently available in the USA	Type 1 diabetes	Signs of hypo- or hyperglycaemia (blood glucose level)	Mostly administered through injections (subcutaneous or IV) U-100 EXCEPT pen device containing U-300 insulin glargine	Individualise dose based on metabolic needs and frequent monitoring of blood glucose Total daily insulin requirements are generally between 0.5 and 1 U/kg/day Most individuals with type 1 diabetes should be treated with multiple daily insulin (MDI) injections or continuous subcutaneous insulin infusion (CSII)
Sulfonylureas Glimepiride Glipizide Micronised glyburide Glibenclamide, gliclazide (immediate release 80 mg and modified release [MR] 60 mg and 30 mg [(2 × 30 mg is equivalent to 80 mg] (Australian Medicines Handbook Pty Ltd 2016)	Stimulates the pancreas to release more insulin, right after a meal and then over several hours	Type 2 diabetes	Low blood glucose, occasional skin rash, irritability, upset stomach	Might cause low blood glucose *Gliclazide:* immediate release 80 mg and modified release (MR) 60 mg and 30 mg (2 × 30 mg MR is equivalent to 80 mg immediate release) (Australian Medicines Handbook Pty Ltd 2016)	Take with a meal once or twice a day

Continued

TABLE 8.4 Common drugs used for diabetes mellitus—cont'd

Drug group/name	Mechanism of action	Indications	Common side effects	Practice points	Common adult dosage range
Biguanides Metformin	Decreases amount of glucose released from liver	Type 2 diabetes	Gas, diarrhoea, upset stomach symptoms Nausea, vomiting, fatigue, loss of appetite, shortness of breath – all signs of lactic acidosis	Loss of appetite usually disappears after several weeks of treatment Does not cause hypoglycaemia	**Metformin:** Usually taken twice a day with breakfast and evening meal **Metformin extended release:** usually taken once a day in the morning
Thiazolidinediones Pioglitazone Rosiglitazone	More sensitivity to insulin activity Increases the amount of glucose taken up by muscle cells and keeps the liver from overproducing glucose	Type 2 diabetes	May cause oedema (fluid retention) Increased risk of congestive heart failure	Does not cause low blood sugar when used alone May improve blood fat levels	Usually taken once a day; take at the same time each day
Combination products Glibenclamide/metformin 1.25 mg/250 mg 2.5 mg/500 mg 5 mg/500 mg Rosiglitazone/metformin 2 mg/500 mg 4 mg/500 mg 2 mg/1000 mg 4 mg/1000 mg Sitagliptin/metformin Vildagliptin/metformin (50 mg/500 mg) (50 mg/850 mg) (50 mg/1000 mg)	Combinations taken when metformin alone is unable to control blood glucose levels Makes the body more sensitive to insulin activity and promoting insulin production in the pancreas	Type 2 diabetes	*Glibenclamide/metformin:* sweating, shaking, palpitations, confusion *Rosiglitazone/metformin:* rapid weight increase, shortness of breath *Sitagliptin/metformin:* nausea, vomiting, stomach upset, diarrhoea, constipation, headache, weakness, back pain, joint or muscle pain, a metallic taste in the mouth, or cold symptoms such as runny or stuffy nose, sneezing and sore throat *Vildagliptin/metformin:* skin irritation, joint pain, low blood glucose, diarrhoea	Regular monitoring of kidney and liver function Vitamin B12 monitoring every 2–3 years	Usually taken twice a day at the same time each day

Hypoglycaemia occurs when the blood glucose level drops below normal. It may occur when there is an imbalance between medication and food input or when there is insulin or glucose lowering medication overdose. It can also occur following a skipped meal and/or becoming involved in more physical activity. Signs and symptoms of hypoglycaemia include: sweating, shakiness, weakness, hunger, dizziness, headache, blurred vision, heart palpitations, slurred speech, drowsiness, confusion and seizures.

Type 1 diabetes mellitus

The type of drug intervention in diabetes is entirely dependent on the type of diabetes (see Table 8.4).

Type 1 DM is caused by a lack of insulin production when the beta-islet cells in the islets of Langerhans in the pancreas have ceased to function. The therapy for type 1 diabetes, therefore, is exogenous insulin replacement. There are three broad categories of insulin used in the treatment of type 1 DM: short-acting (including ultra-short acting), long-acting and ultra-long acting. Insulin is not orally absorbed intact, but is digested to its component amino acids and cannot be reconstructed to insulin due to beta-islet cell dysfunction. Therefore, insulin must currently be injected subcutaneously, although inhaled insulin dose forms are currently available in the USA (Davis 2008).

Many type 1 diabetics maintain appropriate glucose levels by using insulin pumps. These pumps only use short-acting insulin on a 'basal/bolus' regimen. A small basal dose of insulin is continuously infused (subcutaneously) with a bolus administered when the patient eats something, based on the carbohydrate content of the meal. Infusion pumps have been shown to be as effective as intensive multiple injection therapy, and require fewer injections during each day.

Type 2 diabetes mellitus

Type 2 DM is caused by insulin resistance, where the pancreas is still producing insulin, but that insulin is not sufficient for physiological needs and/or is not stimulating its receptors effectively. A range of drug classes with various mechanisms of action are used to combat this condition, and sometimes exogenous insulin is utilised.

Oral therapy is preferred for type 2 DM and there are multiple mechanisms used to target various aspects of glucose metabolism to:

*   increase insulin secretion (sulfonylureas, dipeptidyl peptidase-4 [DPP4] inhibitors, glucagon-like peptide-1 (GLP1) analogues)
*   increase insulin sensitivity (metformin, thiazolidinediones [glitazones])
*   decrease hepatic glucose output (metformin, glitazones)
*   reduce glucagon production (DPP4 inhibitors, GLP1 analogues)
*   delay gastric emptying (slow glucose absorption) (GLP1 analogues)
*   inhibit intestinal enzymes responsible for liberating glucose from food (acarbose)

+ inhibit renal tubule reabsorption of glucose (increase renal excretion) (dapaglifozin).

Oral medications are combined to gain control of blood glucose while minimising side effects for the patient and utilising different mechanisms of action (see Table 8.4).

Gestational diabetes

Gestational diabetes is treated with insulin as insulin does not cross the placenta and is therefore a better option in pregnancy (Simmons et al. 2007). (For further details refer to Chapter 4.)

■ Bone metabolism and calcium balance

Osteoporosis

Osteoporosis is the most common metabolic bone disorder and is most prevalent in post-menopausal women. It is reported that women over 50 years of age in developed countries have a greater than 40% chance of sustaining an osteoporotic fracture in their remaining lifetime and a 20% chance of sustaining a fractured hip. The mortality rate associated with sustaining a fractured hip is 20% (Howe et al. 2011). Osteoporosis, meaning 'porous bones', describes a state whereby bones lose an excessive amount of their protein and mineral content, particularly calcium. This ultimately results in a reduction in the density of bone tissue and hence leads to an increased risk of fracture. Osteopenia refers to bone density that is lower than normal peak density but not low enough to be classified as osteoporosis.

Pharmacological management for osteoporosis

Bone is in a dynamic state of resorption and formation. The medications used for osteoporosis aim to increase bone formation and/or slow bone resorption in order to change this balance and produce a net bone density gain. Drugs of various classes are utilised to treat osteoporosis and, while different classes can be indicated for different body areas (e.g. hip, spine etc.), they all fall into the following mechanistic categories (Table 8.5):

+ drugs that slow bone resorption (bisphosphonates, cinacalcet [reduces PTH secretion])
+ drugs that reduce osteoclast activity (denusomab, raloxifene, salcatonin)
+ drugs that increase bone formation (vitamin D, calcium, teriparatide)
+ drugs that slow bone resorption and increase bone formation (strontium).

Drug choice is usually based on co-morbidities, severity of osteoporosis and other patient-specific factors (Swaim, Barner & Brown 2008); see Table 8.5.

Osteoporosis and osteopenia occur in the older population and may also be associated with pain and polypharmacy issues. For further details on these topics please refer to the specific chapters: pain, refer to Chapter 7; polypharmacy, refer to Chapter 11.

TABLE 8.5 Common drugs used for osteoporosis/osteopenia

Drug group/name	Mechanism of action	Indications	Common side effects	Practice points	Common adult dosage range
Bisphosphonates Alendronate Ralendronate Etidronate Zolendronic acid (injected)	Bisphosphonates inhibit mineralisation or resorption of the bone Act as enzyme-resistant analogues of pyrophosphate, which normally inhibits mineralisation in the bone	Commonly used for the prevention and treatment of osteopenia and osteoporosis	Heartburn, irritation of the throat to the oesophagus Headache, constipation, diarrhoea and wind Muscle and joint pain	Bisphosphonates are not usually recommended for people with severe kidney disease Required to sit or stand for ½ hour after taking the medication and must be taken on an empty stomach at least ½ hour before any food or drinks are consumed (except water)	Effect is dose dependent and due to the reduction of the turnover of bone by inhibiting recruitment and promoting apoptosis of osteoclasts Usually given orally; can also be given IV 35 mg once a week (this is the dose approved for prevention; the official dose for treatment is 70 mg/week)
Denosumab Raloxifene	Denusomab assists with reducing bone resorption Raloxifene mimics some of the beneficial effects of oestrogen	For treatment of osteoporosis in postmenopausal women	*Denosumab:* skin rash *Raloxifene:* hot flushes, leg cramps, muscle spasms, swelling in hands, feet and legs or flu-like symptoms	*Denosumab:* injection every 6 months *Raloxifene:* may need to be taken in conjunction with supplementary calcium if daily calcium intake is inadequate	**Denosumab:** 60 mg every 6 months **Raloxifene:** 60 mg once a day

Continued

TABLE 8.5 Common drugs used for osteoporosis/osteopenia—cont'd

Drug group/name	Mechanism of action	Indications	Common side effects	Practice points	Common adult dosage range
Vitamin D Calcium Teriparatide	Increases bone formation	Treatment of post-menopausal women with osteoporosis at high risk for fracture. Increase of bone mass in men with primary or hypogonadal osteoporosis at high risk for fracture. Treatment of men and women with osteoporosis associated with sustained systemic glucocorticoid therapy at high risk for fracture		*Teriparatide:* applies to the following strength(s): 750 mcg/3 mL; 600 mcg/2.4 mL	**Teriparatide:** 20 mcg subcutaneously once a day into the thigh or abdominal wall
Strontium	Slows bone resorption and increases bone formation	Treatment of osteoporosis, to slow bone resorption and increase bone formation	Nausea, diarrhoea, headache and skin irritation. *Very rarely:* Blood clot, fever, swollen glands	Patients with a heart/circulatory condition should only take this medication if alternatives are not available. Should be taken on an empty stomach at least 2 hours after eating	2 g sachets for dilution in water

---

PHYSIOTHERAPY PRACTICE POINTS: OSTEOPOROSIS

Aerobic exercise, weight-bearing exercise and resistance training have been demonstrated to preserve bone mass and stimulate bone growth in patients with osteoporosis (Howe et al. 2011). Physiotherapists are therefore essential members of the treating team for patients with known osteoporosis (Baert et al. 2015; Giangregorio et al. 2015; He & Wang 2014; Schröder et al. 2014). The physiotherapist working in primary care may be the first clinician to note an increase in incidence of low impact fractures in a patient, and therefore the need for onward referral for further investigations/management.

Osteogenesis imperfecta

Osteogenesis imperfecta (OI) is a rare hereditary condition characterised by an increased fracture rate. In addition to their diagnosis of OI, these patients may have scoliosis, joint hypermobility and muscular hypotonia. OI is an autosomal dominant disease causing a defect in the gene that produces type 1 collagen (an important building block of bone). The bones in OI are therefore fragile and susceptible to fractures. There is no cure for OI although bisphosphonates are drugs valuable in the treatment of OI symptoms, particularly in children, due to their ability to increase the strength and density of the bone (Bartl et al. 2007; Harrington, Sochett & Howard 2014).

PHYSIOTHERAPY PRACTICE POINTS: OSTEOGENESIS IMPERFECTA

Along with medication management an essential component of treatment of OI is physiotherapy to improve strength and motor function and maximise bone density. Since patients with OI are often deconditioned and have poor muscle mass following prolonged periods of immobilisation during the management of fractures, physiotherapy treatment must be carefully graded. A treatment program may include resistance training and weight-bearing exercise (Hoyer-Kuhn et al. 2014).

Parathyroid disease

The parathyroid glands, situated on the thyroid gland in the neck (see Figure 8.1) produce parathyroid hormone (PTH), which maintains the calcium and phosphorus balance in the body. Excess PTH can cause hyperparathyroidism with an increase in blood calcium; hypoparathyroidism, where there is a decrease in PTH, produces a decrease in blood calcium and an increase in phosphorus.

Primary hyperparathyroidism (i.e. an increase in PTH) may be caused by enlarged parathyroid glands or radiation to the head and neck. Secondary hyperparathyroidism is usually due to medical conditions that cause low blood calcium levels or increased phosphate levels.

Symptoms of hyperparathyroidism include: bone pain or tenderness; depression and forgetfulness; feeling tired, ill and weak; fragile bones of the limbs and spine; increased amount of urine produced; and polyuria, kidney stones, nausea and loss of appetite (see Tables 8.1 and 8.2). There is no pharmacological treatment; surgery is recommended to remove the enlarged gland.

Hypoparathyroidism is a rare disorder in which the parathyroid glands in the neck do not produce enough PTH. The blood calcium level falls, and the phosphorus level rises. The most common cause of hypoparathyroidism is injury to the parathyroid glands during thyroid or neck surgery. It may also be caused by radioactive iodine treatment for hyperthyroidism, very low magnesium levels in the blood or an autoimmune attack on the parathyroid glands. Pharmacological replacement therapy is recommended; treatment with twice daily PTH provides a safe and effective alternative to calcitriol therapy and is able to maintain normal serum calcium levels (Sikjaer, Rejnmark & Mosekilde 2011; Winer et al. 2003).

PHYSIOTHERAPY PRACTICE POINTS: PARATHYROID DISEASE

Physiotherapists are not usually directly involved with these patients except in the event that this disease state exists as a co-morbidity with other more commonly treated conditions. When this is the case, care must be taken to grade activities and reduce the incidence of falls since fragile bones may easily lead to fractures.

Metabolic syndrome

Metabolic syndrome is a complex set of clinical signs associated with the metabolic system. The National Heart, Lung and Blood Institute and American Heart Association guidelines advise that a diagnosis of metabolic syndrome can be made when a patient has **three** of the following **five** conditions (Grundy et al. 2004, 2005):

1 fasting glucose $\geq$ 100 mg/dL (or receiving medication for hyperglycaemia)
2 blood pressure $\geq$ 130/85 mm Hg (or receiving medication for hypertension)
3 triglycerides $\geq$ 150 mg/dL (or receiving medication for hypertriglyceridaemia)
4 HDL-C < 40 mg/dL in men or < 50 mg/dL in women (or receiving medication for reduced HDL-C)
5 waist circumference $\geq$ 102 cm in men or $\geq$ 88 cm in women.

PHYSIOTHERAPY PRACTICE POINTS: METABOLIC SYNDROME

Metabolic syndrome has been linked to osteoarthritis and musculoskeletal pain (Yoo et al. 2014). Physiotherapists treating patients with musculoskeletal pain need to be aware of the possibility of metabolic syndrome as a co-morbidity (Cameron et al. 2007; Eckel et al. 2010).

Thyroid disorders

The thyroid, a small butterfly-shaped gland, is situated at the base of the neck (see Figure 8.1) and produces the thyroid hormones. Imbalance in the production of thyroid hormones may arise from dysfunction of the thyroid gland itself, of the pituitary gland, which produces thyroid-stimulating hormone (TSH), or of the hypothalamus, which regulates the pituitary gland via thyrotropin-releasing hormone (TRH). Impairment might be due to hyperthyroidism and hypothyroidism (primarily or secondary). The thyroid gland manufactures hormones that regulate the body's metabolism.

TABLE 8.6 Common signs and symptoms of thyroid disease	
Hypothyroidism	Hyperthyroidism
Fatigue	Tremor
Poor concentration	Nervousness
Dry skin	Fast heart rate
Constipation	Fatigue
Feeling cold	Intolerance for heat
Fluid retention	Increase in bowel movements
Muscle and joint aches	Increased sweating
Depression	Concentration problems
Prolonged or excessive menstrual bleeding	Unintentional weight loss

The common thyroid disorders include Hashimoto's disease, Graves' disease, goitre and thyroid nodules (see Table 8.6).

Hashimoto's disease

Hashimoto's disease is a chronic lymphatic thyroiditis resulting in hypothyroidism. The body's immune system mistakenly attacks and slowly destroys the thyroid gland and its ability to produce hormones. Symptoms of hypothyroidism include: fatigue, depression, constipation, mild weight gain, dry skin and heavy/irregular menstruation.

There is no cure for Hashimoto's disease; treatment is designed to reduce symptoms by giving hormone-replacing medication that raises thyroid hormone levels or lowers TSH levels (Bahn et al. 2011).

Graves' disease

Graves' disease is an autoimmune disorder that results in the hypersecretion of thyroxine. It is the most common cause of hyperthyroidism (Scanlon & Sanders 2010). Symptoms of hyperthyroidism (high level of thyroid hormone) include: weight loss, anxiety, irritability, fatigue, hand tremors, increased or irregular heart rate, excessive sweating, difficulty sleeping, diarrhoea, altered menstrual cycle, bulging eyes and vision problems (Burch, Burman & Cooper 2012).

Since there is no treatment to stop the immune system from attacking the thyroid gland and causing it to overproduce hormones, the focus of the treatment is mainly to reduce symptoms. Beta blockers are prescribed to control rapid heart rate, anxiety and sweating. Treatments to reduce the effect of the hormone (such as anti-thyroid medications to prevent the thyroid from producing excessive amounts of hormone) are available. Other treatments include radioactive iodine to destroy all or part of the thyroid and/or surgery to remove the thyroid gland. Occasionally, the treatment for hyperthyroidism induces hypothyroidism.

Goitre

Goitre is a non-cancerous enlargement of the thyroid gland. The most frequent cause of goitre is iodine deficiency in the diet. Occasionally, goitre induces hyperthyroidism.

Thyroid nodules

Thyroid nodules may develop due to iodine deficiency and Hashimoto's disease. Most are benign, but more rarely they may become cancerous. Most thyroid nodules do not cause any symptoms.

Pharmacological management for thyroid disorders

Hypothyroidism

The synthetic thyroid hormone thyroxine is an oral medication that restores adequate hormone levels, reversing the signs and symptoms of hypothyroidism. Treatment with thyroxine is usually lifelong, although the dosage may alter. Dose adjustments should be made upon significant changes in body weight, with ageing and with pregnancy; thyroid-stimulating hormone (TSH) assessment should be performed 4–6 weeks after any dosage change.

Hyperthyroidism

The goal of the therapy is to reduce the free hormone level in the blood and to decrease the pathological symptoms. There several ways to achieve this aim:

- Radioactive iodine is taken orally. It is absorbed by the thyroid gland, and causes the gland to shrink and as such reduces hormone production. Occasionally, it may lead to hypothyroidism, requiring replacement therapy with thyroxine.
- Anti-thyroid medications include propylthiouracil and carbimazole.
- Symptoms usually begin to improve in 6–12 weeks, but treatment with anti-thyroid medications typically continues for at least a year and often longer. These drugs can cause serious liver damage, sometimes leading to death.
- Beta blockers are used to treat high blood pressure and reduce a rapid heart rate and palpitations. Side effects may include fatigue, headache, upset stomach, constipation, diarrhoea or dizziness.

PHYSIOTHERAPY PRACTICE POINTS: THYROID DISORDERS

Due to the high prevalence of thyroid disorders many patients will present with a thyroid disorder as a co-morbidity. Physiotherapists therefore need to be aware of the clinical presentation and medication management of these conditions and the potential physical impact the signs and symptoms might have on physiotherapy treatment (see Table 8.6).

■ Adrenal disorders

The adrenal glands are small glands located on top of each kidney (see Figure 8.1). They produce hormones including the sex hormones and cortisol. Cortisol helps the body to respond to stress and has other important functions. Adrenal gland disorders may cause hyperfunction or hypofunction, and may be congenital or acquired (see Tables 8.1 and 8.2). The hormones, including the glucocorticoids (e.g. cortisol), mineralocorticoids (e.g. aldosterone), catecholamines (e.g. adrenaline) and adrenal androgens (e.g. dehydroepiandrosterone), regulate several fundamental aspects of human physiology via secretion. Specifically, glucocorticoids help regulate blood sugar, blood pressure, fat and protein metabolism and immunity; mineralocorticoids help regulate kidney and cardiovascular function (maintenance of salt and water balance within the body); catecholamines help regulate the 'fight or flight' response to stress; and adrenal androgens are precursors to sex hormones such as testosterone and oestrogen.

Disordered adrenal function can lead to a barrage of significant complications, including diabetes, high blood pressure, prolonged fatigue and depression. Addison's disease and Cushing's syndrome are two major adrenal gland disorders (Gorman 2013) (see Table 8.7).

Primary adrenal insufficiency (Addison's disease)

Addison's disease occurs when the cortex of the adrenal gland is damaged and does not produce its hormones in adequate quantities. When the origin of adrenal insufficiency is due to an impairment located initially at the adrenal glands, it is termed primary adrenal insufficiency. The most common aetiology is an autoimmune disease that attacks and destroys the adrenal cortex. Other causes of adrenal gland failure might be: tuberculosis, infections of the adrenal glands, spread of cancer to the adrenal glands or bleeding into the adrenal glands that can induce sudden adrenal failure. In Addison's disease, the function of the adrenal cortex progressively declines over time, resulting in glucocorticoid and mineralocorticoid deficiency, as well as reduced levels of dehydroepiandrosterone (DHEA) and androgens (Falorni, Minarelli & Morelli 2013; Johannsson et al. 2015; Puttanna, Cunningham & Dainty 2013).

TABLE 8.7 Common signs and symptoms of adrenal disease

Cushing's disease	Addison's disease
Upper body obesity, round face and neck and thinning arms and legs	Weight loss
Skin problems, such as acne or reddish-blue streaks on the abdomen or underarm area	Weakness
High blood pressure	Extreme fatigue
Muscle and bone weakness	Nausea and/or vomiting
Moodiness, irritability or depression	Low blood pressure
High blood sugar	Patches of darker skin
Slow growth rates in children	Craving for salt
	Dizziness upon standing
	Depression

Secondary adrenal insufficiency

The term secondary adrenal insufficiency is used when the adrenal glands fail to function as a result of pituitary gland impairment (through insufficiency of adrenocorticotropic hormone [ACTH]). Another situation that induces secondary adrenal insufficiency is reduction in the production of the hormone due to long-term corticosteroid treatment.

Adrenal hyperfunction (Cushing's syndrome)

When the blood levels of cortisol are elevated for a prolonged time, Cushing's syndrome may develop. Characteristic signs of this syndrome are the development of a rounded 'moon' face as well as weight gain, especially around the trunk, arms and legs. The skins stretches, bruises appear, hirsutism (abnormal hair growth) develops and muscles become weak. In addition, hyperglycaemia and osteoporosis may develop. Individuals with Cushing's syndrome may also suffer from mood disorders such as anxiety and depression. In children, excess cortisol can lead to stunted growth.

The adrenal glands may also produce high blood levels of cortisol due to excess secretion of ACTH from the pituitary gland. A common cause for this syndrome is a pituitary gland tumour. Increased cortisol levels might also be due to ACTH secretion from ectopic tumours. Over-treatment with glucocorticoid medications is the most common cause of Cushing's syndrome (Lacroix et al. 2015).

Pharmacological management for adrenal diseases

Addison's disease

Addison's disease is treated by replacing the deficient hormones. Hydrocortisone, which is a synthetic glucocorticoid, is one of the most common cortisol replacement therapies. In acute illnesses, such as an adrenal crisis, intravenous hydrocortisone and saline should be administered immediately to prevent potentially life-threatening complications. Since cortisol levels are highest in the mornings and lowest in the evenings it is difficult to administer an optimal dosing regimen that mimics the natural circadian rhythm; hence there is risk of over-treatment, which can lead to hypertension. Aldosterone and fludrocortisone can also be orally administered.

Cushing's syndrome

Cushing's syndrome is treated by administration of drugs that prevent steroid production or that suppress the release of ACTH from pituitary or ectopic tumours. Mifepristone was approved by the US Food and Drug Administration (FDA) in 2012 for the treatment of high blood sugar in people with Cushing's syndrome. The antifungal drug ketoconazole inhibits several steps in steroid synthesis within the adrenal cortex and may directly inhibit ACTH secretion from the pituitary gland. However, prolonged treatment with ketoconazole might induce adrenal crisis. Mitotane is used to treat patients with tumours of the adrenal cortex. The action of mitotane is to prevent the production of steroids by interfering with enzymes involved in the conversion of cholesterol to various other steroid hormones.

PHYSIOTHERAPY PRACTICE POINTS: ADRENAL DISORDERS

Physiotherapists are often involved with patients receiving long-term corticosteroid treatment, such as clients with multiple sclerosis, and therefore it is important they are aware of this possible complication, in addition to the problem of osteoporosis caused by long-term corticosteroid treatment. Other drugs that inhibit the synthesis of steroids in the adrenal cortex (e.g. the antifungal drug ketoconazole) can also impair adrenal hormone production.

Pituitary gland syndromes

The pituitary gland is a pea-sized gland situated at the base of the brain (see Figure 8.1). The pituitary gland produces hormones that affect the growth and functions of all the other glands in the body (see Tables 8.1 and 8.2). Pituitary disorders include: acromegaly, growth hormone deficiency and inappropriate ADH secretion/diabetes insipidus (also known as syndrome of inappropriate ADH secretion [SIADH]).

Pineal gland disorders

The pineal gland is a small organ in the brain (see Figure 8.1) that produces melatonin (a sleep-regulating hormone) (see Table 8.1). For a more detailed discussion of sleep disorders, see Chapter 10.

Disorders of the pineal gland are generally manifested by abnormal secretion of melatonin. This may occur when a person is exposed to excess light during the night or not enough light during the day. A pineal gland disorder may also result from jet lag or changes in time zones. People who are working in shifts may suffer from disorders of the pineal gland as well because of disturbed circadian rhythm. Poor vision disrupts the melatonin cycle as well, and in blind people circadian rhythm is often imbalanced because of lack of feedback concerning the beginning of the day and beginning of the night. Pineal gland disorders may occur due to deficiency or excess production of melatonin (Macchi & Bruce 2004).

In the case of melatonin deficiency, insomnia may occur. In addition, the affected person may suffer from increased anxiety and a disturbance of their immune system. Increased levels of the oestrogen/progesterone ratio as well as decreased basal temperature may also be caused by melatonin deficiency. Overproduction of melatonin is another manifestation of pineal gland disorders and is associated with seasonal affective disorder (SAD), lowered oestrogen/progesterone ratio, low thyroid and adrenal function and hypotension. Apart from abnormal production of melatonin, the pineal gland may be affected by tumours such as gliomas, germ cell tumours and pineal cell tumours. Symptoms of these tumours include headaches, seizures, nausea, vomiting, disturbed memory and visual problems.

Pharmacological management for pineal gland disorders

Melatonin is available in Australia in two forms – over the counter (OTC) and prescription only. The prescribed form is more effective as the OTC products are homeopathic and therefore extremely dilute. According to the principles of homeopathy, the extreme dilution should enhance wakefulness, rather than causing sleep. Melatonin may be used to treat insomnia such as in patients with post-traumatic brain injury.

PHYSIOTHERAPY PRACTICE POINTS: PINEAL GLAND DISORDERS

Although not directly involved in the treatment of patients with pineal gland disorders, as indicated these complications may arise as an indirect result of other conditions. Therefore, the treating physiotherapist may be the first allied health professional who observes these signs and, as such, must be aware of such possible complications.

Table 8.8 contains an overview of drugs commonly used to treat disorders of the thyroid, adrenal, pituitary and pineal glands.

TABLE 8.8 Overview of common drugs used in other endocrine disorders

Gland	Common drugs used
Thyroid disorders	*Hypo:* synthetic thyroid hormone levothyroxine *Hyper:* radioactive iodine
Adrenal disorders	*Hypo:* hydrocortisone *Hyper:* drugs that prevent steroid production or that suppress the release of ACTH from pituitary or ectopic tumours (e.g. mifepristone, ketoconazole, mitotane)
Pituitary disorders	Specific hormone replacement therapy as required
Pineal gland disorders	Melatonin

ACTH, adrenocorticotropin hormone.

References

Alberti, K.G.M.M., Zimmet, P., Shaw, J., 2007. International Diabetes Federation: a consensus on type 2 diabetes prevention. Diabetic Medicine 24 (5), 451–463.

Australian Medicines Handbook Pty Ltd, 2016. *Australian Medicines Handbook* (online). Australian Medicines Handbook Pty Ltd, Adelaide. [Internet] <https://amhonlineamhnetau.ezp01.library.qut.edu.au> (accessed 24.03.16.).

Baert, V., Gorus, E., Mets, T., et al., 2015. Motivators and barriers for physical activity in older adults with osteoporosis. Journal of Geriatric Physical Therapy 38 (3), 105–114.

Bahn, R.S., Burch, H.B., Cooper, D.S., et al., 2011. Hyperthyroidism and other causes of thyrotoxicosis: management guidelines of the American Thyroid Association and American Association of Clinical Endocrinologists. Endocrine Practice 17 (3), 456–520.

Barr, E.L.M., Zimmet, P.Z., Welborn, T.A., et al., 2007. Risk of cardiovascular and all-cause mortality in individuals with diabetes mellitus, impaired fasting glucose, and impaired glucose tolerance: The Australian Diabetes, Obesity, and Lifestyle Study (AusDiab). Circulation 116 (2), 151–157.

Bartl, R., Frisch, B., von Tresckow, E., et al., 2007. Osteogenesis Imperfecta (OI). In: Bisphosphonates in Medical Practice. Springer, Berlin, pp. 117–120.

Burch, H.B., Burman, K.D., Cooper, D.S., 2012. A 2011 survey of clinical practice patterns in the 'management of Graves' disease. Journal of Clinical Endocrinology & Metabolism 97 (12), 4549–4558.

Cameron, A.J., Magliano, D.J., Zimmet, P.Z., et al., 2007. The metabolic syndrome in Australia: prevalence using four definitions. Diabetes Research and Clinical Practice 77 (3), 471–478.

Davis, S.N., 2008. The role of inhaled insulin in the treatment of type 2 diabetes. Journal of Diabetes and its Complications 22 (6), 420–429.

Dietrich, J.W., Landgrafe, G., Fotiadou, E.H., 2012. TSH and thyrotropic agonists: key actors in thyroid homeostasis. Journal of Thyroid Research 2012, 351864.

Eckel, R.H., Alberti, K.G.M.M., Grundy, S.M., et al., 2010. The metabolic syndrome. Lancet 375 (9710), 181–183.

Falorni, A., Minarelli, V., Morelli, S., 2013. Therapy of adrenal insufficiency: an update. Endocrine 43 (3), 514–528.

Fekete, C., Lechan, R.M., 2014. Central regulation of hypothalamic–pituitary–thyroid axis under physiological and pathophysiological conditions. Endocrine Reviews 35 (2), 159–194.

Giangregorio, L.M., McGill, S., Wark, J.D., et al., 2015. Too fit to fracture: outcomes of a Delphi consensus process on physical activity and exercise recommendations for adults with osteoporosis with or without vertebral fractures. Osteoporosis International 26 (3), 891–910.

Gorman, L.S., 2013. The adrenal gland: common disease states and suspected new applications. Clinical Laboratory Science 26 (2), 118–125.

Greenstein, B., Wood, D., 2011. The Endocrine System at a Glance, third ed. Wiley-Blackwell, Chichester.

Grundy, S.M., Brewer, H.B., Cleeman, J.I., et al., 2004. Definition of metabolic syndrome: report of the National Heart, Lung, and Blood Institute/American Heart Association Conference on scientific issues related to definition. Circulation 109 (3), 433–438.

Grundy, S.M., Cleeman, J.I., Daniels, S.R., et al., 2005. Diagnosis and management of the metabolic syndrome: an American Heart Association/National Heart, Lung, and Blood Institute scientific statement. Circulation 112 (17), 2735–2752.

Harrington, J., Sochett, E., Howard, A., 2014. Update on the evaluation and treatment of osteogenesis imperfecta. Pediatric Clinics of North America 61 (6), 1243–1257.

He, C.Q., Wang, P., 2014. Arguments and debates about physical therapies for osteoporosis and osteoarthritis. Journal of Sichuan University (Medical Science Edition) 45 (1), 102–106.

Houshyar, J., Bahrami, A., Aliasgarzadeh, A., 2015. Effectiveness of insulin glargine on recovery of patients with diabetic ketoacidosis: a randomized controlled trial. Journal of Clinical and Diagnostic Research 9 (5), OC1–OC5. doi:10.7860/JCDR/2015/12005.5883.

Howe, T.E., Shea, B., Dawson, L.J., et al., 2011. Exercise for preventing and treating osteoporosis in postmenopausal women. Cochrane Database of Systematic Reviews (7), CD000333, doi:10.1002/14651858.CD000333.pub2.

Hoyer-Kuhn, H., Semler, O., Stark, C., et al., 2014. A specialized rehabilitation approach improves mobility in children with osteogenesis imperfecta. Journal of Musculoskeletal and Neuronal Interactions 14 (4), 445–453.

Johannsson, G., Falorni, A., Skrtic, S., et al., 2015. Adrenal insufficiency: review of clinical outcomes with current glucocorticoid replacement therapy. Clinical Endocrinology 82 (1), 2–11.

Lacroix, A., Feelders, R.A., Stratakis, C.A., et al., 2015. Cushing's syndrome. Lancet 386 (9996), 913–927.

Li, W., Liu, Y., Lu, X., et al., 2015. A cross-sectional study of breath acetone based on diabetic metabolic disorders. Journal of Breath Research 9 (1), 016005. doi:10.1088/1752-7155/9/1/016005.

Macchi, M.M., Bruce, J.N., 2004. Human pineal physiology and functional significance of melatonin. Frontiers of Neuroendocrinology 25 (3–4), 177–195.

McEwen, B.S., 2000. Allostasis and allostatic load: implications for neuropsychopharmacology. Neuropsychopharmacology 22 (2), 108–124.

McEwen, B.S., Wingfield, J.C., 2010. What is in a name? Integrating homeostasis, allostasis and stress. Hormones and Behavior 57 (2), 105–111.

Puttanna, A., Cunningham, A.R., Dainty, P., 2013. Addison's disease and its associations. BMJ Case Reports doi:10.1136/bcr-2013-010473.

Scanlon, V.C., Sanders, T., 2010. Essentials of Anatomy and Physiology, sixth ed. F.A. Davis, Philadelphia.

Schröder, G., Knauerhase, A., Kundt, G., et al., 2014. New aspects of physical therapy for osteoporosis: a randomized clinical trial. Osteologie 23 (2), 123–132.

Sikjaer, T., Rejnmark, L., Mosekilde, L., 2011. PTH treatment in hypoparathyroidism. Current Drug Safety 6 (2), 89–99.

Simmons, D., Eaton, S., Shaw, J., et al., 2007. Self-reported past gestational diabetes mellitus as a risk factor for abnormal glucose tolerance among Australian women. Diabetes Care 30 (9), 2293–2295.

Swaim, R.A., Barner, J.C., Brown, C.M., 2008. The relationship of calcium intake and exercise to osteoporosis health beliefs in postmenopausal women. Research in Social and Administrative Pharmacy 4 (2), 153–163.

Taylor, J.D., Fletcher, J.P., Mathis, R.A., et al., 2014. Effects of moderate versus high-intensity exercise training on physical fitness and physical function in people with type 2 diabetes: a randomized clinical trial. Physical Therapy 94 (12), 1720–1730.

Taylor, J.D., Fletcher, J.P., Tiarks, J., 2009. Impact of physical therapist-directed exercise counseling combined with fitness center-based exercise training on muscular strength and exercise capacity in people with type 2 diabetes: a randomized clinical trial. Physical Therapy 89 (9), 884–892.

Winer, K.K., Ko, C.W., Reynolds, J.C., et al., 2003. Long-term treatment of hypoparathyroidism: a randomized controlled study comparing parathyroid hormone-(1–34) versus calcitriol and calcium. The Journal of Clinical Endocrinology & Metabolism 88 (9), 4214–4220.

Yoo, J.J., Cho, N.H., Lim, S.H., et al., 2014. Relationships between body mass index, fat mass, muscle mass, and musculoskeletal pain in community residents. Arthritis & Rheumatology 66 (12), 3511–3520.

Haematological system

Anthony Hall, Jacqueline Reznik, Ofer Keren, Iftah Biran

OBJECTIVES

This chapter will discuss the role that medications have in the supplementary management of the most common haematological disorders encountered (treated) by physiotherapists. By the end of this chapter (including cross-referencing with other relevant chapters) the reader should have an understanding of:

♦ the major classification of haematological disorders according to structure, location, signs and symptoms

♦ pharmacotherapy options for the major haematological disorders

♦ routes of administration and major contraindications and precautions of some of the medications used in haematological disorders

♦ any potential impact of these medications on physiotherapeutic management.

■ Introduction

The haematological system can be divided into cells that are seen within the circulating blood and also their precursors found within the bone marrow (Figure 9.1).

The pluripotent stem cell is responsible for initial differentiation into lymphoid or myeloid precursor cells before differentiation into the lineal blast cells, which is followed by the progress of mature cells into the peripheral blood. In normal healthy individuals immature cells are not seen within the peripheral blood (below the dotted line in Figure 9.1) although with increased stress, for example during an infection, the more mature precursors may appear (e.g. neutrophil 'band' or 'stab' cells secondary to infection).

The haematological system can be described in terms of:

♦ red blood cells or erythrocytes and their precursors
♦ white blood cells or leukocytes and their precursors divided into:

  ● myelocyctes

    ▪ neutrophils

    ▪ basophils

    ▪ eosinophils

  ● lymphocytes and functional derivatives

    ▪ B cells

    ▪ T cells

  ● platelets and their precursor cells

  ● aqueous and protein elements of blood – clotting factors, immunoglobulins, complement etc.

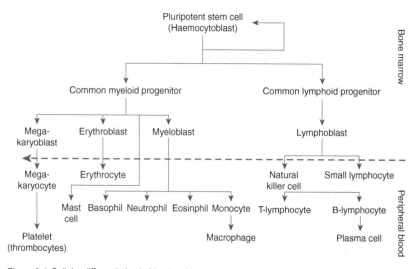

Figure 9.1 Cellular differentiation in blood and bone marrow.

Haematological disorders usually occur following:

- over- or under-production of the various components of the haematological system
- mal-production such as in thalassaemia and leukaemia

or

- secondary to the effects of hormones and other control mechanisms on these systems.

Red blood cell disorders

Abnormal erythrocytes (genetic or acquired)

Haemoglobinopathies

Transport of oxygen from the lungs to the tissues is ensured by the function of the highly specialised haemoglobin molecule (Hb), which is contained within the red blood cells. The normal function and total amount of Hb depend upon its adequate synthesis and precise structure (Figure 9.2). If these conditions are not met and the erythrocytes carry either a decreased amount of Hb or an Hb variant that may present with abnormal properties, a group of conditions collectively termed the haemoglobinopathies may present (Kohne 2011).

Haemoglobin is a specialised protein that can exist in two forms: oxyhaemoglobin and deoxyhaemoglobin. The oxygenated form is the molecule that carries oxygen around the body. Each red blood cell contains ~640 million molecules of haemoglobin. Haemoglobin A, the form most commonly found in

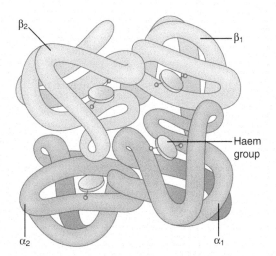

Figure 9.2 A haemoglobin molecule is made up of two alpha and two beta globin chains and four haem groups.
Reproduced with permission from: Provan, D., Newland, A., Syndercombe Court, D., 2015. Haematology. In: Naish, J., Syndercombe Court D. (Ed.), Medical Sciences, second ed., Elsevier Saunders, pp. 567-611, Fig. 12.7.

adults, is made up of four polypeptide chains, two α chains and two β chains $(\alpha_2\beta_2)$. Small amounts of haemoglobin A2, which contains two α chains and two δ chains, are also found in adults, whereas foetal haemoglobin (haemoglobin F) contains a pair of α chains and two γ chains. A switch from the production of haemoglobin F to haemoglobin A usually occurs at 3–6 months after birth. Approximately 65% of the synthesis of haemoglobin occurs in the erythroblast and 35% in the reticulocyte stages of red blood cell maturation. Synthesis occurs in the mitochondria under the control of a key rate-limiting enzyme, α-aminolaevulinic acid (ALA) synthetase. Vitamin B6 (pyridoxal phosphate) is a coenzyme to this reaction that is stimulated by erythropoietin. Ultimately, protoporphyrin combines iron in the ferrous state to form haem, which then combines with a tetramer of four globin chains for each haem molecule.

Methaemoglobulinaemia

This is a clinical condition where the circulating haemoglobin is present with iron in the oxidised ferric state. This may occur because of either a hereditary deficiency of nicotinamide-adenine dinucleotide (NADH) diaphorase or the inheritance of the structurally abnormal haemoglobin M. In this condition the patient will display cyanosis since they are unable to carry sufficient oxygen to the tissues of the body.

Pharmacological management

Treatment of methaemoglobulinaemia involves the administration of oxygen and the dye methylene blue, which restores the iron to its normal reduced, or ferrous, state.

Some drugs that can cause methaemoglobulinaemia include: trimethoprim, sulfonamides and sulfones; local anaesthetics such as prilocaine; and medications such as metoclopramide.

Thalassaemia

This includes a heterogeneous group of genetic disorders that result in a reduction in the synthesis of the α and β polypeptide chains, which in turn results in anaemia. People with a thalassaemia trait in one gene are known as carriers or are said to have thalassaemia minor. Clinically, the condition can be divided into: hydrops fetalis; β-thalassaemia, which is often transfusion dependent; thalassaemia intermedia; and thalassaemia minor, which is often an asymptomatic carrier condition.

α-Thalassaemias are usually caused by gene deletions. As an individual normally inherits the genes for four α-polypeptide chains, the deletion of all four genes is necessary to completely suppress α chain synthesis, as in hydrops foetalis. The α-chain is essential for the normal function of foetal haemoglobin, so this failure leads to foetal death in utero. Three α-chain gene deletions leads to haemoglobin H disease with moderately severe microcytic, hypochromic anaemia and splenomegaly. Two α-chain gene deletions is termed thalassaemia intermedia, and a single α-chain gene deletion is termed thalassaemia trait. The α-thalassemia trait is usually not associated with anaemia.

β-Thalassaemia major is also known as Mediterranean anaemia. Excess α-chains precipitate in erythroblasts and mature red cells, causing severe ineffective erythropoiesis and haemolysis. The greater the α chain excess, the greater the anaemia. Production of γ-chains helps to 'mop up' excess α-chains and ameliorate the condition (Yu et al. 2016).

Thalassaemia may be found in a particular genetic distribution as shown in Figure 9.3.

The impact of immigration has made this disease important in the Australian setting.

Pharmacological management

The treatment of patients exhibiting anaemia caused by thalassaemia requires frequent blood transfusions, which may then lead to iron overload (see the section below, 'Haemochromatosis').

Sickle cell disease

Another variant on the haemoglobin molecule is haemoglobin S ($\alpha_2^{A}\beta_2^{S}$ haemoglobin). Haemoglobin S is insoluble and forms crystals when in a low oxygen tension environment. Deoxygenated sickle haemoglobin polymerises into long chains and causes the erythrocyte molecule to deform into a 'sickle' shape, hence the name of this condition. Sickle erythrocytes can cause occlusion of microcirculation, do not carry oxygen and may cause infarction of organs involved. Clinical features of a sickle cell crisis, when this occurs, may be a severe haemolytic anaemia with painful vasculature-occlusive events. These crises arise when patients experience changes in oxygen tension such as accompany infections, changes in blood pH (acidosis) and dehydration or deoxygenation (altitude, operations, exposure to cold, violent exercise etc). Infarcts can occur in a variety of body tissues including bone (hips, shoulders and vertebrae), lungs and spleen.

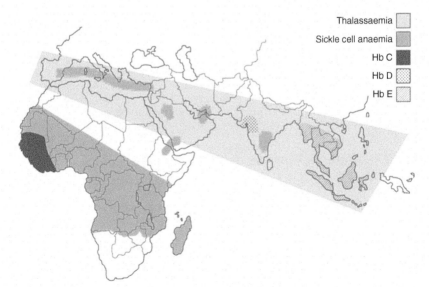

Figure 9.3 Geographical distribution of haemoglobinopathies.
Adapted with permission from: Hoffbrand A.V., Pettit J.E., 1993. Essential Haematology, third ed. Blackwell Scientific, Oxford, Fig. 26-3.

The geographical distribution of sickle cell anaemia (HbS) is shown in Figure 9.3.

Pharmacological management

Treatment of sickle cell crises is mainly preventative although supplementation with folic acid and good general nutritional and hygiene support may reduce episodes. Patients commonly develop functional asplenia[1] and are prone to infections, especially from organisms with capsules such as *Pneumococcus* bacteria.

Prophylactic oral penicillin and pneumococcal vaccination are common interventions in such patients.

Haemoglobin C and haemoglobin E diseases

Two other haemoglobinopathies, involving haemoglobin C (HbC) and haemoglobin E (HbE), are worthy of mention. HbC is a genetic defect of haemoglobin, found frequently in West Africa, involving the substitution of lysine for glutamic acid in the β-globin chain. Patients with HbC present with signs and symptoms similar to those with sickle cell disease.

HbE is the commonest haemoglobin variant seen in South East Asia and the homozygous state only presents as very mild microcytic anaemia.

It is of interest to note that there is evidence that individuals with α-thalassaemia, HbC and HbE have some protection against the malaria parasite.

PHYSIOTHERAPY PRACTICE POINTS: HAEMOGLOBINOPATHIES

The signs and symptoms of the haemoglobinopathies are vague pain, jaundice, enlarged spleen, mild-to-moderate anaemia and some haemorrhaging. Paediatric physiotherapists may see some of the genetic forms and should be aware of the possible signs and symptoms in order to prevent confusion with other conditions.

The treating physiotherapist must also be aware and concerned with fatigue in this patient group, as it might be related to bleeding (i.e. gastrointestinal tract bleeding) or anaemia. Whenever fatigue is encountered, physiotherapists should try to assess whether it is within their clinical expectations of the patient or whether it is exaggerated and might be related to the above-mentioned conditions.

Anaemia/reduced number of erythrocytes

Anaemia is not a disease in itself but a symptom/disorder related to another disease process.

Anaemia is usually either associated with the underproduction of red blood cells, due to their loss from the peripheral blood (secondary to bleeding), or secondary to the lack of various nutrients required for their normal development or an increase in red blood cell destruction (haemolysis).

---

[1]Asplenia refers to the absence of normal spleen function and is associated with some serious infection risks.

Pharmacological management

Differentiation of the red blood cell is controlled by the glycoprotein hormone erythropoietin. This hormone is produced by interstitial fibroblasts in the peritubular capillary cells of the kidney and hepatic perisinusoidal cells in response to changes in oxygenation. As oxygenation of these tissues drops they secrete erythropoietin to stimulate erythrocyte production. Erythropoietin, in cooperation with various other growth factors (e.g. IL-3, IL-6), glucocorticoids and stem cell factor (SCF), stimulates the activity of erythrocyte colony-forming units and increases the production of erythrocytes.

If renal function begins to diminish there can be a failure in the production of red blood cells and the patient may experience anaemia of chronic kidney disease. Patients experiencing this problem may be given injections of recombinant erythropoietin to stimulate red blood cell production and reverse this anaemia.

Erythropoietin may also be used to stimulate red blood cell proliferation where bone marrow failure occurs, such as myelodysplasia, and where anaemia may occur subsequent to the bone marrow suppression often experienced during the treatment of cancer.

Macrocytic anaemia

The two important nutritional elements that are necessary for the proper formation of haemoglobin are folic acid and vitamin B12. Deficiencies in either can result in inhibition of the differentiation of the erythrocyte and the production of enlarged erythroid macrocytes (mean corpuscular volume [MCV] >100). Identification of the deficient nutrient and its appropriate supplementation should correct the condition.

Pharmacological management

Folic acid supplementation of 5 mg is given daily for 3–6 months with potential maintenance.

Vitamin B12 requires the presence of gastric intrinsic factor (GIF) in gastric fluid for normal gut absorption. An antibody may form against GIF leading to chronic vitamin B12 deficiency or pernicious anaemia. Vitamin B12 supplementation is normally given by the parenteral route (i.e. as an injection or infusion) to avoid this.

Vitamin B12 (hydroxocobalamin) 1 mg is administered intramuscularly (IM) daily for 3 days, weekly for 3 weeks, monthly for 3 months and then every 3 months.

Iron deficiency

Ferrous iron is necessary for the creation of the 'haem' elements of haemoglobin. Chronic iron deficiency in the diet or chronic loss of iron from body stores can lead to microcytic anaemia in which the red blood cell becomes smaller because of the deficiency in its haemoglobin content. Identification of the cause of the deficiency and its appropriate management, followed by increased supplementation, may lead to correction of this form of anaemia (see Tables 9.1 and 9.2).

At risk groups for iron deficiency include:

+ infants and young children – particularly premature and low birth weight babies
+ teens – if underweight or have chronic illness; teenage girls with heavy menstruation
+ women – of child-bearing age due to menstruation; pregnant women
+ adults – if internal bleeding (e.g. intestinal bleeding) is present
+ patients receiving kidney dialysis treatment
+ patients post gastric bypass surgery
+ people with certain eating patterns or habits (e.g. diets that exclude fish and meat; low-fat diet over a prolonged period; high-fibre diet).

Pharmacological management

Iron absorption through the gastrointestinal tract (GIT) is limited to about 1–2 mg/day, sufficient to balance the normal loss of iron through the GIT of ~1 mg/day. Oral absorption can be enhanced slightly by maintaining the iron as a reduced ferrous ion rather than ferric ion. This can be achieved by coadministration with ascorbic acid, but this also enhances the adverse effects of oral administration.

Iron deficiency anaemia presents as a microcytic anaemia (MCV <80 and mean corpuscular haemoglobin [MCH] reduced).

Using ferrous sulfate, approximately 100 mg of elemental iron are required.

Consider parenteral iron (intramuscular or intravenous) only where patients do not respond to oral supplementation or oral therapy is inappropriate. All parenteral forms carry with them the risk of anaphylactic reactions. Intramuscular injections are painful and may stain the skin and are not considered to be any safer than IV iron. Intravenous iron is often preferred in patients with chronic kidney disease (CKD) (Table 9.1).

PHYSIOTHERAPY PRACTICE POINTS: ANAEMIA

The most common symptom of anaemia is fatigue; other signs and symptoms include shortness of breath, dizziness, headache, coldness of hands and feet, pale skin and chest pain. All physiotherapists should be aware of these signs and symptoms and the possibility of their patient being anaemic. If anaemia is suspected, the relevant tests will reveal the possible underlying cause and the correct treatment may then be implemented. Patients with fatigue may have difficulty in becoming active with a rapid tachycardia response (Table 9.2).

Haemochromatosis

Haemochromatosis (too much iron) is a relatively common genetic disorder affecting about 1 in 200 Australians of European origin and involving the HFE gene. Symptoms generally occur after the age of 40 and may include fatigue, abdominal pain and joint aches, although iron overload may produce no symptoms but still be causing organ damage. The organs most commonly affected include the liver, heart, pancreas, joints and sex organs. Treatment commonly involves bloodletting, the removal of one to two units of blood in a manner similar to a blood donation.

TABLE 9.1 Common drugs used in iron deficiency disorders

Iron salt	Formulation	Elemental iron content	Common adult, child dosage range
Oral iron			
Ferrous sulfate	200 mg tablets	35 mg	1 tablet tds
Ferrous sulfate	30 mg/mL	6 mg elemental iron/mL	Child: 0.5–1 mL/kg Adult: 15–30 mL/d
Ferrous sulfate CR	325 mg	105 mg	1–2 daily
Ferrous fumarate	200 mg	65.7 mg	1 tablet b/tds
Iron polymaltose	370 mg	100 mg	1–2 daily
Iron polymaltose	37 mg/mL	10 mg/mL	0.3–0.6 mL/kg (child) 10–20 mL daily (adult)
Iron with vitamin C			
Ferrous sulfate + vit C SR	325/500 mg	105 mg	1–2 tablets daily
Iron with folic acid			
Ferrous sulfate + folic acid	270 mg + 300 mcg	87.4 mg	1–2 capsules daily
Ferrous fumarate +folic acid	310 mg + 350 mcg	100 mg	1–2 tablets daily
Ferrous sulfate + folic acid CR	250 mg + 300 mcg	80 mg	1–2 tablets daily
Parenteral iron			
Iron sucrose	20 mg/mL, 5-mL vial	20 mg/mL	See product datasheet
Ferric carboxymaltose	50 mg/mL, 2-mL vial	50 mg/mL	See product datasheet
Iron polymaltose	50 mg/mL, 2-mL vial Avoid IM injections	50 mg/mL	See product datasheet

CR, controlled release; SR, sustained release.

Iron acts as a toxin to nuclear function, so excess accumulation of iron may occur in the myelodysplastic disorders refractory anaemia with ring sideroblasts (sideroblastic anaemia) and polycythaemia rubra vera.

Pharmacological management

Affected patients may require treatment to try and chelate the iron before it is incorporated into their tissues in toxic quantities. The traditional agent has been parenterally administered: desferrioxamine but more recently two oral products, deferasirox and deferiprone, have been introduced.

Iron overload conditions can also occur associated with repeat red blood cell infusions (such as in thalassaemia; each unit of infused packed red blood cells contains the equivalent of about 250 mg of elemental iron) or in inherited conditions such as haemochromatosis.

TABLE 9.2 Ferrous compounds used for chronic Iron deficiency

Medication class/drug group	Mechanism of action	Indications for therapeutic use	Common side effects	Practice points	Common adult dosage range
Ferrous compounds[2]	Iron replacement	Used as iron replacement in microcytic, hypochromic anaemia	Constipation, gastrointestinal upset	Anaemia will increase feelings of fatigue and tiredness Iron therapy may be indicated for this but only where anaemia is associated with iron deficiency If patients are complaining of fatigue despite iron replacement refer back to their GP	~100–200 mg elemental iron/day

---

PHYSIOTHERAPY PRACTICE POINTS: HAEMOCHROMATOSIS

Although signs and symptoms of haemochromatosis may vary depending upon the severity of the disease, common signs and symptoms include joint pain, fatigue, general weakness, weight loss and stomach pain. Physiotherapists, particularly those involved in treating patients with musculoskeletal problems, must therefore be aware of the possible clinical signs and symptoms occurring with these disorders and, when necessary, refer these patients to the appropriate specialist.

◼ White blood cell disorders

Leukocyte pathologies

Leukocytes or white blood cells respond normally to changes within the body that occur in response to conditions such as infections.

The presence of immature cells in the peripheral blood indicates that the differentiation of mature blood cells within the bone marrow is being stressed. The presence of blast cells would be considered abnormal and may indicate a major blood disease such as leukaemia.

Acute leukaemia is suggested when large numbers of blast cell precursors (immature cells) emerge from the bone marrow into the peripheral blood. Leukaemias can present with an increase in blast cell precursors from any of the cell lines. Chronic leukaemias are suggested when large numbers of apparently mature blood cells are seen.

Chronic myeloid leukaemia may present with an increase in any of the cell lines despite the name (Figure 9.4).

---

[2]See also Table 9.1.

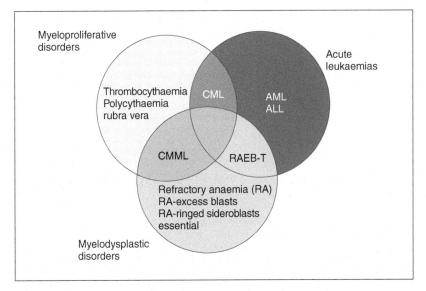

Figure 9.4 Relationship between myelodysplastic, myeloproliferative and leukaemic diseases. ALL, acute lymphoblastic leukaemia; AML, acute myeloid leukaemia; CML, chronic myeloid leukaemia; CMML, chronic myelomonocytic leukaemia; RAEB-T, refractory anaemia with excess blasts in transformation.

Pharmacological management

The main treatment used for leukaemia is chemotherapy, which may be administered in conjunction with stem cell transplantation. Treatment for each leukaemia is different, and is beyond the scope of this handbook. See relevant oncological textbooks.

PHYSIOTHERAPY PRACTICE POINTS: LEUKAEMIA

Physiotherapists involved in the care of this group of patients must be aware of all the possible side effects of chemotherapy and implement any physical treatments with caution. They should be particularly cognisant of those patients who develop infections and might be treated in isolation.

■ Platelet disorders and clotting disorders

Platelet disorders

Platelets are derived in the bone marrow from thrombocyte precursors, in particular the megakaryocyte. This cell fragments to release small particles called the platelets. The platelet is responsible for stopping bleeding by aggregating with other platelets in response to thromboxane in order to plug damaged blood vessels.

Insufficient platelet numbers or impaired platelet function can lead to excessive bleeding. The most common form of platelet insufficiency is the condition called idiopathic thrombocytopenic purpura (ITP). In this condition the platelet becomes recognised by the immune system as 'foreign' to the body and is consumed by immunoglobulin/complement within splenic tissue.

Pharmacological management

Treatment of ITP is similar to other autoimmune diseases and is dependent upon the platelet count. At platelet counts $>60 \times 10^3$/microlitre management may be just observational since significant bleeding is rare at this level. However, as platelet counts drop treatment may be indicated. First-line treatment is often with high dose corticosteroids: 60 mg oral prednisolone per day or methylprednisolone 1 g intravenously. Further treatment may be required including surgical splenectomy although the effects of this may be reduced by the generation of splenic tissue elsewhere within the body.

Other treatment options include other immune suppressant therapy with azathioprine, cyclosporin or methylphenidate or inhibiting antiplatelet immunoglobulin activity by infusions of non-specific immunoglobulin G (IgG) from 'normal' donors.

An abnormal increase in the number of platelets is termed essential thrombocythaemia and may be associated with increased risk of thrombosis including stroke. Treatment is aimed at reducing platelet numbers using cytotoxic medication such as hydroxyurea. Hydroxyurea inhibits DNA synthesis by interfering with the conversion of ribonucleotides to deoxyribonucleotides, interfering more with differentiation of cells than their replication. Utilisation of these agents is recommended for specialist use only.

PHYSIOTHERAPY PRACTICE POINTS: PLATELET DISORDERS

Physiotherapy within this patient group may lead to joint and muscular trauma and cause bleeding in susceptible patients. However, in those patients who are immobile, physiotherapy may be vital in the prevention of the formation of thrombi (i.e. deep vein thrombosis in the calves). The physiotherapist should be aware of these possibilities and find the appropriate level of physical activation.

Clotting disorders

The haemostasis response of the body is fast localised and carefully controlled. It involves many clotting factors normally present in plasma (Table 9.3) as well as substances released by platelets and injured tissue cells.

The clotting cascade

Blood clots are usually formed to stop leakage from damaged blood vessels. The first step in the formation of a clot involves the aggregation of platelets to form a platelet plug, and this initiates a cascade of chemical reactions that leads to the conversion of prothrombin to thrombin followed by the activation of fibrinogen to form long fibrin threads that bind the platelet plug and initiate healing of the

TABLE 9.3 **Clotting factors**

I	Fibrinogen	VIII	Antihaemophilic factor
II	Prothrombin	IX	Christmas factor
III	Thromboplastin	X	Stuart-Prower factor
IV	Calcium	XI	Plasma thromboplastin antecedent
V	Proaccelerin	XII	Hageman factor
VI	Same as factor V	XIII	Fibrin-stabilising factor
VII	Proconvertin		

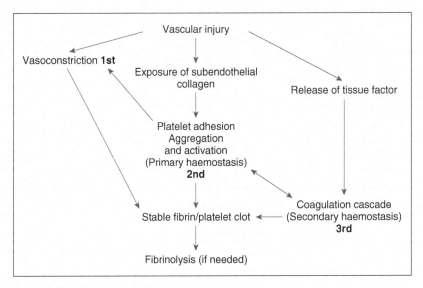

Figure 9.5 Three steps in the clotting cascade.

damaged blood vessel. The process involves a complex interaction between platelets, clotting and fibrinolytic processes, the blood vessel endothelium, inflammatory and pro-inflammatory mediators and white blood cells (see Figures 9.5, 9.6, 9.7 and 9.8).

Anticoagulant medications

Anticoagulant medications are used initially to treat and then to maintain patients after an acute thrombosis (Gage et al. 2001; Lip et al. 2010, 2011) (Figure 9.9). They may also be used to prevent cardiovascular complications after acute myocardial infarction with ST elevations (STEMI) and ST-segment elevation in acute coronary syndromes (STEACS), prevent thrombotic strokes in at-risk patients following atrial fibrillation, and after transient ischaemic attacks (TIAs)

Text continued on p. 266

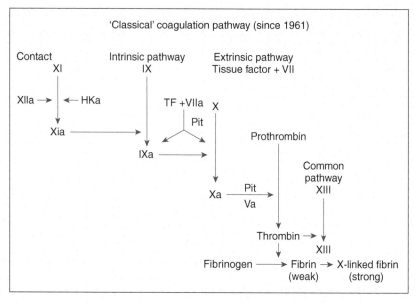

Figure 9.6 'Classical' coagulation pathway.

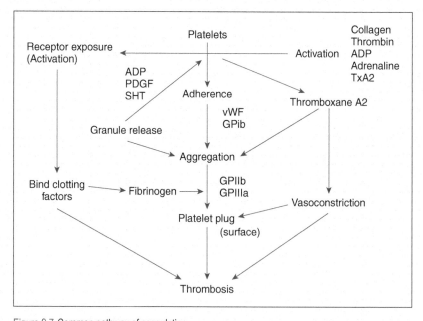

Figure 9.7 Common pathway of coagulation.
ADP, adenosine di-phosphate; GPIb, glycoprotein 1b; GPIIb, glycoprotein 2b; GPIIIb, glycoprotein 3b; PDGF, platelet-derived growth factor; TxA2, thromboxane A2; vWF, von Willebrand Factor; 5HT, serotonin.

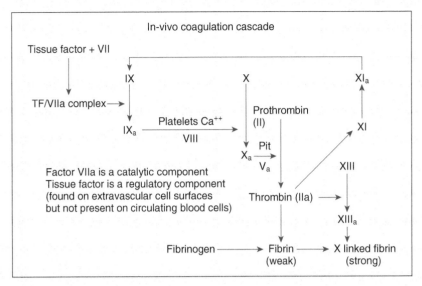

Figure 9.8 Blood coagulation pathways in vivo showing the central role played by thrombin.

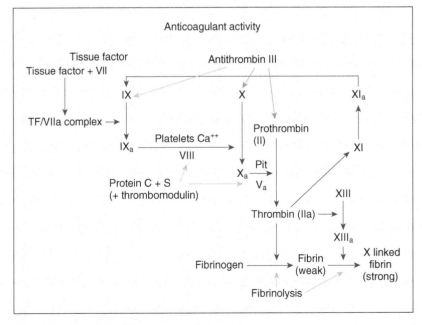

Figure 9.9 Anticoagulant activity.

and ischaemic strokes. Tools such as $CHADS_2$ and CHA_2DS_2-VASc have been designed to help assess clinical need for anti-coagulation and tools such as HAS-BLED to assess major bleeding risk (see Tables 9.4A, 9.4B and 9.4C).

TABLE 9.4A CHADS$_2$

	Factor	Score If 'Yes'
C	History of coronary heart failure	+1
H	History of hypertension	+1
A	Age > or = 75 years	+1
D	History of diabetes mellitus	+1
S	History of previous stroke or TIA symptoms	+2

- *Score of 0: no anticoagulant recommended; 0.8–3.2% annual risk of stroke, antithrombotic therapy may be sufficient.*
- *Score of 1: recommend use of CHA2DS2-VASc.*
- *Score of >2: significant risk of stroke – anticoagulant recommended; 5.9% annual risk when score 2–3, 18.2% annual risk when score 3–6.*

Adapted from: Gage B.F., Waterman A.D., Shannon W., et al., 2001. Validation of clinical classification schemes for predicting stroke: results from the National Registry of Atrial Fibrillation. Journal of the American Medical Association 285 (22), 2864–2870.

TABLE 9.4B CHA$_2$DS$_2$-VASc

	Factor	Score
C	History of coronary heart failure	+1
H	History of hypertension	+1
A	Age <65 years 65–74 years >75 years	0 +1 +2
D	History of diabetes mellitus	+1
S	History of previous stroke or TIA symptoms	*2
VASc	History of vascular disease	+1

- *Score of 0: low risk of thromboembolic events.*
- *Score of 1: immediate risk low (0.6% at 1 year).*
- *Score of >2: high risk (3% rate at 1 year).*

Adapted with permission from: Lip G.Y.H., Nieuwlaat R., Pisters R., et al., 2010. Refining clinical risk stratification for predicting stroke and thromboembolism in atrial fibrillation using a novel risk factor-based approach: The Euro Heart Survey on atrial fibrillation. Chest 137 (2), 263–272.

TABLE 9.4C HAS-BLED

	Factor	Score
H	History of • hypertension • renal disease (SCr >200 micromol/L) • liver disease (cirrhosis or bilirubin >2 × URL)	+1 +1 +1
A	Age > 65 years	+1
S	History of stroke	+1
B	History of major bleeding episode or predisposition to bleeding	+1
L	Labile INR (time in therapeutic range <60%)	+1
E	Medication use predisposing to bleeding (e.g. antiplatelet agents or NSAIDs)	+1
D	Alcohol or drug use history	+1

Score of 0: low risk of major bleeding episode (1%/patient/year). The number of bleeds/100 patient years increased from 1.13 for a HAS-BLED score of '0' to 1.88 for a score of '2', 3.74 for a score of '3', 8.7 for a score of '4' and 12.5 for a score of '5' (Pisters et al. 2010).
Adapted with permission from: Lip G.Y., Frison L., Halperin J.L., et al., 2011. Comparative validation of a novel risk score for predicting bleeding risk in anticoagulated patients with atrial fibrillation: the HAS-BLED (Hypertension, Abnormal Renal/Liver Function, Stroke, Bleeding History or Predisposition, Labile INR, Elderly, Drugs/Alcohol Concomitantly) score. Journal of the American College of Cardiology 57 (2), 173–180.

Warfarin

Warfarin was first identified by the Wisconsin Alumni Research Foundation (WARF) in 1941 following the autopsy of a cow that had died after eating spoiled sweet clover hay, which contains the chemical dicoumarol. This was found to be an inhibitor of vitamin K epoxide reductase, which recycles oxidised vitamin K1 to a reduced form after it has been carboxylated and inactivates several coagulation factors (II, VII, IX and X, particularly II [prothrombin] and VII). Its anticoagulant effects therefore can be reversed by administering vitamin K1.

The effects of warfarin build slowly over 2–5 days following a single dose because of the half-lives ($t\frac{1}{2}$) of the different coagulation factors. Warfarin therapy is controlled by using the International Normalised Ratio or INR, which is derived from the ratio of the measured prothrombin time to the result from a known standard. The normal therapeutic range for INR used in most situations is between 1.5 and 2.5. For patients with ongoing risk of thrombosis, such as patients with prosthetic heart valves, an INR range of 3–4 may be necessary.

Warfarin is used therapeutically as an isomeric mixture of R- and S-warfarin. It should be noted that warfarin has multiple interactions. The most important drug interactions associated with warfarin are those with drugs involving CYP2C9, 2C19 and 3A4 metabolic enzymes. In particular, inhibitors or inducers of CYP2C9 will significantly affect a patient's response to warfarin.

Novel oral anticoagulants

The novel oral anticoagulants (NOACs), rivaroxaban and apixaban, work by selectively inhibiting Factor Xa; dabigatran is a direct thrombin inhibitor that blocks the conversion of fibrinogen to fibrin. The quoted advantage of NOACs over warfarin is the absence of the need to monitor the INR, so that the patient does not have to undergo frequent blood tests and dose changes. However, there is no means of identifying either over- or under-coagulation and, as yet, no easy antidote is available should a patient experience a severe haemorrhagic complication.

Heparin
Heparin is a highly sulfonated glycosaminoglycan. It is an injectable anticoagulant that binds to the enzyme inhibitor antithrombin III, producing conformational changes that inactivate thrombin and Factor Xa. Other agents termed low-molecular-weight (LMW) heparins (enoxaparin, dalteparin and tinzaparin) are active more specifically as inhibitors of Factor Xa. Heparin and the LMW heparins are all administered parenterally, heparin as a continuous infusion in patients with thrombosis or subcutaneously for prophylaxis. The LMW heparins are all administered by intermittent subcutaneous injection.

Thrombolytic medications
These are medications that break down or dissolve clots and are used following acute myocardial infarctions (AMIs), after thrombotic strokes or following massive venous thromboembolism.

Tissue plasminogen activators
Four agents are available in Australia: alteplase, reteplase, tenectoplase and the somewhat old-fashioned urokinase. These agents work by converting plasminogen to plasmin, which then catalyses the breakdown of fibrin.

PHYSIOTHERAPY PRACTICE POINTS: ANTICOAGULANT MEDICATIONS

The major adverse effects of these anticoagulation medications are to increase the risk of haemorrhage and occasional allergic reactions.

Due to the potential impact of the anticoagulation therapy the treating physiotherapist should be observant of any sign of bleeding (i.e. bruising marks, haematomas) that might be related to physical activity in general and physiotherapy procedures in particular. Whenever these are encountered physiotherapists can verify with patients their adherence to the therapy (anticoagulants or replacement coagulation products).

Other agents affecting haemostasis
Protamine is a drug that is used to reverse the effects of heparin. It combines with heparin to form a stable and inactive complex. Tranexamic acid is available in both oral and parenteral forms and inhibits the breakdown of the clot by inhibiting the binding of plasminogen and plasmin to fibrin. It may be used to reduce excessive bleeding following minor surgery, heavy menstrual bleeds or following hip and knee arthroplasty. See Table 9.5 for details of medications used in clotting disorders.

TABLE 9.5 Medications used in clotting disorders

Medication class/drug group	Mechanism of action	Indications for therapeutic use	Common side effects	Practice points	Common adult dosage range
Anticoagulants Warfarin NOACs Heparin and low-molecular-weight heparins	Vitamin K antagonist Direct factor X antagonists Factor X antagonists	Post thrombotic stroke, CVA prevention in AF, treatment of VTE	Easy bruising, bleeding (nose bleeds etc)	Physiotherapists may observe bruising, bleeding or may cause bruising if conducting manual therapy Avoid dry needling in patients on any anticoagulant therapy	**Warfarin**: 1–5 mg/day
Tranexamic acid	Inhibits thrombus breakdown	Hereditary angioedema, reduces bleeding after minor surgery or hip or knee arthroplasty, in heavy menstrual bleeding	Increased risk of VTE	Watch for unexplained lower limb pain or SOB	1–4.5 g/day
Protamine	Used as antidote to heparin; combines with heparin to form stable inactive complex	Heparin, dalteparin or enoxaparin overdose	May cause severe haemorrhage May cause excessive tiredness	Observe for easy bruising or bleeding	Up to 50 mg

AF, atrial fibrillation; CVA, cardiovascular accident; SOB, shortness of breath; VTE, venous thromboembolism.

PHYSIOTHERAPY PRACTICE POINTS:
OTHER AGENTS AFFECTING HAEMOSTASIS

Since the use of this medication, however, is associated with an increased risk of venous thromboembolism, the treating physiotherapist should be aware of this possible complication and adjust the level of physical activity appropriately.

Haemophilia

Haemophilia is a group of genetic disorders that impair the body's ability to control blood clotting (see Table 9.6). Haemophilia A (factor VIII deficiency) is present in about 1 in 5,000–10,000 male births and haemophilia B (factor IX deficiency) occurs in around 1 in 20,000–34,000 male births. As with other recessive sex-linked, X chromosome disorders, haemophilia is more likely to occur in males than females. Females are almost exclusively asymptomatic carriers of the disorder and are able to inherit the defective gene from either their mother or father, or it may be a new mutation. Although it is not impossible for a female to have haemophilia, it is unusual. The severity of haemophilia is classified as mild in patients with more than 5% clotting factor, moderate for between 1% and 5% and severe for those with less than 1%. In severe haemophiliacs even a minor injury can result in blood loss lasting days or weeks. In areas such as the cerebral cortex or joint spaces, this blood loss can be fatal or permanently disabling (Sona & Muthu Lingam 2010).

TABLE 9.6 Comparison of signs and symptoms of common bleeding disorders

Type	Symptoms
Haemophilia A	Spontaneous bleeding to joints, muscles and soft tissues; haemarthrosis; deep muscle haematomas; intracranial bleeding in the absence of major trauma; neonatal cephalohematoma or intracranial bleeding Prolonged oozing or renewed bleeding after initial bleeding stops following tooth extractions, mouth injury or circumcision Prolonged bleeding or renewed bleeding following surgery or trauma; unexplained GI bleeding or haematuria, menorrhagia (especially at menarche), prolonged nosebleeds (especially recurrent and bilateral) Excessive bruising, especially with firm subcutaneous haematomas
Haemophilia B	Same clinical symptoms as haemophilia A
Haemophilia C	Mostly the same as those of mild haemophilia; individuals are not likely to bleed spontaneously, and haemorrhage normally occurs after trauma or surgery Certain procedures carry an increased risk of bleeding such as dental extractions, tonsillectomies, surgery in the urinary and genital tracts and nasal surgery Joint, muscle and soft tissue bleeds are uncommon
Von Willebrand disease (vWD)	Usually signs are mild or even absent Abnormal bleeding associated with vWD: recurrent and prolonged nosebleeds, bleeding from the gums, increased menstrual flow, excessive bleeding from a cut or following a tooth extraction or other dental procedure, blood in the stool or urine, bleeding from shaving with a razor or other similarly minor injury Other possible signs include: easy bruising, bruises with lumps that form underneath the skin

Von Willebrand disease (vWD) is the most common hereditary coagulation abnormality described in humans, although it can also be acquired as a result of other medical conditions. It arises from a qualitative or quantitative deficiency of von Willebrand factor (vWF), a multimeric protein that is required for platelet adhesion (Favaloro 2015).

In general, coagulation disorders are treated by administering either drugs that stimulate the release of the deficient factor or its replacement.

Pharmacological management

◆ Factor concentrates
  ● plasma-derived concentrates
  ● recombinant factors
◆ Cryoprecipitates
  ● prepared from pooled blood and contain factor VIII, von Willebrand factor and factor XIII
◆ Fresh frozen plasma (FFP)
◆ Desmopressin (DDAVP)
  ● temporary increases in both vWF and Factor VIII can be achieved using desmopressin.
◆ Factor VIII inhibitor bypass activity (FEIBA)
◆ Recombinant activated factor VIIa (rFVIIa)
◆ Adjuvant therapies
  ● tranexamic acid
  ● fibrin sealant
  ● antispasmodic analgesics (avoid aspirin because it will increase the bleeding by inhibiting platelet aggregation)
  ● corticosteroids
  ● calcium alginate
  ● second generation NSAIDs such as celebrex
  ● opioid analgesics

PHYSIOTHERAPY PRACTICE POINTS: HAEMOPHILIA

The major group of patients treated by physiotherapists with disorders of the haematological system is those with haemophilia. The benefits of physiotherapy and rehabilitation for people with haemophilia are well documented (Blamey et al. 2010; Buzzard 2007; Negrier et al. 2013; Wittmeier & Mulder 2007). Having early treatment post a muscle or joint bleed, strengthening key muscle groups and protecting joints from adverse effects of repeated haemorrhages are measures provided by physiotherapy, which plays a key role in maintaining quality of life in this patient group. Rehabilitation in conjunction with the availability of replacement coagulation products in haemophiliac patients in the developing countries has led to a substantial decrease in both the mortality and morbidity rates among the haemophiliac population (Blamey et al. 2010). Also, some sports programs require physiotherapy orientation, protective gear and timing with prophylaxis (factors and other measures) to help prevent a bleed. Similarly, manual therapy and the close patient contact that is required can enable the physiotherapist to identify clinical signs and symptoms that might be associated with haematological disorders.

TABLE 9.7 Coagulopathy of liver disease

Test	Mild hepatocellular injury	Severe hepatocellular injury	Cirrhosis	Vitamin K deficiency
PT	Prolonged, N	Prolonged	Prolonged	Prolonged
PTT	Prolonged, N	Prolonged	Prolonged in severe cirrhosis	Prolonged in severe deficiency
Factor VII	Reduced, N	Reduced	Reduced	Reduced
Factors II,IX, X	N	Reduced	Reduced	Reduced
D-dimers	N	Increased	Increased	N
FDPs	N	Increased	Increased	N
Platelets	N	Reduced	Reduced	N
ATIII	N	N	Reduced	N
TT	N	Prolonged	Prolonged	N
Factor VIII	N	Reduced	Reduced	N

ATIII, antithrombin III; FDPs, fibrin degradation products; N, normal; PT, prothrombin time; PTT, partial thromboplastin time; TT, thrombin time.

Clotting factors and liver disease

Since all clotting factors and associated proteins are manufactured in the liver, changes in clotting function may be associated with liver disease (Table 9.7).

■ Lymphatic system disorders

Lymphoedema/oedema

The function of the lymphatic system is to transport lymph – fluid that is formed from collection of the interstitial fluid through lymph capillaries. The lymphatic system includes a network of lymph ducts, lymph vessels and lymph nodes that enable the movement of lymph from tissues to the bloodstream. The lymph fluids contain protein, fats (which may be responsible for its milky appearance), infection fragments and white blood cells. The lymph is collected through lymph capillaries that constitute a network through the whole body, and one of its major functions is to rid the body of unwanted materials such as toxins and waste, as well as some blood substances. The lymphatic system includes lymph nodes that serve as 'filters' for unwanted substances including bacteria, and therefore it has an important function in immune activity and inflammation processes. The lymphatic system also has the ability to 'capture' metastatic cancer cells that are transported via the lymphatic system. Inflammation that might be induced by infections and/or cancer can cause lymph node enlargement.

Oedema develops from an increase in the existing interstitial fluid. It may be caused by over-production or by decreased absorption of the interstitial fluid, such as in chronic venous hypertension. Under these circumstances capillary filtration is increased and lymphatic drainage also increases to meet the demand until such time as the flow exceeds the maximum capacity of the lymphatics, when oedema will develop. Persistent high lymphatic flow in this situation leads to damage of the lymphatic system, which then exacerbates the oedema.

Lymphoedema is a chronic swelling resulting from failure of lymphatic drainage. The term primary lymphoedema is related to lymphoedema due to an intrinsic genetic abnormality of the lymphatic system (possibly an inherited entity). Secondary lymphoedema is related to lymphatic failure as a result of damage to a primarily intact system post surgery, radiotherapy, infection (such as cellulitis), immobilisation and/or trauma.

The usual symptoms of lymphoedema might include aching/pain, feeling of heaviness and tightness, abnormal sensations (e.g. itching, prickling, numbness, pins and needles), gross swelling, skin changes such as redness and irregularity.

Pharmacological management

Pharmacological management might involve antibiotics if there are elements of cellulitis. Diuretics and corticosteroids might be used to reduce oedema, especially associated with cancer. Pain should treated by analgesics[3]. High dosages of diuretics (e.g. furosemide at a dosage of 240 mg per day) may also be used in some cases.

PHYSIOTHERAPY PRACTICE POINTS: LYMPHOEDEMA

The most effective treatment for both primary and secondary lymphoedema in both the long and short term is complex physical therapy (CPT). This is therapy consisting of lymphatic massage, skin care and compressive garments in combination with carefully graded exercise. CPT is usually given for 1 hour every day for several weeks. It mechanically improves lymphatic drainage and induces the reduction of the oedema through specialised massage techniques. The principal element is to soften the areas of hard oedema and increase the mobility of the limb. Physiotherapists treating this patient group must take great precautions with skin care and hygiene since these patients are extremely prone to infections (Gradalski, Ochalek & Kurpiewska 2015; Lu et al. 2015; Rockson 2016).

Disorders of plasma proteins and immunoglobulins

Blood plasma is made up of ~90% water and contains more than 100 dissolved solutes including nutrients, gases, hormones, wastes and products of cell activity, ions and proteins. The major protein found in plasma is albumin, accounting for about 55% of all proteins present. Albumin is the major contributor to maintaining the osmotic pressure of plasma. Globulins make up 38% and are important in the transport of metal ions, hormones and lipids. Fibrinogen comprises 7% and the remaining 1% is represented by enzymes (including clotting factors), proenzymes and hormones.

Plasma cell disorders are a diverse group of disorders of unknown aetiology that are characterised by a disproportionate proliferation of a single clone of B

---

[3]See Chapter 7.

cells and the presence of a structurally and electrophoretically homogeneous monoclonal immunoglobulin or polypeptide subunit in serum, urine or both.

Complications of plasma cell proliferation and monoclonal immunoglobulin protein (M-protein) include:

+ autoimmune damage to the organs
+ impaired immunity
+ bleeding tendency
+ secondary amyloidosis
+ osteoporosis[4], hypercalcaemia, anaemia and pancytopenia.

Pharmacological management

The pharmacological treatments for this group of disorders are beyond the scope of this handbook; the reader is referred to some of the recent literature (Chaulagain & Comenzo 2013; Li & Zhou 2013).

PHYSIOTHERAPY PRACTICE POINTS: DISORDERS IN PLASMA PROTEINS AND IMMUNOGLOBULINS

Many of these patients will be treated in isolation and may be immobile for long periods. It is important to maintain an adequate level of exercise in order to avoid complications arising from immobilisation. Due to the nature of these diseases and the high risk of infections because of the impaired immune system of the patient, precautions must be taken to avoid any contamination of the patient.

■ References

Blamey, G., Forsyth, A., Zourikian, N., et al., 2010. Comprehensive elements of a physiotherapy exercise programme in haemophilia: a global perspective. Haemophilia : The Official Journal of the World Federation of Hemophilia 16 (Suppl. 5), 136–145.

Buzzard, B.M., 2007. Physiotherapy, rehabilitation and sports in countries with limited replacement coagulation factor supply. Haemophilia : The Official Journal of the World Federation of Hemophilia 13 (Suppl. 2), 44–46.

Chaulagain, C.P., Comenzo, R.L., 2013. New insights and modern treatment of AL amyloidosis. Current Hematologic Malignancy Reports 8 (4), 291–298.

Favaloro, E.J., 2015. Recent advances in laboratory-aided diagnosis of von Willebrand disease. Expert Opinion on Orphan Drugs 3 (9), 975–995.

Gage, B.F., Waterman, A.D., Shannon, W., et al., 2001. Validation of clinical classification schemes for predicting stroke: results from the National Registry of Atrial Fibrillation. Journal of the American Medical Association 285 (22), 2864–2870.

Gradalski, T., Ochalek, K., Kurpiewska, J., 2015. Complex decongestive lymphatic therapy with or without Vodder II manual lymph drainage in more severe chronic postmastectomy upper limb lymphedema: a randomized noninferiority prospective study. Journal of Pain and Symptom Management 50 (6), 750–757.

Kohne, E., 2011. Hemoglobinopathies: clinical manifestations, diagnosis, and treatment. Deutsches Ärzteblatt International 108 (31–32), 532–540.

---

[4]See Chapter 8 for more detail.

Li, J., Zhou, D.B., 2013. New advances in the diagnosis and treatment of POEMS syndrome. British Journal of Haematology 161 (3), 303–315.

Lip, G.Y., Frison, L., Halperin, J.L., et al., 2011. Comparative validation of a novel risk score for predicting bleeding risk in anticoagulated patients with atrial fibrillation: the HAS-BLED (Hypertension, Abnormal Renal/Liver Function, Stroke, Bleeding History or Predisposition, Labile INR, Elderly, Drugs/Alcohol Concomitantly) score. Journal of the American College of Cardiology 57 (2), 173–180.

Lip, G.Y.H., Nieuwlaat, R., Pisters, R., et al., 2010. Refining clinical risk stratification for predicting stroke and thromboembolism in atrial fibrillation using a novel risk factor-based approach: The Euro Heart Survey on atrial fibrillation. Chest 137 (2), 263–272.

Lu, S.R., Hong, R.B., Chou, W., et al., 2015. Role of physiotherapy and patient education in lymphedema control following breast cancer surgery. Therapeutics and Clinical Risk Management 11, 319–327.

Negrier, C., Seuser, A., Forsyth, A., et al., 2013. The benefits of exercise for patients with haemophilia and recommendations for safe and effective physical activity. Haemophilia : The Official Journal of the World Federation of Hemophilia 19 (4), 487–498.

Pisters, R., Lane, D.A., Nieuwlaat, R., et al., 2010. A novel user-friendly score (HAS-BLED) to assess 1-year risk of major bleeding in patients with atrial fibrillation: the Euro Heart Survey. Chest 138 (5), 1093–1100.

Rockson, S.G., 2016. Lymphedema. Vascular Medicine 21 (1), 77–81.

Sona, P.S., Muthu Lingam, C., 2010. Hemophilia: an overview. International Journal of Pharmaceutical Sciences Review and Research 5 (1), 18–26.

Wittmeier, K., Mulder, K., 2007. Enhancing lifestyle for individuals with haemophilia through physical activity and exercise: the role of physiotherapy. Haemophilia : The Official Journal of the World Federation of Hemophilia 13 (Suppl. 2), 31–37.

Yu, T.T., Nelson J., Streiff M.B., et al., 2016. Risk factors for venous thromboembolism in adults with hemoglobin SC or Sβ+ thalassemia genotypes. Thrombosis Resesearch 141, 35–38.

Mental health

Iftah Biran, Jacqueline Reznik

OBJECTIVES

This chapter will discuss the most common psychiatric conditions treated by physiotherapists, and the role that medications have in their management. By the end of this chapter the reader should have an understanding of:

* the major classification of mental disorders
* treatment options for the major mental disorders
* groups of major medications used to treat mental disorders and their modes of action
* usual dosages, routes of administration and major contraindications and precautions of these medications
* mental disorders that present with symptoms that deserve the attention of the physiotherapist and any potential impact of medications on physiotherapeutic management.

OVERVIEW

Psychotropic medication
Antipsychotics
Anxiolytics (anti-anxiety drugs)
Antidepressants
Mood stabilisers

Clinical syndromes and pharmacological management
Schizophrenia spectrum and other psychotic disorders
Bipolar and related disorders
Depressive disorders
Anxiety disorders
Obsessive–compulsive and related disorders

Trauma- and stress-related disorders
Somatic symptom and related disorders
Insomnia

Psychiatric disorders with sensory motor deficits and psychopharmacological management
Psychiatric disorders with sensory motor deficits
Major sensory and motor side effects of psychopharmacological interventions

■ Introduction

Mental disorders, along with neurological and substance use disorders, account for a substantial proportion of the disease burden worldwide. They are the leading cause for years lived with disability and a leading cause of mortality (Charlson et al. 2015; Whiteford et al. 2015).

Current psychiatric practice approaches mental disorders based on the biopsychosocial model. This model, as suggested in the late 1970s by Engel (1977), stresses the importance of a psychosocial approach to the classic biological medical model (i.e. psychiatric impairments should be evaluated in a holistic view that integrates the pathology as well as function from the perspective of biological, psychological and social factors rather than purely in biological-medical terms). Although its applicability to psychiatric practice is at times debatable, this approach is still of importance (Adler 2009; Alvarez, Pagani & Meucci 2012). According to this model, interventions should include not only biological input (psychopharmacological) but also psycho/social interventions (i.e. social rehabilitation programs [Mueser et al. 2010]) and psychotherapeutic interventions (Huhn et al. 2014). Biological interventions are not only confined to the use of chemical substances but also include brain activation interventions (i.e. treating resistant depression with electroconvulsive therapy or with transcranial magnetic stimulation [Fitzgerald 2013]), brain surgery (i.e. capsulotomy for obsessive–compulsive disorder [Lapidus et al. 2013]), deep brain stimulation for depression (Fitzgerald 2013; Luigjes et al. 2013) and pharmacological management, which are the topics of this chapter (see Table 10.1).

How is a specific pharmacological intervention chosen? Multiple factors influence the prescribing patterns of psychotropic medications. Among them are the patient's symptoms profile, patient's diagnosis, professional guidelines, official indications and prescriber's profession, attitudes and beliefs (see Table 10.2).

TABLE 10.1 Therapeutic interventions in psychiatry

Intervention mode	Examples
Social interventions	Social rehabilitation, social skills training, supported employment, family psychoeducation (Mueser et al. 2010; Lecomte et al. 2014)
Psychological interventions	Psychodynamic psychotherapy, cognitive behavioural therapy, dialectical behavioural therapy, interpersonal psychotherapy, supportive psychotherapy (Gabbard 2009)
Biological interventions	Brain activation – electroconvulsive therapy, repetitive transcranial magnetic stimulation (Fitzgerald 2013) Psychosurgery – capsulotomy, vagus nerve stimulation, deep brain stimulation (the last two are invasive activation procedures) (Lapidus et al. 2013; Luigjes et al. 2013) Psychopharmacology

TABLE 10.2 Factors affecting the choice of a psychotropic medication	
Domain	Factors
Prescriber factors	Evidence-based decision Acquaintance with professional guidelines Awareness of approved indications Familiarity with certain medications 'Courage' to prescribe off-label indications Prescriber's profession (primary care doctor, psychiatrist, physiotherapist etc) Pharmaceutical industry promotion
Patient factors	Diagnosis Symptoms Previous exposure Beliefs
Medication factors	Side effects profile Concurrent medications (interaction evaluation) Availability Pricing Reimbursement/government subsidy

This chapter opens with a brief summary of the major psychotropic medications. This is followed by a description of conditions that warrant therapy and therapeutic options for these conditions. The text follows the American diagnostic nomenclature (DSM) (American Psychiatric Association 2013) and the Australian approved indications as specified in the MIMS registry (available on the MIMS website, http://www.mims.com.au). The chapter concludes by describing psychiatric conditions with somatic signs, as patients with such presentations are often encountered in the physiotherapist's practice.

■ Psychotropic medication

The mode of action of most psychotropic medications is through interaction with neurotransmitters and their binding sites.[1] Traditionally, most psychotropic medications are classified into the following four groups: 1) antipsychotics (neuroleptics), 2) anxiolytics/anti-anxiety/sedative medications, 3) antidepressants and 4) mood stabilisers. Many psychiatric and psychopharmacological textbooks still follow this categorisation (Stahl 2008). However, it is becoming less and less relevant as drugs from one class are prescribed to treat disorders related to another class (i.e. antipsychotics as mood stabilisers or antidepressants, mood stabilisers as antidepressants, antidepressants as anti-anxiety medications). Aside from these four groups drugs from other groups, such as sleep medication, can be used to treat specific conditions. See Table 10.3 for an overview of the major psychotropic medication groups and their relevance to the physiotherapist.

The following is a brief overview of each drug group.

---

[1]See Chapter 1 for a review of pharmacodynamics and Chapter 6 on the neurological system.

TABLE 10.3	Overview of medications used to treat psychiatric conditions		
General category	**Specific group**	**Relevance for physiotherapists**	**Where addressed**
Drugs used for psychiatric disorders	Antipsychotics	+++ (frequent motor side effects)	This chapter
	Anxiolytics	+++ (can decrease muscular tone)	This chapter
	Antidepressants	+	This chapter
	Mood stabilisers	+	This chapter and Chapter 6
Adjuvant drugs			
Drugs used for specific conditions	Sleep medications	+	This chapter (with anxiolytics)
	Anti-Parkinsonian drugs (for motor side effects)	+++	Chapter 6

Antipsychotics

Most antipsychotics exert their effect through modulation of dopamine activity as implied by the 'dopamine hypothesis', which emerged in the 1950s with the design of chlorpromazine and is still of relevance today (Ban 2007; Stahl 2009). According to this hypothesis, psychosis is related to dopamine overactivity in the mesolimbic dopamine pathway, and treatment of psychotic disorders is based on D_2 dopamine receptor blockade (i.e. decreasing the effect of the pathological overactivity of dopamine at these sites). The classic antipsychotics, referred to as first-generation antipsychotics, share this mechanism. Although most antipsychotics antagonise the D_2 receptor to some extent, it is well established that many other neurotransmitters play a role in psychosis and its therapy. Accordingly, some of the second-generation antipsychotics block the serotonin 5-HT_2 receptor as well as the D_2 receptor. However, their effect on the D_2 receptor is not as strong as that of the first-generation antipsychotics. While first-generation antipsychotics cause more motor extrapyramidal side effects due to their effect on D_2 receptors and the following blockade of the nigrostriatal dopaminergic pathway, the second-generation antipsychotics cause more metabolic side effects (since their receptor profile is not specific only to emotional/behavioural/psychiatric manifestations). See Table 10.4 for a list of antipsychotics by group and Table 10.5 for a description of the major side effects of the antipsychotic drugs and their management.

Antipsychotics are used to treat psychotic disorders as well as mania, depression in the context of bipolar disorders, mood shifts (as mood stabilisers), anxiety, agitation and behavioural impairments.

Most antipsychotics are delivered orally; however, a few formulations are delivered also as intramuscular injection either for acute therapy or as long-term therapy for patients who do not comply with therapy.

TABLE 10.4 Antipsychotic medications by group

Drug group/specific drugs	Common adult dosage range	Mechanism of action	Major group side effects [a]
First-generation antipsychotics			
Chlorpromazine hydrochloride	*Oral:* 75–800 mg/day	D_2 blockade	Motor side effects
Droperidol	*IM:* 5–20 mg IV formulations with different doses are available		Conduction blocks Neuroleptic malignant syndrome Hyperprolactinaemia
Flupenthixol decanoate	*IM:* 12.5–100 mg/3–6 weeks		
Fluphenazine decanoate	*IM:* 12.5–25 mg/month		
Haloperidol	*Oral:* 2–100 mg/day (An injectable form is available, usually used for acute indications: 2–10 mg IM or IV)		
Haloperidol decanoate	*IM:* 50–100 mg/month		
Pericyazine	*Oral:* mild/moderate, 15–30 mg/day; severe, 25–75 mg/day		
Trifluoperazine hydrochloride	*Oral:* 2–6 mg/day (outpatients), up to 20 mg/day (inpatients)		
Zuclopenthixol	*Oral:* acute, up to 75 mg/day; chronic, 20–40 mg/day		
Zuclopenthixol acetate	*IM:* up to 150 mg per injection (maximum 4 doses/4 weeks)		
Zuclopenthixol decanoate	*IM:* 200–400 mg/2–4 weeks		
Second-generation antipsychotics			
Amisulpride	*Oral:* 400–1200 mg/day	Various mechanisms and sites: D_2 receptor, serotonin 5-HT_2 receptor and some other receptors	Metabolic syndrome
Aripiprazole	*Oral:* 10–30 mg/day		Conduction blocks Motor side effects
Aripiprazole monohydrate	*IM:* 400 mg/month		Neuroleptic malignant syndrome
Asenapine	*Oral:* 5–20 mg/day		Hyperprolactinaemia
Clozapine	*Oral:* 200–900 mg/day		Clozapine, which is a highly effective
Lurasidone	*Oral:* 40–160 mg/day		antipsychotic, requires special
Olanzapine	*Oral:* 5–20 mg/day		blood count monitoring due to the
Olanzapine pamoate monohydrate	*IM:* 150–405 mg every 2 weeks		risk of neutropenia (see Table 10.12
Paliperidone	*Oral:* 3–12 mg/day		later)
Paliperidone palmitate	*IM:* 25–150 mg/month		

TABLE 10.4 **Antipsychotic medications by group—cont'd**

Drug group/specific drugs	Common adult dosage range	Mechanism of action	Major group side effects [a]
Quetiapine	*Oral:* 150–800 mg/day (both immediate and sustained release formulations)		
Risperidone	*Oral:* 4–6 mg/day *IM:* 50 mg every 2 weeks		
Ziprasidone	*Oral:* 80–160 mg/day *IM:* 10–20 mg every 2 hours up to 40 mg/day; up to 3 days		

[a]*The common and most disturbing side effects for each group are underlined.*
IM, intramuscular; IV, intravenous.

Anxiolytics (anti-anxiety drugs)

Gamma-aminobutyric acid (GABA) is a major inhibitory neurotransmitter. Enhancement of its effect leads to reduced activation of the central nervous system and a concomitant decrease in anxiety. Most anxiolytics are benzodiazepines and they exert their effect through the $GABA_A$ receptor (a chloride channel) by enhancing the effect of GABA. Benzodiazepines are used widely and for a variety of indications. Aside from their use in treating anxiety, they are used for insomnia, for stopping seizures, as muscle relaxants and for alcohol withdrawal syndrome. Major side effects are the development of dependence and tolerance, and therefore the use of benzodiazepines should be limited to short periods only. Other common side effects are drowsiness, memory impairment, cognitive changes, impaired psychomotor skills, falls and respiratory compromise. Therefore, this class of drugs is not generally recommended for elderly people. In some cases a paradoxical reaction with arousal, agitation and aggression can occur (Howard et al. 2014). Although most benzodiazepines share the same mechanisms and effects, they differ on the time course of their action and the clinician can select a compound based on its temporal effect (see Table 10.6). This section also includes the 'z-drugs' (called as such as most of their names start with a 'z'). Z-drugs are used as hypnotics and, although non-benzodiazepine in structure, they have similar effects to benzodiazepines as they bind to the GABA–benzodiazepine receptor complex and are therefore included here. Z-drugs are usually more tolerable than benzodiazepines. However, they can cause behavioural impairments such as sleep walking and sleep eating (Olson 2008).

Antidepressants

The current conceptualisation of depression is still dominated by the 'monoamine deficiency hypothesis', according to which imbalance in aminergic transmission

TABLE 10.5 Adverse effects and management of antipsychotic medications

Adverse effect	Characteristics	Management
Cardiac conduction abnormalities	QT interval[2] prolongation with the risk of ventricular arrhythmia and/or sudden cardiac death; increased risk with various antipsychotics both first- and second-generation (Fanoe et al. 2014; Wu, Tsai & Tsai 2015)	Electrocardiography (ECG) testing (Shah, Aftab & Coverdale 2014) Consider dose reduction, switch to a drug with no effect on QT interval (Fanoe et al. 2014)
Motor side effects (Divac et al. 2014)	Parkinsonism (tremor, rigidity, bradykinesia) Acute dystonia (sustained abnormal postures and muscle spasm) Akathisia (restlessness and pacing) Tardive dyskinesia – highly debilitating abnormal involuntary movements, usually facial More common following the use of first-generation antipsychotics	Treatment options are: anticholinergic drugs that counteract the dopaminergic motor effect (benzhexol hydrochloride, benztropine mesylate), reduce dosage, switch to another medication (i.e. a 2nd generation antipsychotic with fewer extrapyramidal side effects)
Neuroleptic malignant syndrome	A life-threatening situation caused by both first- and second-generation anti-psychotics Altered mental state, muscle rigidity, tremor, tachycardia, hyperpyrexia, leukocytosis and elevated serum creatine phosphokinase (CPK) (Sahoo, Agarwal & Biswas 2014)	Admission to intensive care unit Discontinuation of antipsychotic drug Treatment options are: bromocriptine, levodopa, amantadine, rotigotine, dantrolene, lisuride, apomorphine, non-ergot dopamine agonists; in severe cases electroconvulsive therapy can be administered (Frucht 2014)
Hyperprolactinaemia (Wong-Anuchit 2016)	Hyperprolactinaemia is secondary to inhibition of tuberoinfundibular dopaminergic pathways It is caused by most of the first-generation antipsychotics but only by a few of the second-generation such as amisulpride, paliperidone and risperidone Prominent symptoms are galactorrhoea, gynaecomastia and sexual dysfunction	Switch to another antipsychotic Prescribe dopamine agonists such as bromocriptine; this should be done with great caution as dopamine agonists might exacerbate psychosis
Metabolic syndrome	Weight gain, type 2 diabetes, dyslipidaemia, cardiovascular disease Highest with second-generation antipsychotics, especially olanzapine, clozapine and risperidone (Gautam & Meena 2011; Young, Taylor & Lawrie 2015)	Monitor cardio-metabolic risk factors (weight, height and waist circumference measurement, blood glucose, lipid profile and blood pressure) Lifestyle interventions and education Switch antipsychotic Drugs for metabolic illness Bariatric surgery if indicated (Lambert 2011; Saravane et al. 2009)

Adapted from: Young, S.L., Taylor, M., Lawrie, S.M., 2015. '"First do no harm." A systematic review of the prevalence and management of antipsychotic adverse effects'. Journal of Psychopharmacology 29 (4), 353–62. Buchanan, R.W., Kreyenbuhl, J., Kelly, D.L., et al., 2010. The 2009 schizophrenia PORT psychopharmacological treatment recommendations and summary statements. Schizophrenia Bulletin 36 (1), 71–93.

---

[2]The QT interval (ECG parameter) represents the time of ventricular activity including both depolarisation and repolarisation.

TABLE 10.6 Major benzodiazepines and z-drugs prescribed for mental health indications (in alphabetical order)

Drug	Common adult dosage range	Mental health indication(s)	Duration of effect[a]	Equivalent dose[b] (lorazepam = 1)
Alprazolam	0.5–4 mg/day	Anxiety, panic disorder, phobia	Short acting	0.5
Bromazepam	6–9 mg/day	Anxiety	Intermediate acting	3 (Bezchlibnyk-Butler et al. 2014)
Clobazam	10–30 mg/day	Anxiety	Long acting (Janicak, Marder & Pavuluri 2011)	20
Clonazepam	Maximum 20 mg/day; most mental health indications – maximum 4 mg/day	FDA approved for anxiety disorders Approved in Australia for seizure disorders only	Intermediate acting	0.25 (Bezchlibnyk-Butler et al. 2014)
Diazepam	Maximum 45 mg/day	Anxiety	Long acting	10
Flunitrazepam	0.5–2 mg/day	Hypnotic	Intermediate acting	1
Lorazepam	1–10 mg/day	Anxiety	Intermediate acting	1
Nitrazepam	2.5–10 mg/day	Hypnotic	Intermediate acting	10
Oxazepam	60–120 mg/day	Anxiety	Intermediate acting	10
Temazepam	7.5–30 mg/day	Hypnotic	Intermediate acting	20
Triazolam	0.125–0.5 mg/day	Hypnotic	Short acting	0.5
Z-drugs				
Eszopiclone	1–3 mg/day	Hypnotic	Short acting	Not applicable
Zaleplon	5–20 mg/day	Hypnotic	Short acting	Not applicable
Zolpidem	5–10 mg/day	Hypnotic	Short acting; there is a sustained release formulation	Not applicable
Zopiclone	5–20 mg/day	Hypnotic	Short/ intermediate acting	Not applicable

[a]Adapted from: Bezchlibnyk-Butler, K.Z., Jeffries, J.J., Procyshyn, R.M., et al., 2014. *Clinical Handbook of Psychotropic Drugs,* twentieth ed. Hogrefe Publishing, Boston, MA.
[b]Adapted from: Ashton, H., 1994. Guidelines for the rational use of benzodiazepines. When and what to use. Drugs 48 (1), 25–40.

(mainly serotonergic and noradrenergic) and the associated 'chemical imbalance' play a critical role in the emergence of depression. This hypothesis relies heavily on the fact that most classes of antidepressants affect monoaminergic transmission (Massart, Mongeau & Lanfumey 2012). The antidepressants are grouped into the following major groups: selective serotonin reuptake inhibitors (SSRIs), selective noradrenaline reuptake inhibitors (SNRIs), tricyclic antidepressants (TCAs) and mono-amine oxidase inhibitors (MAO-Is) as well as a few other minor groups. SSRIs are prescribed more often than all other classes (Abbing-Karahagopian et al. 2014), and SSRIs and TCAs account for more than 90% of all antidepressants prescribed (Exeter, Robinson & Wheeler 2009). Antidepressants are indicated for depression, anxiety disorders and obsessive–compulsive disorders. See Table 10.7 for an overview of the various antidepressants.

TABLE 10.7 Antidepressants according to pharmacological groups

Group	Mechanism	Practice points and common side effects
SSRIs (Thronson & Pagalilauan 2014) Citalopram Escitalopram Fluoxetine Fluvoxamine Paroxetine Sertraline	SSRIs increase the extracellular level of serotonin by blocking the serotonin transporter	Delayed effect – Response within 2–3 weeks Common side effects are gastrointestinal discomfort, headaches, weight gain, sexual dysfunction, sleep disturbances, falls and bleeding tendency Some drugs are more activating (e.g. escitalopram) while some are more sedating (e.g. paroxetine) Paradoxically, there might be increased suicidality, especially in young adults (<24 years old) There is a risk of hyponatraemia, seizures and serotonin syndrome (a life-threatening toxic state caused by increased intrasynaptic serotonin and characterised by altered mental status, autonomic dysfunction and neuromuscular hyperactivity) (Volpi-Abadie, Kaye & Kaye 2013) Citalopram and escitalopram might elongate the QT interval (see footnote 2 on page 282)
SNRIs (Thronson & Pagalilauan 2014) Desvenlafaxine Duloxetine Venlafaxine	SNRIs increase the extracellular level of both serotonin and norepinephrine	More activating than the SSRIs Duloxetine is also indicated for diabetic peripheral neuropathy Similar side effects pattern to the SSRIs; the main adverse reactions include nausea, dizziness and diaphoresis Desvenlafaxine is a major active metabolite of venlafaxine

TABLE 10.7 Antidepressants according to pharmacological groups—cont'd

Group	Mechanism	Practice points and common side effects
TCAs (Gillman 2007) Amitriptyline Clomipramine Dothiepin Doxepin Imipramine Nortryptiline Trimipramine	TCAs block both serotonin and norepinephrine transporters	High incidence of anticholinergic effects (dry mouth, urinary retention, blurred vision, constipation, cognitive impairment) and cardiotoxicity Consider avoiding in elderly population due to anticholinergic, sedative and orthostatic effects Amitriptyline is effective for pain disorders Both amitriptyline and doxepin are highly sedating and can be used to alleviate insomnia in depressed patients
MAO-Is (Shulman, Herrmann & Walker 2013) Phenelzine Tranylcypromine Moclobemide	MAO inhibition prevents breakdown of monoamine neurotransmitters such as serotonin, epinephrine, norepinephrine and dopamine Phenelzine and tranylcypromine are irreversible inhibitors of the enzyme while moclobemide is reversible (reversible inhibition of mono-amine oxidase, RIMA)	Highly effective in depression However, may cause hypertensive crisis in combination with sympathomimetic agents or tyramine-containing food substances Require a strict diet with no tyramine; foods to avoid are: aged cheeses, tap beer and fermented foods among a long list of other food substances; for a comprehensive list see the dietetic recommendations by Holden (2015) As moclobemide is a reversible and selective inhibitor of the MAO enzyme it has fewer dietary restrictions
Other Compounds Agomelatine (Gahr 2014; Whiting & Cowen 2013)	Melatonergic (MT1/MT2) agonists Serotonergic (5-HT2c) antagonists	Positive effects on sleep Minimal sexual side effects Risk of hepatotoxicity
Bupropion	Norepinephrine dopamine reuptake inhibitor (NDRI)	Not approved for depression in Australia – only approved for smoking cessation Highly epileptogenic
Mianserin Mirtazapine	Noradrenergic and specific serotonergic antidepressant (NaSSA)	Highly sedating Mirtazapine can cause QT-interval prolongation in patients with heart disease and in combination with QT-prolonging agents (see footnote 2 on page 282)
Reboxetine Atomoxetine	Noradrenaline reuptake inhibitor (NARI)	Atomoxetine is approved only for attention deficit hyperactivity disorder (ADHD)
Vortioxetine (Dhir 2013)	Serotonin modulator/ stimulator	A novel drug, unique in its ability to reverse cognitive decline in depressive patients

MAO-Is, monoamine oxidase inhibitors; SNRIs, serotonin norepinephrine reuptake inhibitors; SSRIs, selective serotonin reuptake inhibitors; TCAs, tricyclic antidepressants.

Mood stabilisers

The definition of the term 'mood stabiliser' is not clear. Following a lithium-inspired definition, a mood stabiliser is a drug that has efficacy in mania, depression and in preventing both of these presentations (Keck & McElroy 2003). This section describes lithium and the anticonvulsants used in bipolar disorders. Some antipsychotics are also used as mood stabilisers and are described in previous sections.

Lithium

Lithium is an ion whose introduction as an agent in mania prevention was suggested in 1949 by the Australian psychiatrist John Frederick Joseph Cade (Cade 1949). Its mechanism as a mood stabiliser is not certain. Suggested mechanisms are alterations in ion transport and signal transduction pathways, among others. Although lithium is still one of the most potent drugs available in the prevention of mood episodes (Severus et al. 2014), it has many side effects and a narrow therapeutic index leading to a high risk of toxicity.

Anticonvulsants

Currently three anticonvulsants are used as mood stabilisers: carbamazepine, valproate and lamotrigine (approved in Australia for seizure disorders only). While both valproate and carbamezapine are effective at 'treating from above' (i.e. reducing manic symptoms), lamotrigine is effective at 'treating from below' (i.e. improving depressive symptoms) (Stahl 2008) (see Table 10.8).

TABLE 10.8 Mood stabilisers

Initial medical workup	Monitoring	Common adult dosage ranges and levels	Major adverse effects
		Lithium	
Electrolytes Thyroid function Renal function Calcium Parathyroid hormone Pregnancy test ECG Weight measurement	Levels (2–6 months): Thyroid function Renal status	*Immediate release preparations*: Acute: 1500–2000 mg/day (serum levels: 0.5–1.2 mmol/L) Chronic: 500–1000 mg/day (serum levels: 0.4–1.0 mmol/L); start 500–100 mg/day *Extended release preparations*: Acute: 1800 mg/day Chronic: 900–1200 mg/day	Multiple adverse effects including: tremor, impaired renal function/polyuria, polydipsia (nephrogenic diabetes insipidus), diarrhoea, nausea, weight gain, thyroid impairment, acne, rash, alopecia, leucocytosis, ECG changes Toxicity – neurological (tremor, ataxia, dysarthria, delirium, tremor, memory problems), and gastrointestinal signs Can be fatal

TABLE 10.8 Mood stabilisers—cont'd

Initial medical workup	Monitoring	Common adult dosage ranges and levels	Major adverse effects
		Carbamazepine	
Liver function Blood count	Blood level Liver function Blood count	400–1600 mg/day; start 100–200 mg/day	CNS (e.g. dizziness, ataxia, fatigue, diplopia), hepatic, hyponatraemia, severe hypersensitivity reactions (Stevens–Johnson syndrome, drug rash with eosinophilia and systematic symptoms [DRESS]), suicidality and worsening of depression
		Lamotrigine	
Baseline creatinine	Eye examinations	100–200 mg/day; start 25 mg/day, increase dosage by 25 mg/day every 2 weeks *Adjunct to valproic acid:* Start 12.5 mg/day, increase dosage by 12.5 mg every 2 weeks	Serious rash that can develop to multiorgan failure (Stevens–Johnson syndrome) or toxic epidermal necrolysis (higher risk with concurrent therapy with valproic acid; higher risk at beginning of therapy and rapid dose escalation) Benign rash, sedation, visual impairment, dizziness, ataxia, headache, tremor, insomnia, fatigue, gastrointestinal complaints Suicidality and worsening of depression
		Valproate	
Liver function Blood count	Blood level Liver function Blood count	750–1500 mg/day; start 600 mg/day	Sedation, tremor, gastrointestinal complaints, abnormal liver function, hepatic failure (rare), pancreatitis (rare), thrombocytopenia, suicidality and worsening of depression

Adapted with permission from: Thronson, L.R., and Pagalilauan, G.L., 2014. Psychopharmacology. The Medical Clinics of North America 98 (5), 927–58.

■ Clinical syndromes and pharmacological management

This chapter follows the mental disorder classification of the *Diagnostic and Statistical Manual of Mental Disorders*, fifth edition (DSM-5) (American Psychiatric Association 2013) and the Australian drug registry (available on the MIMS website, http://www.mims.com.au). Other sources are used and referenced where appropriate.

DSM-5 groups the mental disorders into 21 categories (see Box 10.1). Addressing the pharmacological interventions applied to all of these groups is beyond the scope of this chapter. Instead, the focus is on the following DSM-5 categories: 1) psychotic disorders, 2) bipolar and related disorders, 3) depressive disorders, 4) anxiety disorders, 5) obsessive–compulsive and related disorders and 6) trauma- and stressor-related disorders. There are two reasons for this. Firstly, their high prevalence and impact worldwide in general, and in Australia and New Zealand in particular. Three of the 25 leading causes for disability-adjusted life-years in both Australia and New Zealand are: 1) depressive disorders, 2) schizophrenia (one of the psychotic disorders) and 3) anxiety disorders, which include, according to the *International Statistical Classification of Diseases and Related Health Problems* (ICD-10; World Health Organization 1992) and previous editions of the DSM (American Psychiatric Association 2000), the various anxiety disorders, trauma- and stressor-related disorders as well as

---

BOX 10.1 DSM-5 categories of mental disorders

Neurodevelopment disorders	Sleep–wake disorders
Schizophrenia spectrum and other psychotic disorders	Sexual dysfunction
Bipolar and related disorders	Gender dysphoria
Depressive disorders	Disruptive, impulse-control and conduct disorders
Anxiety disorders	Substance-related and addictive disorders
Obsessive–compulsive and related disorders	Personality disorders
Trauma- and stressor-related disorders	Paraphilic disorders
Dissociative disorders	Other mental disorders
Somatic symptom and related disorders	Medication-induced movement disorders and other adverse effects of medications
Feeding and eating disorders	Other conditions that may be a focus of clinical attention
Elimination disorders	Sexual dysfunction

Adapted from: American Psychiatric Association. 2013. *Diagnostic and Statistical Manual of Mental Disorders (DSM 5)*, fifth ed. American Psychiatric Association, Washington, DC.

obsessive–compulsive disorders (Australian Bureau of Statistics 2009; Institute for Health Metrics and Evaluation 2010a, 2010b; Slade et al. 2009). Secondly, the majority of psychotropic agents are aimed at treating psychotic disorders, anxiety disorders (including obsessive–compulsive disorders and trauma- and stressor-related disorders) and affective disorders (depressive disorders and bipolar disorders).

The various sleep disorders as specified in DSM 5 are beyond the scope of this handbook. However, a small section is devoted to insomnia, which is highly prevalent within this patient group (Cunnington, Junge & Fernando 2013). This chapter also addresses somatic symptoms and related disorders. Patients suffering from these disorders, which are signified by bodily manifestations of psychiatric origin, are often treated in rehabilitation programs and referred to physiotherapists. Although there are no specific pharmacological interventions for these disorders, some principles regarding psychopharmacological management will be discussed.

The majority of the disorders listed in this chapter do not have a reliable laboratory test, and therefore a definite diagnosis is hard to establish unless a categorical diagnostic system (a set of symptoms that define a disorder) is applied. Relying on a categorical diagnostic approach and treating only patients who meet specific diagnostic criteria might deprive many patients from symptomatic relief. Accordingly, a high percentage of subjects with mental disorders are treated with off-label medications[3] in a dimensional non-DSM categorical approach, and many psychotropic agents are prescribed off-label and according to specific symptoms (Biondi & Pasquini 2015; Kharadi et al. 2015; Mark 2010; Rajendran, Sajbel & Hartman 2012; Raven & Parry 2012; Widiger & Samuel 2005). This can be demonstrated in the management of patients with borderline personality disorder. A patient may be treated with antidepressants for depressive symptoms, mood stabilisers for emotional lability, antipsychotics for irritability or transient psychotic symptoms, all of which might not reach the threshold for any of the relevant diagnoses (Stoffers et al. 2010).

Schizophrenia spectrum and other psychotic disorders

Psychotic disorders are characterised by abnormalities in one or more of the following five domains: delusions, hallucinations, disorganised speech, disorganised or abnormal motor behaviour and negative symptoms. The first four domains lead to positive symptomatology while the fifth domain, as implied by its name, leads to negative symptoms (see Table 10.9).

Schizophrenia is the prototype of these disorders and is defined by impairment in at least two of the above domains, lasting for more than a month and leading to a functional impairment, with some signs lasting for at least 6 months. Schizophrenia and the other psychotic disorders are described briefly in Table 10.10.

The mainstay of pharmacological management for psychotic disorders in general and schizophrenia in particular is first-generation and second-generation

---

[3] Approved medications but not for the specific use employed.

TABLE 10.9 The key features that define psychotic disorders

Domain	Description
Delusions	Fixed beliefs held with conviction despite conflicting evidence
Hallucinations	Perceptual experience without external stimuli
Disorganised thinking	Impaired thinking process as judged by the subject's speech
Disorganised/abnormal motor behaviour	Abnormal motor movements ranging from diminished motor output to agitation; an extreme variant is catatonia
Negative symptoms	Diminished emotional expression, decreased motivation, diminished speech output, decreased social interactions

TABLE 10.10 Schizophrenia and other psychotic disorders

Disorder	Description
Schizophrenia	Impairment in at least 2 of the 5 psychotic domains listed in Table 10.9, lasting for more than 1 month and leading to a functional impairment, with some signs lasting for at least 6 months
Schizoaffective disorder	Hybrid of an affective disorder with schizophrenia, in which a major mood episode develops simultaneously with psychotic symptoms The psychotic symptoms are compatible with the diagnosis of schizophrenia (2 out of the 5 psychotic domains listed in Table 10.9); however, for at least 2 weeks in the course of the disorder there were delusions or hallucinations without a major mood episode
Brief psychotic disorder	A psychotic episode limited to 1 month duration
Schizophreniform disorder	A psychotic episode limited to 6 months duration
Delusional disorder	Occurrence of delusions without other substantial psychotic signs
Substance-/medication-induced psychotic disorder	Occurrence of hallucinations and/or delusions following substance intoxication or an exposure to medications
Psychotic disorder due to another medical condition	Occurrence of hallucinations and/or delusions related to another medical condition
Other specified psychotic disorder	Patient has symptoms characteristic of schizophrenia spectrum disorders; the symptoms do not fill the full criteria of any of the disorders in the group; however, a specific related disorder can be specified
Unspecified psychotic disorder	Patient has symptoms characteristic of schizophrenia spectrum disorders; the symptoms do not fill the full criteria of any of the disorders in the group and a specific related disorder is not specified
Catatonia	Catatonia is not an independent disease entity but rather a condition that can accompany a psychotic disorder, a bipolar disorder, a depressive disorder or other mental disorders as well as a medical condition; it is regarded as a specifier (feature) of the specific disorder The essential features of catatonia are psychomotor disturbances ranging from retarded activity to hyperactivity The diagnosis of catatonia is established by the occurrence of at least 4 symptoms from a list of 12 aberrant motor symptoms (stupor, mutism, posturing, catalepsy, waxy flexibility, agitation, stereotypy, grimacing, echolalia, echopraxia, mannerism, negativism)

antipsychotics. Schizoaffective disorders are treated with antipsychotics, mood stabilisers (e.g. lithium, which is rarely used) and antidepressants (Murru et al. 2011). Table 10.11 lists the approved medications for the various psychotic presentations (e.g. schizophrenia, schizophrenia-related psychoses, schizoaffective disorders, secondary psychoses). The management of psychoses related to affective disorder is discussed further in the text. Some issues regarding the choice of an antipsychotic and its administration route are discussed in Table 10.12.

For dosage ranges and routes of administration see Table 10.4.

Bipolar and related disorders

Bipolar disorders are characterised by periods of elevated mood and periods of depression. The 'building blocks' of these disorders are manic episodes, hypomanic episodes and major depressive episodes (see Table 10.13).

Table 10.14 describes the major disorders in this category.

Treating bipolar disorders is aimed at the current episode (either manic/hypomanic or depressive) and at stabilising and preventing the occurrence of further episodes. The major drugs used are lithium, anti-epileptics and antipsychotics. The use of antidepressants for the treatment of depressive episodes is controversial as these medications can cause a switch from a depressive episode to a manic/hypomanic episode (McInerney & Kennedy 2014), and currently pharmacological interventions for bipolar depression are relatively limited (Frye et al. 2014). Table 10.15 lists the different psychotropic drugs approved for bipolar disorders.

TABLE 10.11 Psychotropic agents in schizophrenia and related disorders

Condition	Approved antipsychotics – 1st generation	Approved antipsychotics – 2nd generation
Schizophrenia	Chlorpromazine hydrochloride, droperidol, flupenthixol decanoate, fluphenazine, haloperidol, trifluoperazine hydrochloride, zuclopenthixol	Amisulpiride, aripiprazole, aripiprazole monohydrate, asenapine, clozapine, lurasidone, olanzapine, olanzapine pamoate monohydrate, paliperidone, paliperidone palmitate, quetiapine, risperidone, ziprasidone
Schizoaffective disorder		Paliperidone
Schizophrenia-related psychoses	Chlorpromazine hydrochloride, droperidol, flupenthixol, haloperidol, trifluoperazine hydrochloride	Amisulpiride, olanzapine, risperidone, ziprasidone
Secondary psychoses (e.g. following brain damage)	Droperidol, haloperidol, trifluoperazine hydrochloride	
Psychoses in general	Droperidol, haloperidol decanoate, pericyazine, zuclopenthixol	

TABLE 10.12 Choosing an antipsychotic medication

'Issue'	Clinical recommendations
First- or second-generation antipsychotic?	The common practice is initiating therapy with a second-generation antipsychotic such as risperidone, olanzapine, quetiapine, amisulpride or aripiprazole (see the Australian and New Zealand guidelines [Royal Australian and New Zealand College of Psychiatrists 2005]) This is probably due to the lower risk of extrapyramidal side effects and not due to superiority in alleviating negative symptoms (Attard & Taylor 2012)
Which second-generation antipsychotic to prescribe first?	Olanzapine is somewhat more efficacious compared with aripiprazole, quetiapine, risperione and ziprazidone and is second only to clozapine (Leucht et al. 2009); however, its serious metabolic side effects should be considered
When to prescribe clozapine?	Clozapine is unique in its effect in the treatment resistant population and is usually reserved as a third-line drug due to its dangerous haematological side effects (Attard & Taylor 2012; Royal Australian and New Zealand College of Psychiatrists 2005)
Long-acting or short-acting antipsychotic formulations?	Long-acting formulations (first-generation: flupenthixol decanoate, haloperidol decanoate, zuclopenthixol decanoate; second-generation: olanzapine pamoate, risperidone depot) are used to improve compliance in patients with low adherence to therapy regimen (Kulkarni & Reeve-Parker 2015)
Are there specific interventions for negative symptoms in schizophrenia?	Negative symptoms are generally treatment resistant Clozapine, amisulpride and asenapine can be of benefit (Davis, Horan & Marder 2014)
How to treat catatonia?	Catatonia is treated with either benzodiazepines (in particular lorazepam) or electroconvulsive therapy Antipsychotics are relatively contraindicated and might cause deterioration in the patient's condition Catatonia is an acute life-threatening condition and requires hospitalisation and immediate intervention (Sienaert et al. 2014).

Depressive disorders

The hallmark of depressive disorders is the occurrence of depressed mood, which can be both acute and dramatic as in major depressive disorder or chronic as in persistent depressive disorder. Table 10.16 lists the various disorders in this category.

Current pharmacological interventions in treating depression modulate aminergic transmission (noradrenergic, serotonergic or dopaminergic). Therapy can follow general guidelines or be tailored and individualised to the patient (Malhi et al. 2013).

Most guidelines and treating protocols recommend starting with an SSRI. If the outcome of this intervention is not satisfactory, the clinician may choose to add an antidepressant from another group or switch to another antidepressant, either an SSRI or from another group. In severe resistant cases therapy can be augmented with lithium or T_3 (thyroid hormone), electroconvulsive therapy (ECT) can be administered and MAO-A inhibitors can be used. Psychotherapy

TABLE 10.13 The building blocks of mood disorders

Episode type	Description
Manic episode	A distinct period of at least 1 week with abnormally and persistently elevated, expansive or irritable mood with increased activity During this episode at least 3 of the following 7 criteria are observed: 1) inflated self-esteem, 2) decreased sleep, 3) talking more than usual, 4) racing thoughts, 5) distractability, 6) increased goal-directed activity, 7) involvement in activities that might have painful consequences Manic episodes have severe consequences and often lead to hospitalisation A mixed manic episode is a manic episode accompanied by some features of a depressive episode; psychotic or catatonic features can accompany a manic episode (see the section 'Schizophrenia spectrum and other psychotic disorders')
Hypomanic episode	Hypomanic episodes are similar to manic episodes but are briefer (up to 4 days) and less severe A mixed hypomanic episode is a manic episode accompanied by some features of a depressive episode
Major depressive episode	Major depressive episodes are a period of at least 2 weeks with either depressed mood or inability to enjoy life accompanied by some of the following symptoms: problems in eating and sleeping, psychomotor agitation or retardation, impaired concentration, low energy, guilt feelings and feeling of worthlessness, suicidal thoughts A mixed major depressive episode is a depressive episode accompanied with some features of a manic episode; psychotic or catatonic features can accompany a major depressive episode (see the section 'Schiozphrenia spectrum and other psychotic disorders')

can be added to therapy in any stage. Table 10.17 illustrates a treating algorithm based on the Sequenced Treatment Alternative to Relieve Depression (STAR*D) trial, a large scale, long-term study assessing depression treatments in both primary and specialty care (Sinyor, Schaffer & Levitt 2010). This study is of major importance in the current approach to treating depression and is therefore included here, although neither bupropion nor buspirone, which were prescribed in this study, are indicated for depression in Australia.

Personalised and individually tailored therapy is based on multiple parameters including patients' previous therapy and the profile of the patients' symptoms. The clinician chooses the antidepressant based on its side effects profile, doing this in an attempt to relieve the bothersome symptoms (i.e. a sedating SSRI such as paroxetine for a patient with severe insomnia; an activating NARI such as reboxetine for an obtunded patient with psychomotor retardation) (Malhi et al. 2013). There is some evidence for prescribing certain antidepressants for specific subtypes of major depressive disorder (i.e. MAO-A inhibitors for atypical depression, characterised by significant weight gain, hypersomnia, sensitivity to interpersonal rejection and leaden paralysis [Shulman, Herrmann & Walker 2013]). Discontinuation of the therapy should be done gradually, to minimise 'discontinuation syndrome'.

TABLE 10.14 Bipolar and related disorders

Disorder	Description
Bipolar I	The diagnosis requires at least one manic episode; depressive episodes are not required although most patients experience or will experience a major depressive episode as well
Bipolar II	Patients must meet the criteria for a current or past hypomanic episode as well as current or past major depressive episode; a manic episode was never experienced
Cyclothymic disorder	Patients suffer from substantial and distinct mood swings with either depressive or manic symptoms; however, these episodes never meet the full criteria of a major depressive episode, manic episode or hypomanic episode
Substance-/ medication-induced bipolar disorder	Manic-/hypomanic-like episode with or without depressed mood following substance intoxication or an exposure to medications An exception is the occurrence of a manic or hypomanic episode following the use of antidepressants, which might suggest a 'true' bipolar disorder
Bipolar disorder due to another medical condition	Manic-/hypomanic-like episode related to another medical condition
Other specified bipolar and related disorder	The patient has symptoms characteristic of bipolar and related disorders; the symptoms do not fill the full criteria of any of the disorders in the group; however, a specific related disorder can be specified
Unspecified bipolar and related disorder	The patient has symptoms characteristic of bipolar and related disorders; the symptoms do not fill the full criteria of any of the disorders in the group and a specific related disorder is not specified

TABLE 10.15 Psychotropic agents used to treat bipolar disorders

Group	Drug	Common adult dosage range	Comments
		Acute mania	
Lithuim	Lithium carbonate	500–2000 mg/day	Monitor lithium levels
First-generation antipsychotics	Chlorpromazine	75–800 mg/day	Indicated for mania with psychosis
	Droperidol	5–25 mg/day	Intramuscular
	Haloperidol	2–100 mg/day	
	Zuclopenthixol acetate	Up to 150 mg per injection (maximum 4 doses/4 weeks)	

TABLE 10.15 Psychotropic agents used to treat bipolar disorders—cont'd

Group	Drug	Common adult dosage range	Comments
Second-generation antipsychotics	Aripiprazole	15–30 mg/day	+/– Lithium or valproate Manic episode +/– mixed features
	Asenapine	5–20 mg/day	+/– Lithium or valproate Manic episode +/– mixed features
	Quetiapine	200–800 mg/day	+/– Lithium or valproate Manic episode +/– mixed features
	Olanzapine	5–20 mg/day	+/– Lithium or valproate Manic episode +/– mixed features
	Risperidone	2–6 mg/day	
	Ziprasidone	Up to 80 mg/day	Manic episode or manic episode with mixed features
Anticonvulsants	Carbamazepine	400–1600 mg/day	
	Valproate	750–1500 mg/day	
Bipolar depression			
Second-generation antipsychotic	Quetiapine	50–600 mg	This is the only medication approved for bipolar depression in Australia; in other parts of the world lurasidone and olanzapine/fluoxetine combinations are approved for this indication (Frye et al. 2014)
Maintenance			
Lithium	Lithium carbonate	500–2000 mg	Maintenance usually 500–1000 mg/day Monitor lithium levels
Second-generation antipsychotics	Aripiprazole	15–30 mg/day	Can be used as monotherapy
	Asenapine	5–20 mg/day	+/– lithium or valproate
	Quetiapine	300–800 mg/day	+/– lithium or valproate
	Olanzapine	5–20 mg/day	
	Risperidone	50 mg every 2 weeks	Long-acting depot
Anticonvulsants	Carbamezapine	400–1600 mg/day	
	Lamotrigine	200 mg/day	Slow titration due to severe rash (Stevens–Johnson syndrome), especially when combined with valproate
	Valproate	750–1500 mg/day	

TABLE 10.16 Depressive disorders according to DSM 5

Disorder	Description
Major depressive disorder	Patients who have had one or more major depressive episodes (see Table 10.13 for description of a major depressive episode) without the occurrence of a manic or hypomanic episode Psychotic features can accompany the clinical presentation
Persistent depressive disorder (dysthymia)	Persistent mood lasting for at least 2 years (in adults); the occurrence of a major depressive episode during this period does not exclude this diagnosis
Premenstrual dysphoric disorder (PMDD)	Symptoms of depression and anxiety that appear in most of the menstrual cycles in the week before menses and improve within a few days after menses
Disruptive mood dysregulation disorder	This childhood disorder is characterised by a combination of temper outbursts with irritable and angry mood; it is included among the depressive disorders as children with this disorder are at risk for developing depressive disorders
Substance-/ medication-induced depressive disorder	Depression-like episode following substance intoxication or an exposure to medications
Depressive disorder due to another medical condition	Depression-like episode as a direct consequence of another medical condition
Other specified depressive disorder	The patient has symptoms characteristic of depression and the symptoms do not fill the full criteria of any of the disorders in the group; however, a specific related disorder can be specified
Unspecified depressive disorder	The patient has symptoms characteristic of a depressive disorder; the symptoms do not fill the full criteria of any of the disorders in the group and a specific related disorder is not specified

TABLE 10.17 Depression treating algorithm based on STAR*D

Level	Intervention
Level 1	Citalopram (SSRI)
Level 2 – Augmentation	Buspirone[a]/bupropion (NDRI)/cognitive behavioural therapy
Level 2 – Switch	Bupropion (NDRI)/venlafaxine (SNRI)/sertraline/cognitive behavioural therapy
Level 3 – Augmentation	Lithium/T_3
Level 3 – Switch	Nortriptyline (TCA)/mirtazapine (NaSSA)
Level 4	Tranylcypromine (MAO-I)/venlafaxine (SNRI) + mirtazapine (NaSSA)

[a]*Buspirone is an anxiolytic drug with serotonergic activity (Loane & Politis 2012).*
MAO-I, mono-amine oxidase A inhibitor; NARI, noradrenaline reuptake inhibitor; NaSSA, noradrenergic and specific serotonergic antidepressant; NDRI, noradrenaline dopamine reuptake inhibitor; SNRI, serotonin noradrenaline reuptake inhibitor; SSRI, selective serotonin reuptake inhibitor; TCA, tricyclic antidepressant.

Table 10.18 lists the various antidepressants used for depressive disorders.

Anxiety disorders

Anxiety can be a normal reaction to stress. However, in anxiety disorders this reaction is exaggerated and may cause impairment to the function and wellbeing of the individual. Table 10.19 describes the various anxiety disorders. Anxiety disorders are treated by a combination of anxiolytics, usually benzodiazepines, antidepressants and psychological interventions (CBT). Benzodiazepines have a direct and a fast effect. However, due to their addictive potential and the developing tolerance to their effect, they are not indicated for long-term use. This is in contrast to the antidepressants, which take time to build their effect and do not carry the risk of tolerance and addiction. Antipsychotics can also be used to relieve anxiety. Table 10.20 lists the approved drugs for these disorders (in Australia).

Obsessive–compulsive and related disorders

This group of disorders share together intrusive thoughts accompanied by time-consuming repetitive behaviours. These disorders cause significant anxiety. The prototype of these disorders, obsessive–compulsive disorder, was included in the previous version of DSM in the section of anxiety disorders (American Psychiatric Association 2000). The disorders are described in Table 10.21.

Obsessive–compulsive disorder is regarded as a serotonergic disorder (Westenberg, Fineberg & Denys 2007) and treated accordingly with various SSRIs and with clomipramine (see Table 10.22), a highly serotonergic TCA. The dosage required to treat obsessive–compulsive disorder is usually higher than that required for depression and the response time is longer. Refractory cases might need dose elevation, off-label augmentation with antipsychotic medications, switch to a SNRI or combination with CBT (Fineberg et al. 2013, 2015; Soomro 2012). CBT for obsessive–compulsive disorder is based on exposure and response prevention, a technique in which patients are exposed to the thoughts, images and situations that make them anxious, and are required to not react by the compulsive behaviour (McKay et al. 2015). There is no clear-cut literature regarding whether combination therapy of CBT with an SSRI improves symptoms compared with each treatment alone (Soomro 2012).

There are no approved medications for the treatment of body dysmorphic disorder, hoarding disorder, trichotillomania and skin picking disorder. However, many studies suggest a similar strategy as with obsessive–compulsive disorder (Dougherty et al. 2006; Fang, Matheny & Wilhelm 2014; Keuthen et al. 2015; Mataix-Cols 2014; Rothbart & Stein 2014; Spiegel & Finklea 2009).

Trauma- and stress-related disorders

The hallmark of this group of disorders is the emergence of psychiatric reaction following exposure to trauma or stress. Reactive attachment disorder and disinhibited social engagement disorder follow childhood neglect by an adult caregiver. As there are no indicated pharmacological interventions for these childhood disorders and as the mainstay of therapy is psychosocial, they are described here only in brief (Zeanah & Gleason 2015). Posttraumatic stress

Text continued on p. 301

TABLE 10.18 Psychotropic agents used to treat depressive disorder

Group	Drug	Common adult dosage range
	Major depression	
SSRI	Citalopram	Up to 40 mg/day
	Escitalopram	10–20 mg/day
	Fluoxetine	20–80 mg/day
	Fluvoxamine	50–150 mg/day
	Paroxetine	20–50 mg/day
	Sertraline	50–200 mg/day
TCA	Amitriptyline	50–150 mg/day (hospitalised patients 100–300 mg/day)
	Clomipramine	25 mg/day
	Doxepin	30–300 mg/day
	Imipramine	25–200 mg/day
	Nortriptyline	25–100 mg/day
	Trimipramine	50–100 mg/day (hospitalised patients 75–300 mg/day)
	Dothiepin	25–200 mg daily
SNRI	Desvenlafaxine	50–400 mg/day
	Duloxetine	60 mg/day
	Venlafaxine	75–225 mg/day
NaSSA	Mianserin hydrochloride	30–120 mg/day
	Mirtazapine	15–60 mg/day
MAO inhibitors	Phenelzine (irreversible)	15–90 mg/day
	Tranylcypromine (irreversible)	10–30 mg/day
	Moclobemide (reversible)	300–600 mg daily
Other	Agomelatine (melatonergic)	25–50 mg daily
	Reboxetine (NARI)	4–10 mg daily
	Vortioxetine (serotonin modulator and stimulator)	5–20 mg daily
	Chlorpromazine (first-generation antipsychotic used for psychotic depression)	75–800 mg daily
	Premenstrual dysphoric disorder	
SSRI	Fluoxetine	20 mg daily (14 days before to 1st full day of menses)
	Sertraline	50–150 mg daily (14 days before to 1st full day of menses)

MAO, mono-amine oxidase; NARI, noradrenaline reuptake inhibitor; NaSSA, noradrenergic and specific serotonergic antidepressant; SNRI, serotonin noradrenaline reuptake inhibitor; SSRI, selective serotonin reuptake inhibitor; TCA, tricyclic antidepressant.

TABLE 10.19 Anxiety disorders

Disorder	Description
Separation anxiety disorder	A predominantly childhood diagnosis in which the individual experiences excessive anxiety when separated from home or from an attachment figure
Selective mutism	The individual, despite normal language abilities, fails to speak in certain situations, usually of social nature; this condition lasts for more than a month and leads to impaired social, educational and occupational achievements
Specific phobia	Exaggerated and unreasonable fear related to exposure to an object, place or situation such as certain animals, insects, closed places, elevator rides and heights Exposure to such stimuli can cause an immediate anxiety response such as panic attack and end in avoidance behavior; this pattern interferes with the individual's daily life
Social anxiety disorder (social phobia)	Marked fear or anxiety related to social situations in which others might scrutinise the individual, leading to avoidance of such situations
Panic disorder (and panic attacks)	Panic disorder is characterised by recurrent panic attacks A panic attack is an episode of intense fear, developing within minutes and during which at least 4 of the following 13 symptoms occur: palpitations, sweating, trembling/shaking, shortness of breath, feeling of choking, chest pain, nausea/abdominal distress, dizziness, paraesthesiae, de-realisation (feelings of unreality)/depersonalisation (feeling detached from oneself), fear of 'going crazy' and fear of dying Some panic attacks are followed by at least 1 month of a behavioural change (avoidance of situations perceived as related to the attacks) and persistent concern or worry The attacks are not attributable to other anxiety disorders Panic attacks can occur in other anxiety disorders; in these instances they are recorded as a specifier of the disorder
Agoraphobia	A long-standing fear of more than 6 months duration related to being alone or away from home in situations such as a bus ride, standing in line, being in open spaces (i.e. parking lot), being in enclosed places (i.e. shopping malls, cinema) The fear leads the individual to avoid such situations; if unable to avoid the situation, the individual might suffer from anxiety and fear
Generalised anxiety disorder	A pattern of more than 6 months duration of excessive worrying about issues such as health concerns, finance and the wellbeing of family members This is accompanied by physical and mental complaints (restlessness, muscle tension, being easily fatigued, impaired concentration, sleep disturbances, irritability) and leads to significant distress and impaired functioning
Substance-/medication-induced anxiety disorder	Anxiety or panic attacks following the use of a certain medication or substance
Anxiety disorder due to another medical condition	Anxiety or panic attacks developing as a direct outcome of another medical condition
Other specified anxiety disorder	The patient has symptoms characteristic of an anxiety disorder and these symptoms do not fill the full criteria of any of the disorders in the group; however, a specific related disorder can be specified
Unspecified anxiety disorder	The patient has symptoms characteristic of an anxiety disorder; the symptoms do not fill the full criteria of any of the disorders in the group and a specific related disorder is not specified

TABLE 10.20 Common adult dosage ranges for psychotropic agents used to treat anxiety disorders

Drug	Anxiety general	General anxiety disorder	Panic disorder	Phobia	Social anxiety
Benzodiazepines					
Alprazolam	0.5–4 mg/day		Maximum 10 mg/day	Maximum 10 mg/day	
Bromazepam	6–9 mg/day				
Clozabam	10–30 mg/day				
Diazepam	Maximum 45 mg/day				
Lorazepam	1–10 mg/day				
Oxazepam	60–120 mg/day				
Antidepressants – SSRIs					
Escitalopram		10–20 mg/day			10–20 mg/day
Paroxetine		20–50 mg/day	40–60 mg/day		20–50 mg/day
Sertraline			50 mg/day		50 mg/day
Antidepressants – SNRIs					
Duloxetine		30–120 mg/day			
Venlafaxine		75–225 mg/day	37.5–75 mg/day		75–225 mg/day
Antidepressants – TCA					
Clomipramine				100–150 mg/day	
Antipsychotics					
Quetiapine		50–300 mg/day			
Peryciazine	Maximum 75 mg/day				
Trifluoperazine	2–6 mg/day (outpatients) Maximum 20 mg/day (inpatients)				

SNRI, serotonin noradrenaline reuptake inhibitor; SSRI, selective serotonin reuptake inhibitor; TCA, tricyclic antidepressant.

TABLE 10.21 Obsessive–compulsive and related disorders

Disorder	Description
Obsessive–compulsive disorder	The patient suffers from a combination of obsessions and compulsions that are time-consuming and cause significant distress Obsessions are thoughts, images or urges that at some time are felt as intrusive and the patient tries to suppress or ignore them Compulsions are behaviours or mental acts that are performed to reduce anxiety related to obsessions Common obsessions are those related to contamination, symmetry, forbidden/taboo thoughts and harm
Body dysmorphic disorder	Patients believe unjustifiably that they have a flaw in their body and devote much time attending their body (i.e. looking at a mirror, grooming, skin picking and/or comparing their appearance with others)
Hoarding disorder	Continuous accumulation of objects, regardless of their actual value There is 1) a perceived need to save the objects and 2) distress associated with discarding them The accumulated objects congest and clutter the living areas ending in significant distress and impairment
Trichotillomania (hair-pulling disorder)	Recurrent hair pulling and repeated attempts to decrease or stop this behaviour
Excoriation (skin-picking) disorder	Recurrent skin picking resulting in skin lesions with repeated attempts to decrease or stop this behaviour
Substance-/ medication-induced obsessive–compulsive and related disorder	Obsessive–compulsive and related disorder-like symptoms (obsessions, compulsions, skin picking, hair pulling, body-focused behaviours) following substance intoxication or an exposure to medications
Obsessive–compulsive and related disorder due to another medical condition	Obsessive–compulsive and related disorder-like symptoms due to another medical condition
Other specified obsessive–compulsive and related disorder	The patient has symptoms characteristic of an obsessive–compulsive and related disorder and these symptoms do not fill the full criteria of any of the disorders in the group; however, a specific related disorder can be specified
Unspecified obsessive–compulsive and related disorder	The patient has symptoms characteristic of an obsessive–compulsive and related disorder; the symptoms do not fill the full criteria of any of the disorders in the group and a specific related disorder is not specified

disorder (PTSD) and acute stress disorder follow a severe trauma, and adjustment disorders follow an identifiable stressor such as business difficulties or marital problems. The disorders are listed in Table 10.23.

The pharmacological management of posttraumatic stress disorders may include antidepressants, antipsychotics, anti-anxiety medications and antihypertensive drugs (used to alleviate arousal and nightmares). See Table 10.24 for a detailed description.

Regarding acute stress disorders, there are no indicated pharmacological interventions. In addition, there is a major controversy as to whether interventions

TABLE 10.22 Psychotropic agents indicated for obsessive–compulsive disorders

Group	Drug	Common adult dosage range
SSRI	Escitalopram	10–20 mg/day
	Fluoxetine	20–80 mg/day
	Fluvoxamine	100–300 mg/day
	Paroxetine	40–60 mg/day
	Sertraline	50–200 mg/day
TCA	Clomipramine	100–150 mg/day

SSRI, selective serotonin reuptake inhibitor; TCA, tricyclic antidepressant.

TABLE 10.23 Trauma- and stressor-related disorders

Disorder	Description
Reactive attachment disorder	Following childhood neglect and insufficient care the child is inhibited toward the adult caregiver and does not seek comfort from them
Disinhibited social engagement disorder	Following childhood neglect and insufficient care the child is disinhibited and fails to show normal shyness in the company of unfamiliar adults
Posttraumatic stress disorder	Following involvement or exposure to severe trauma the patient has multiple symptoms including re-experiencing the trauma through dreams, flashbacks and distressing memories; avoidance of stimuli related to the trauma; negative alterations in cognition or mood (i.e. amnesia to the event, negative beliefs, detachment from others, inability to experience positive emotions, emotional numbing); alterations in arousal and reactivity such as irritability, increased startle response, impaired concentration, hypervigilance All of these might be accompanied by dissociative symptoms (depersonalisation – feeling detached from oneself; de-realisation – experiencing reality as unreal) and last longer than 1 month
Acute stress disorder	Similar to posttraumatic stress disorder but in a more acute time course (3 days to 1 month) following exposure to the trauma
Adjustment disorders	Following an identifiable stressor, the patient suffers from anxiety, depressed mood, conduct disturbances or any combination of the aforementioned Adjustment disorders start within 3 months from the onset of the stressor and should resolve by 6 months following its termination Stressors vary from acute stressors such as death of a loved one, moving, divorce, retirement and accident to chronic stressors such as unemployment, financial difficulties, chronic illness and illness of a relative (Maercker et al. 2012) A comprehensive list of stressors with their severity ranking can be found in the Holmes and Rahe Stress Scale (Holmes & Rahe 1967)
Other specified trauma- and stressor-related disorder	The patient has symptoms characteristic of trauma- and stressor-related disorders and these symptoms do not fill the full criteria of any of the disorders in the group; however, a specific related disorder can be specified
Unspecified trauma- and stressor-related disorder	The patient has symptoms characteristic of trauma- and stressor-related disorders; the symptoms do not fill the full criteria of any of the disorders in the group and a specific related disorder is not specified

TABLE 10.24 Psychotropic agents used to treat posttraumatic stress disorders

Group	Drugs	Comments
Antidepressants	SSRIs: Paroxetine (20–50 mg/day)	SSRIs are the only group of drugs with a substantial body of evidence supporting their use in PTSD; SNRIs such as venlafaxine may also be of use (Sullivan & Neria 2009)
Atypical antipsychotics	Quetiapine, clozapine, risperidone	Reserved for complex and treatment resistant cases There is some data suggesting that risperidone is the antipsychotic of choice (Ipser & Stein 2012)
Hypnosedatives	Benzodiazepines (i.e. diazepam, temazepam, alprazolam)	Used to reduce anxiety and treat insomnia; there is little evidence for the effectiveness of benzodiazepines (Sullivan & Neria 2009; Ipser & Stein 2012)
Antihypertensive drugs	Clonidine (alpha-2-adrenergic agoist), prazosin (alpha-1-adregnergic agonist), propranolol (beta-blocker)	Used to reduce physiological arousal Prazosin is used to reduce nightmares (Bajor, Ticlea & Osser 2011)

PTSD, posttraumatic stress disorder; SNRI, serotonin noradrenaline reuptake inhibitor; SSRI, selective serotonin reuptake inhibitor.
Based on the Australian Centre for Posttraumatic Mental Health, 2013. Australian Guidelines for the Treatment of Acute Stress Disorder and Posttraumatic Stress Disorder <*http://www.phoenixaustralia.org*> (accessed 7.04.15).

at the acute stage, such as the use of benzodiazepines to relieve anxiety, are beneficial or harmful as they might increase the chances of developing posttraumatic stress disorder (Gelpin et al. 1996). Of interest is that early administration of glucocorticoids such as hydrocortisone may help in the prevention of posttraumatic stress disorder by helping in memory consolidation (Zohar et al. 2011). Weaker evidence suggests the early use of the beta blocker propranolol (Gardner & Griffiths 2014; Hoge et al. 2012).

PHYSIOTHERAPY PRACTICE POINTS: ADJUSTMENT DISORDERS

Adjustment disorders are of special interest in the practice of physiotherapy. Recent physical illness can lead to a maladaptive psychological emotional response culminating in an adjustment disorder. The prevalence of adjustment disorders in consultation liaison psychiatry is very high and can reach, in certain populations, up to 35% (Okamura et al. 2000). In the acutely ill it is almost three times as prevalent as depressive disorders (13.7%, 5.1% respectively) (Silverstone 1996). The physiotherapist, while treating these patients and addressing their somatic rehabilitation, is in a crucial position and can help in early diagnosis and intervention. The patients can be treated symptomatically for anxiety, insomnia and depressive mood with benzodiazepines and antidepressants (Casey 2009; Casey & Bailey 2011).

Somatic symptom and related disorders

All disorders in this group share the prominence of somatic symptoms that are related to psychological factors. Individuals suffering from these disorders usually present to primary care and general medical settings and therefore are of great relevance to the physiotherapist. Table 10.25 describes this group of disorders.

TABLE 10.25 Somatic symptom and related disorders

Disorder	Description
Somatic symptom disorder	The patient suffers from at least one distressing somatic symptom and is excessively occupied with it; this is manifested by disproportionately thinking about the symptom and its severity, exaggerated anxiety related to the symptom and overly immersing oneself in behaviours related to the symptom (i.e. multiple doctor visits and consultations) The duration of the disorder must be at least 6 months In those cases with a significant pain component a 'pain specifier' is added to the diagnosis
Illness anxiety disorder	An excessive anxiety and preoccupation with being ill or having a major medical condition despite the lack of evidence for such a disorder; the patient might either perform multiple health-related behaviours (tests, medical encounters) or adopt an opposite behaviour and avoid medical encounters, clinics and hospitals Unlike somatic symptom disorder the patient does not experience a specific symptom or medical condition but is rather anxious about acquiring it
Conversion disorder (functional neurological symptom disorder)	Patients with this disorder suffer from a neurological deficit or symptom that is incompatible with a neurological or medical condition and cannot be explained by an organic cause; the deficit can be either motor, sensory, seizure-like, impairment in gait, impairment in speech or mixed; a psychological stressor can accompany the presentation This is in contrast with previous editions of the DSM, in which a psychological factor or conflict was required for the diagnosis of this disorder; in this regard DSM-5 is less committed to psychoanalytical thinking, according to which these disorders are a conversion of a psychodynamic conflict into a somatic symptom (American Psychiatric Association 2000; Freud 1910) These disorders are of special interest for the physiotherapist. See further discussion in this section
Psychological factors affecting another medical condition	A physical symptom or illness is adversely affected by a psychological or behavioural factor; clinical examples are a patient with diabetes who manipulates the dosage of insulin in order to lose weight or a patient who refrains from a medical test due to denial of his illness or anxiety
Factitious disorder	Patients simulate symptoms and falsify a medical or psychological condition, not only for a secondary gain (an obvious external reward) but rather for a primary psychologically motivated gain (adopting a sick role)
Other specified somatic symptom and related disorder	A somatic symptom and related disorder-like presentation in which the symptoms are characteristic for a specific disorder but do not meet the criteria for this disorder
Unspecified somatic symptom and related disorder	A somatic symptom and related disorder-like presentation that does not meet the criteria for any of the disorders and a specific disorder cannot be specified

The mainstay of therapy for these disorders is psychotherapy in various forms (psychodynamic, CBT), hypnosis and rehabilitation programs. The use of psychotropic drugs is limited to treating concomitant depression or anxiety. There is only minimal evidence for the application of new generation antidepressants such as the SSRIs (Kleinstauber et al. 2014). However, in somatic disorders with a significant component of pain, it is advisable to choose antidepressants with some pain modulation features such as an SNRI (Somashekar, Jainer & Wuntakal 2013).

PHYSIOTHERAPY PRACTICE POINTS: CONVERSION DISORDERS

Conversion disorders (functional neurological symptom disorder) are common in the physiotherapist's practice and can account for up to 10% of the caseload in certain clinical settings (Edwards, Stone & Nielsen 2012). A psychological minded approach is highly recommended, as the way patients with these disorders are approached has high impact on their prognosis (Nielsen et al. 2015). A combination of physiotherapy and psychotherapy is recommended for a large proportion of patients (de Schipper et al. 2014). Patients with signs of depression or anxiety can benefiet from antidepressants or anxioltyics (Rosebush & Mazurek 2011).

Insomnia

Insomnia is a common disorder with multiple aetiologies. It is defined as a difficulty in falling asleep, staying asleep or early morning awakening, leading to dissatisfaction with sleep quantity or quality (American Psychiatric Association 2013). The management of insomnia requires assessment of possible aetiologies (i.e. mental disorders such as depression, current stressors, change of medications) and evaluation of its chronicity, as chronic insomnia is less responsive to pharmacological interventions. Sleep disorders might also be due to various neurological disturbances, in particular posttraumatic brain injury (TBI). Following TBI insomnia is most prevalent during and after the period of posttraumatic amnesia (PTA). PTA symptoms can include excessive daytime sleepiness, extreme drowsiness, delayed sleep phase syndrome, mixed-up sleep patterns (Ouellet, Beaulieu-Bonneau & Morin 2015). Changes in behaviour and environment are the first line in treating sleep difficulties in this patient group. Treatment of insomnia encompasses a wide variety of interventions from cognitive behavioral therapy (CBT) to sleep-inducing medications (Cunnington, Junge & Fernando 2013; Brasure et al. 2015). The first-line medications are benzodiazepines and the Z-drugs; however, due to issues of dependence and tolerance, it is advisable to limit the use of these drugs, especially the benzodiazepines. Other pharmacological options are highly sedating antidepressants or antipsychotics as well as antihistamines, melatonin and orexin (see Table 10.26).

PHYSIOTHERAPY PRACTICE POINTS: INSOMNIA

A large number of patients receiving physiotherapy may also be suffering insomnia for many of the reasons outlined above. As well as an understanding of the pharmacological management of this condition the treating physiotherapist should also attempt to time the patient's physiotherapeutic treatment schedule to coincide with times when the patient will be least tired. In addition it is important to note that sleep plays an important role in the process of procedural learning; it has been implicated in the continued development of motor-skill learning following initial acquisition. Improvement in motor skill performance is known to continue for at least 24 hours following training; accordingly, a good night's sleep can improve the outcome of physiotherapy (Gudberg & Johansen-Berg 2015).

The treating physiotherapist should also be aware of the possible after effects of sleep medications (i.e. tiredness and lethargy the morning after taking the medication).

TABLE 10.26 Pharmacological interventions for insomnia

Group	Drug	Common adult dosage	Approval for insomnia?	Notes
Benzodiazepines	Flunitrazepam	0.5–2 mg/day	+	See previous sections
	Nitrazepam	2.5–10 mg/day	+	See previous sections
	Temazepam	7.5–30 mg/day	+	See previous sections
	Triazolam	0.125–0.5 mg/day	+	See previous sections
Z-drugs	Eszopiclone	1–3 mg/day	+	See previous sections
	Zelplon	5–20 mg/day	+	See previous sections
	Zolpidem	5–10 mg/day	+	See previous sections
	Zopiclone	5–20 mg/day	+	See previous sections
Antidepressants	Amitriptyline	Minimal dosage	Off label	See Table 10.7
	Doxepine	3–10 mg/day	FDA approved for insomnia	See Table 10.7
	Mirtazapine	Minimal dosages	Off label	See Table 10.7
	Trimipramine	Minimal dosages	Off label	See Table 10.7
Antipsychotics	Olanzapine	Minimal dosages	Off label	See Tables 10.4, 10.5
	Quetiapine	Minimal dosages	Off label	See Tables 10.4, 10.5
Antihistamines	Diphenhydramine	25–50 mg/day	+	Marketed with paracetamol and indicated for pain-associated insomnia
	Doxylamine	25–50 mg/day	+	
Miscellaneous	Melatonin	2–3 mg/day	+	Modulating sleep–wake cycle
	Suvorexant	5–20 mg/day	+	Antagonises orexin receptors

Adapted from: Cunnington, D., Junge, M.F., Fernando, A.T., 2013. Insomnia: prevalence, consequences and effective treatment. Medical Journal of Australia 199 (8), S36–40. Brasure, M., MacDonald, R., Fuchs, E., et al., 2015. Management of Insomnia Disorder. Comparative Effectiveness Review No. 159. AHRQ Publication No. 15(16)-EHC027- EF. Agency for Healthcare Research and Quality, Rockville, MD. <www.effectivehealthcare.ahrq.gov/reports/final.cfm>.

■ Psychiatric disorders with sensory motor deficits and psychopharmacological management

The first part of this section describes mental disorders with sensory motor deficits. It is crucial that the physiotherapist be aware of these presentations not only because they can be a target of therapy but also as they can be confused with drug side effects. The second part of this section looks at the major sensory and motor side effects of psychopharmacological interventions.

Psychiatric disorders with sensory motor deficits

Aside from the somatic symptoms and related disorders (see previous section), there are many psychiatric conditions and disorders that are accompanied by motor and sensory symptoms. These might be encountered in non-psychiatric clinical settings and the psychiatric component of the presentation might not be clear from onset. Many of these patients are referred to physiotherapy and the physiotherapist can help in early diagnosis and intervention for these patients. Table 10.27 lists these conditions.

TABLE 10.27 Sensory motor psychiatric presentations

Presentation	Encountered in...
Changes in motor activity (either psychomotor agitation or retardation)	One of the criteria for major depressive disorder is psychomotor agitation and retardation; an extreme case of motor retardation is found in depression with atypical features in which there are heavy, leaden feelings in arms or legs Anxiety disorders with severe agitation
Disorganised motor behaviour	Psychotic disorders
Catatonia	Psychotic disorders Affective disorders
Unexplained neurological deficits and symptoms	Conversion disorder To some extent in panic attack (paraesthesiae, feeling dizzy, unsteady)
Concern about somatic symptoms (present or future)	Somatic symptom disorders Body dysmorphic disorders Illness anxiety disorders
Muscle tension	General anxiety disorders
A general illness with sensory motor deficits leading to psychiatric presentations	Psychiatric conditions 'due to another medical condition' Adjustment disorders secondary to a general illness Posttraumatic stress disorder and acute stress disorder where the stressor is a medical illness with motor sensory deficits (Kiphuth et al. 2014; Vickrey & Williams 2014)
Impairment in the way one's own body is perceived (depersonalisation, impaired body image)	Dissociative disorders Posttraumatic stress disorders Acute stress disorder Psychotic disorders with somatic delusions Eating disorders (patients with eating disorders might have impaired body image[4])

Continued

[4]Further discussion of these disorders is beyond the scope of this chapter.

TABLE 10.27 Sensory motor psychiatric presentations—cont'd

Presentation	Encountered in...
Abnormal/involuntary movements	Tic disorders Motor side effects of antipsychotic drugs Psychotic disorders with delusions of control and hallucinations commanding to perform certain movements Compulsions in obsessive–compulsive disorders Skin picking disorder Trichotillomania

Major sensory and motor side effects of psychopharmacological interventions

PHYSIOTHERAPY PRACTICE POINTS: PSYCHIATRIC DISORDERS WITH SENSORY MOTOR DEFICITS

The pharmacological interventions used to treat mental disorders can influence in various ways both the interaction with patients and their clinical presentation. The table below lists these interactions. More details and specific referencing can be found in the appropriate sections in this chapter and in earlier chapters, in particular Chapter 6. In this section only a brief reference to each is mentioned.

Physiotherapists involved in the treatment of these patients, however, are in a unique position to monitor the possible effects of the drugs and must therefore be aware of all likely side effects. It is important that physiotherapists report all interactions to the treating psychiatrist.

'Domain'	Comment
Cooperation	Many drugs can lead to sedation, decreased energy (e.g. benzodiazepines, some antipsychotics and antidepressants) Impaired cooperation is also caused by drugs that lead to agitation and hyperactivity (e.g. activating antidepressants)
Hypertonicity	First-generation antipsychotics
Hypotonicity	Benzodiazepines[5]
Tremor	Lithium, antipsychotics, mood stabilisers (e.g. lamotrigine, valproate)
Impaired walking	Benzodiazepines[5] can lead to falls
Dizziness	Benzodiazpeines[5], antidepressants (e.g. SNRIs), mood stabilisers (e.g. carbamazepine)
Involuntary movements	Antipsychotics, especially first generation
Bradykinesia	Antipsychotics, especially first generation

SNRI, serotonin noradrenaline reuptake inhibitor.

---

[5]See Chapter 6 for further details on these medications.

References

Abbing-Karahagopian, V., Huerta, C., Souverein, P.C., et al., 2014. Antidepressant prescribing in five European countries: application of common definitions to assess the prevalence, clinical observations, and methodological implications. European Journal of Clinical Pharmacology 70 (7), 849–857.

Adler, R.H., 2009. Engel's biopsychosocial model is still relevant today. Journal of Psychosomatic Research 67 (6), 607–611.

Alvarez, A.S., Pagani, M., Meucci, P., 2012. The clinical application of the biopsychosocial model in mental health: a research critique. American Journal of Physical Medicine & Rehabilitation 91 (13 Suppl. 1), S173–S180.

American Psychiatric Association, 2000. Diagnostic and Statistical Manual: Mental disorders: DSM-IV-TR. American Psychiatric Association, Washington, DC.

American Psychiatric Association, 2013. Diagnostic and Statistical Manual of Mental Disorders (DSM 5), fifth ed. American Psychiatric Association, Washington, DC.

Ashton, H., 1994. Guidelines for the rational use of benzodiazepines. When and what to use. Drugs 48 (1), 25–40.

Attard, A., Taylor, D.M., 2012. Comparative effectiveness of atypical antipsychotics in schizophrenia: what have real-world trials taught us? CNS Drugs 26 (6), 491–508.

Australian Bureau of Statistics, 2009. 4327.0 – National Survey of Mental Health and Wellbeing: Users' Guide, 2007. Australian Bureau of Statistics, Canberra.

Australian Centre for Posttraumatic Mental Health, 2013. Australian Guidelines for the Treatment of Acute Stress Disorder and Posttraumatic Stress Disorder. [Internet] <http://www.phoenixaustralia.org> (accessed 07.04.15.).

Bajor, L.A., Ticlea, A.N., Osser, D.N., 2011. The Psychopharmacology Algorithm Project at the Harvard South Shore Program: an update on posttraumatic stress disorder. Harvard Review of Psychiatry 19 (5), 240–258.

Ban, T.A., 2007. Fifty years chlorpromazine: a historical perspective. Neuropsychiatric Disease and Treatment 3 (4), 495–500.

Bezchlibnyk-Butler, K.Z., Jeffries, J.J., Procyshyn, R.M., et al., 2014. Clinical Handbook of Psychotropic Drugs, twentyth ed. Hogrefe Publishing, Boston, MA.

Biondi, M., Pasquini, M., 2015. Dimensional psychopharmacology in somatising patients. Advances in Psychosomatic Medicine 34, 24–35.

Brasure, M., MacDonald, R., Fuchs, E., et al., 2015. Management of Insomnia Disorder. Comparative Effectiveness Review No. 159. AHRQ Publication No. 15(16)-EHC027- EF. Agency for Healthcare Research and Quality., Rockville, MD. [Internet] <www.effectivehealthcare.ahrq.gov/reports/final.cfm>.

Buchanan, R.W., Kreyenbuhl, J., Kelly, D.L., et al., 2010. The 2009 schizophrenia PORT psychopharmacological treatment recommendations and summary statements. Schizophrenia Bulletin 36 (1), 71–93.

Cade, J.F., 1949. Lithium salts in the treatment of psychotic excitement. Medical Journal of Australia 2 (10), 349–352.

Casey, P., 2009. Adjustment disorder: epidemiology, diagnosis and treatment. CNS Drugs 23 (11), 927–938.

Casey, P., Bailey, S., 2011. Adjustment disorders: the state of the art. World Psychiatry 10 (1), 11–18.

Charlson, F.J., Baxter, A.J., Dua, T., et al., 2015. Excess mortality from mental, neurological and substance use disorders in the Global Burden of Disease Study 2010. Epidemiology and Psychiatric Sciences 24 (2), 121–140.

Cunnington, D., Junge, M.F., Fernando, A.T., 2013. Insomnia: prevalence, consequences and effective treatment. Medical Journal of Australia 199 (8), S36–S40.

Davis, M.C., Horan, W.P., Marder, S.R., 2014. Psychopharmacology of the negative symptoms: current status and prospects for progress. European Neuropsychopharmacology 24 (5), 788–799.

de Schipper, L.J., Vermeulen, M., Eeckhout, A.M., et al., 2014. Diagnosis and management of functional neurological symptoms: the Dutch experience. Clinical Neurology and Neurosurgery 122, 106–112.

Dhir, A., 2013. Vortioxetine for the treatment of major depression. Drugs of Today 49 (12), 781–790.

Divac, N., Prostran, M., Jakovcevski, I., et al., 2014. Second-generation antipsychotics and extrapyramidal adverse effects. BioMed Research International 2014, 656370.

Dougherty, D.D., Loh, R., Jenike, M.A., et al., 2006. Single modality versus dual modality treatment for trichotillomania: sertraline, behavioral therapy, or both? The Journal of Clinical Psychiatry 67 (7), 1086–1092.

Edwards, M.J., Stone, J., Nielsen, G., 2012. Physiotherapists and patients with functional (psychogenic) motor symptoms: a survey of attitudes and interest. Journal of Neurology, Neurosurgery, and Psychiatry 83 (6), 655–658.

Engel, G.L., 1977. The need for a new medical model: a challenge for biomedicine. Science 196 (4286), 129–136.

Exeter, D., Robinson, E., Wheeler, A., 2009. Antidepressant dispensing trends in New Zealand between 2004 and 2007. Australian and New Zealand Journal of Psychiatry 43 (12), 1131–1140.

Fang, A., Matheny, N.L., Wilhelm, S., 2014. Body dysmorphic disorder. Psychiatric Clinics of North America 37 (3), 287–300.

Fanoe, S., Kristensen, D., Fink-Jensen, A., et al., 2014. Risk of arrhythmia induced by psychotropic medications: a proposal for clinical management. European Heart Journal 35 (20), 1306–1315.

Fineberg, N.A., Reghunandanan, S., Brown, A., et al., 2013. Pharmacotherapy of obsessive-compulsive disorder: evidence-based treatment and beyond. Australian and New Zealand Journal of Psychiatry 47 (2), 121–141.

Fineberg, N.A., Reghunandanan, S., Simpson, H.B., et al., 2015. Obsessive–compulsive disorder (OCD): practical strategies for pharmacological and somatic treatment in adults. Psychiatry Research 227 (1), 114–125.

Fitzgerald, P.B., 2013. Non-pharmacological biological treatment approaches to difficult-to-treat depression. Medical Journal of Australia 199 (Suppl. 6), S48–S51.

Freud, S., 1910. The Psychoanalytic View of Psychogenic Disturbance of Vision. Hogarth, London, pp. 209–218.

Frucht, S.J., 2014. Treatment of movement disorder emergencies. Neurotherapeutics 11 (1), 208–212.

Frye, M.A., Prieto, M.L., Bobo, W.V., et al., 2014. Current landscape, unmet needs, and future directions for treatment of bipolar depression. Journal of Affective Disorders 169, S17–S23.

Gabbard, G.O. (Ed.), 2009. Textbook of Psychotherapeutic Treatments. American Psychiatric Publishing, Arlington, VA.

Gahr, M., 2014. Agomelatine in the treatment of major depressive disorder: an assessment of benefits and risks. Current Neuropharmacology 12 (5), 287–398.

Gardner, A.J., Griffiths, J., 2014. Propranolol, post-traumatic stress disorder, and intensive care: incorporating new advances in psychiatry into the ICU. Critical Care : The Official Journal of the Critical Care Forum 18 (6), 698.

Gautam, S., Meena, P.S., 2011. Drug-emergent metabolic syndrome in patients with schizophrenia receiving atypical (second-generation) antipsychotics. Indian Journal of Psychiatry 53 (2), 128–133.

Gelpin, E., Bonne, O., Peri, T., et al., 1996. Treatment of recent trauma survivors with benzodiazepines: a prospective study. The Journal of Clinical Psychiatry 57 (9), 390–394.

Gillman, P.K., 2007. Tricyclic antidepressant pharmacology and therapeutic drug interactions updated. British Journal of Pharmacology 151 (6), 737–748.

Gudberg, C., Johansen-Berg, H., 2015. Sleep and motor learning: implications for physical rehabilitation after stroke. Frontiers in Neurology 6, 241.

Hoge, E.A., Worthington, J.J., Nagurney, J.T., et al., 2012. Effect of acute posttrauma propranolol on PTSD outcome and physiological responses during script-driven imagery. CNS Neuroscience & Therapeutics 18 (1), 21–27.

Holden, K., Meal ideas and menus: avoiding high-tyramine foods made easy. [Internet] <http://www.mc.vanderbilt.edu> (accessed 14.04.15.).

Holmes, T.H., Rahe, R.H., 1967. The Social Readjustment Rating Scale. Journal of Psychosomatic Research 11 (2), 213–218.

Howard, P., Twycross, R., Shuster, J., et al., 2014. Benzodiazepines. Journal of Pain and Symptom Management 47 (5), 955–964.

Huhn, M., Tardy, M., Spineli, L.M., et al., 2014. Efficacy of pharmacotherapy and psychotherapy for adult psychiatric disorders: a systematic overview of meta-analyses. JAMA Psychiatry 71 (6), 706–715.

Institute for Health Metrics and Evaluation, 2010a. Global Burden of Diseases, Injuries, and Risk Factors Study 2010: GBD Profile: Australia. [Internet] <http://www.healthdata.org/sites/default/files/files/country_profiles/GBD/ihme_gbd_country_report_australia.pdf> (accessed 26.03.15.).

Institute for Health Metrics and Evaluation, 2010b. Global Burden of Diseases, Injuries, and Risk Factors Study 2010: GBD Profile: New Zealand. [Internet] <http://www.healthdata.org/sites/default/files/files/country_profiles/GBD/ihme_gbd_country_report_new_zealand.pdf> (accessed 26.03.15.).

Ipser, J.C., Stein, D.J., 2012. Evidence-based pharmacotherapy of post-traumatic stress disorder (PTSD). The International Journal of Neuropsychopharmacology / Official Scientific Journal of the Collegium Internationale Neuropsychopharmacologicum (CINP) 15 (6), 825–840.

Janicak, P.G., Marder, S.R., Pavuluri, M.N., 2011. Principles and Practice of Psychopharmacotherapy, fifth ed. Wolters Kluwer Health, Philadelphia, PA.

Keck, P.E. Jr., McElroy, S.L., 2003. Redefining mood stabilization. Journal of Affective Disorders 73 (1–2), 163–169.

Keuthen, N.J., Tung, E.S., Reese, H.E., et al., 2015. Getting the word out: cognitive–behavioral therapy for trichotillomania (hair-pulling disorder) and excoriation (skin-picking) disorder. Annals of Clinical Psychiatry 27 (1), 10–15.

Kharadi, D., Patel, K., Rana, D., et al., 2015. Off-label drug use in psychiatry outpatient department: a prospective study at a tertiary care teaching hospital. Journal of Basic and Clinical Pharmacy 6 (2), 45–49.

Kiphuth, I.C., Utz, K.S., Noble, A.J., et al., 2014. Increased prevalence of posttraumatic stress disorder in patients after transient ischemic attack. Stroke; a Journal of Cerebral Circulation 45 (11), 3360–3366.

Kleinstauber, M., Witthoft, M., Steffanowski, A., et al., 2014. Pharmacological interventions for somatoform disorders in adults. The Cochrane Database of Systematic Reviews (11), CD010628.

Kulkarni, J., Reeve-Parker, K., 2015. Psychiatrists' awareness of partial- and non-adherence to antipsychotic medication in schizophrenia: results from the Australian ADHES survey. Australasian Psychiatry 23 (3), 258–264.

Lambert, T., 2011. Managing the metabolic adverse effects of antipsychotic drugs in patients with psychosis. Australian Prescriber 34, 97–99.

Lapidus, K.A., Kopell, B.H., Ben-Haim, S., et al., 2013. History of psychosurgery: a psychiatrist's perspective. World Neurosurgery 80 (3–4), S27 e1–S27 e16.

Lecomte, T., Corbiere, M., Simard, S., et al., 2014. Merging evidence-based psychosocial interventions in schizophrenia. Behavioral Sciences 4 (4), 437–447.

Leucht, S., Komossa, K., Rummel-Kluge, C., et al., 2009. A meta-analysis of head-to-head comparisons of second-generation antipsychotics in the treatment of schizophrenia. The American Journal of Psychiatry 166 (2), 152–163.

Loane, C., Politis, M., 2012. Buspirone: what is it all about? Brain Research 1461, 111–118.

Luigjes, J., de Kwaasteniet, B.P., de Koning, P.P., et al., 2013. Surgery for psychiatric disorders. World Neurosurgery 80 (3–4), S31 e17–S31 e28.

Maercker, A., Forstmeier, S., Pielmaier, L., et al., 2012. Adjustment disorders: prevalence in a representative nationwide survey in Germany. Social Psychiatry and Psychiatric Epidemiology 47 (11), 1745–1752.

Malhi, G.S., Hitching, R., Berk, M., et al., 2013. Pharmacological management of unipolar depression. Acta Psychiatrica Scandinavica. Supplementum 443, 6–23.

Mark, T.L., 2010. For what diagnoses are psychotropic medications being prescribed?: a nationally representative survey of physicians. CNS Drugs 24 (4), 319–326.

Massart, R., Mongeau, R., Lanfumey, L., 2012. Beyond the monoaminergic hypothesis: neuroplasticity and epigenetic changes in a transgenic mouse model of depression. Philosophical Transactions of the Royal Society of London. Series B, Biological Sciences 367 (1601), 2485–2494.

Mataix-Cols, D., 2014. Hoarding disorder. New England Journal of Medicine 370 (21), 2023–2030.

McInerney, S.J., Kennedy, S.H., 2014. Review of evidence for use of antidepressants in bipolar depression. The Primary Care Companion for CNS Disorders 16 (5), doi:10.4088/PCC.14r01653.

McKay, D., Sookman, D., Neziroglu, F., et al., 2015. Efficacy of cognitive–behavioral therapy for obsessive–compulsive disorder. Psychiatry Research 225 (3), 236–246.

Mueser, K.T., Pratt, S.I., Bartels, S.J., et al., 2010. Randomized trial of social rehabilitation and integrated health care for older people with severe mental illness. Journal of Consulting and Clinical Psychology 78 (4), 561–573.

Murru, A., Pacchiarotti, I., Nivoli, A.M., et al., 2011. What we know and what we don't know about the treatment of schizoaffective disorder. European Neuropsychopharmacology 21 (9), 680–690.

Nielsen, G., Stone, J., Matthews, A., et al., 2015. Physiotherapy for functional motor disorders: a consensus recommendation. Journal of Neurology, Neurosurgery, and Psychiatry 86 (10), 1113–1119.

Okamura, H., Watanabe, T., Narabayashi, M., et al., 2000. Psychological distress following first recurrence of disease in patients with breast cancer: prevalence and risk factors. Breast Cancer Research and Treatment 61 (2), 131–137.

Olson, L.G., 2008. Hypnotic hazards: adverse effects of zolpidem and other z-drugs. Australian Prescriber 31, 146–149.

Ouellet, M.C., Beaulieu-Bonneau, S., Morin, C.M., 2015. Sleep-wake disturbances after traumatic brain injury. The Lancet. Neurology 14, 746–757.

Rajendran, S., Sajbel, T.A., Hartman, T.J., 2012. Factors involved in making decisions to prescribe medications for psychiatric disorders by psychiatrists: a survey study. The Psychiatric Quarterly 83 (3), 271–280.

Raven, M., Parry, P., 2012. Psychotropic marketing practices and problems: implications for DSM-5. Journal of Nervous and Mental Disease 200 (6), 512–516.

Rosebush, P.I., Mazurek, M.F., 2011. Treatment of conversion disorder in the 21st century: have we moved beyond the couch? Current Treatment Options in Neurology 13 (3), 255–266.

Rothbart, R., Stein, D.J., 2014. Pharmacotherapy of trichotillomania (hair pulling disorder): an updated systematic review. Expert Opinion on Pharmacotherapy 15 (18), 2709–2719.

Royal Australian and New Zealand College of Psychiatrists, 2005. Clinical practice guidelines for the treatment of schizophrenia and related disorders. The Australian and New Zealand Journal of Psychiatry 39 (1–2), 1–30.

Sahoo, M.K., Agarwal, S., Biswas, H., 2014. Catatonia versus neuroleptic malignant syndrome: the diagnostic dilemma and treatment. Industrial Psychiatry Journal 23 (2), 163–165.

Saravane, D., Feve, B., Frances, Y., et al., 2009. Drawing up guidelines for the attendance of physical health of patients with severe mental illness. L'Encephale 35 (4), 330–339.

Severus, E., Taylor, M.J., Sauer, C., et al., 2014. Lithium for prevention of mood episodes in bipolar disorders: systematic review and meta-analysis. International Journal of Bipolar Disorder 2, 15.

Slade, T., Johnston, A., Oakley Browne, M.A., et al., 2009. 2007 National Survey of Mental Health and Wellbeing: methods and key findings. Australian and New Zealand Journal of Psychiatry 43 (7), 594–605.

Shah, A.A., Aftab, A., Coverdale, J., 2014. QTc prolongation with antipsychotics: is routine ECG monitoring recommended? Journal of Psychiatric Practice 20 (3), 196–206.

Shulman, K.I., Herrmann, N., Walker, S.E., 2013. Current place of monoamine oxidase inhibitors in the treatment of depression. CNS Drugs 27 (10), 789–797.

Sienaert, P., Dhossche, D.M., Vancampfort, D., et al., 2014. A clinical review of the treatment of catatonia. Frontiers in Psychiatry 5, 181.

Silverstone, P.H., 1996. Prevalence of psychiatric disorders in medical inpatients. Journal of Nervous and Mental Disease 184 (1), 43–51.

Sinyor, M., Schaffer, A., Levitt, A., 2010. The sequenced treatment alternatives to relieve depression (STAR*D) trial: a review. Canadian Journal of Psychiatry 55 (3), 126–135.

Somashekar, B., Jainer, A., Wuntakal, B., 2013. Psychopharmacotherapy of somatic symptoms disorders. International Review of Psychiatry 25 (1), 107–115.

Soomro, G.M., 2012. Obsessive–compulsive disorder. BMJ Clinical Evidence 2012, pii: 1004.

Spiegel, D.R., Finklea, L., 2009. The recognition and treatment of pathological skin picking: a potential neurobiological underpinning of the efficacy of pharmacotherapy in impulse control disorders. Psychiatry 6 (2), 38–42.

Stahl, S.M., 2008. Essential Psychopharmacology: Neuroscientific basis and practical applications, third ed. Cambridge University Press, Cambridge, UK; New York, NY, USA.

Stahl, S.M., 2009. Multifunctional drugs: a novel concept for psychopharmacology. CNS Spectrums 14 (2), 71–73.

Stoffers, J., Vollm, B.A., Rucker, G., et al., 2010. Pharmacological interventions for borderline personality disorder. The Cochrane Database of Systematic Reviews (6), CD005653.

Sullivan, G.M., Neria, Y., 2009. Pharmacotherapy of PTSD: current status and controversies. Psychiatric Annals 39 (6), 342–347.

Thronson, L.R., Pagalilauan, G.L., 2014. Psychopharmacology. Medical Clinics of North America 98 (5), 927–958.

Vickrey, B.G., Williams, L.S., 2014. Posttraumatic stress disorder after cerebrovascular events: broadening the landscape of psychological assessment in stroke and transient ischemic attack. Stroke; a Journal of Cerebral Circulation 45 (11), 3182–3183.

Volpi-Abadie, J., Kaye, A.M., Kaye, A.D., 2013. Serotonin syndrome. The Ochsner Journal 13 (4), 533–540.

Westenberg, H.G.M., Fineberg, N.A., Denys, D., 2007. Neurobiology of obsessive–compulsive disorder: serotonin and beyond. CNS Spectrums 12 (2 Suppl. 3), 14–27.

Whiteford, H.A., Ferrari, A.J., Degenhardt, L., et al., 2015. The global burden of mental, neurological and substance use disorders: an analysis from the Global Burden of Disease Study 2010. PLoS ONE 10 (2), e0116820.

Whiting, D., Cowen, P.J., 2013. Drug information update: agomelatine. The Psychiatrist 37 (11), 356–358.

Widiger, T.A., Samuel, D.B., 2005. Diagnostic categories or dimensions? A question for the *Diagnostic and Statistical Manual Of Mental Disorders* – fifth edition. Journal of Abnormal Psychology 114 (4), 494–504.

Wong-Anuchit, C., 2016. Clinical management of antipsychotic-induced hyperprolactinemia. Perspectives in Psychiatric Care 52 (2), 145–152. doi:10.1111/ppc.12111.

World Health Organization, 1992. ICD-10 Classifications of Mental and Behavioural Disorders: Clinical Descriptions and Diagnostic Guidelines. World Health Organization, Geneva.

Wu, C.S., Tsai, Y.T., Tsai, H.J., 2015. Antipsychotic drugs and the risk of ventricular arrhythmia and/or sudden cardiac death: a nation-wide case-crossover study. Journal of the American Heart Association 4 (2), e001568. doi:10.1161/JAHA.114.001568.

Young, S.L., Taylor, M., Lawrie, S.M., 2015. 'First do no harm.' A systematic review of the prevalence and management of antipsychotic adverse effects. Journal of Psychopharmacology 29 (4), 353–362.

Zeanah, C.H., Gleason, M.M., 2015. Annual research review: attachment disorders in early childhood – clinical presentation, causes, correlates, and treatment. Journal of Child Psychology and Psychiatry, and Allied Disciplines 56 (3), 207–222.

Zohar, J., Juven-Wetzler, A., Sonnino, R., et al., 2011. New insights into secondary prevention in post-traumatic stress disorder. Dialogues in Clinical Neuroscience 13 (3), 301–309.

Medication issues in the young and the elderly

Ian Heslop, Jacqueline Reznik, Ofer Keren

OBJECTIVES

This chapter will examine issues relating to the use of medication in both the young and the elderly. It will examine differences in drug absorption, distribution, metabolism and excretion in these age groups and discuss the impact of these pharmacokinetic as well as pharmacodynamic changes on the medication management of the patient. Other legal, clinical and therapeutic considerations relating to the use of medications in both age groups will also be addressed. By the end of this chapter (including cross-referencing with other chapters) the reader should have an understanding of:

♦ the pharmacokinetic and pharmacodynamic differences between the young and elderly compared to the standard adult population
♦ some legal and dosing issues relating to medication management in the young and elderly
♦ the issues caused by poor concordance and adherence in the elderly
♦ the problems associated with polypharmacy in the elderly
♦ the potential impact of any of the above issues on physiotherapeutic management.

■ Medication issues in the younger person

Introduction

Compared to adults, some of the physiological processes and metabolic pathways in young children are not fully developed or are immature. This needs to be considered when prescribing medication for children, as it cannot just be automatically assumed that a child is simply a smaller version of an adult who can be dosed with the same medications, only with a 'scaled down dose'. We also need to be aware of the pharmacokinetic and pharmacodynamic differences between children and adults and select and prescribe medications accordingly, using appropriate methods to calculate the dosages. This section will examine some of these age-related pharmacokinetic and pharmacodynamic changes in children and it will also highlight some of the important issues regarding the prescribing of medications to children. However, firstly it is necessary to define the patient groups that we will be discussing in this chapter. Traditionally, various terms are used to classify children based on their age and these are (Sansom 2015)[1]:

Preterm newborn infant – born before 37 weeks' gestation

Term newborn infant – born from 37 weeks' gestation

Neonate – birth to 28 days

Infant – 28 days to 1 year

Young child – toddler – 1 to 3 years

Young child – preschool – 3 to 5 years

Older child – 5 to 12 years

Adult – over 12 years or weighing 40–50 kg is generally considered as an adult for dose calculations.

Legal issues relating to the use of medicines in children

Some registered medicines used in paediatric clinical practice lack indications for use in children and are therefore used 'off-label'. This means that the medication is being used for an unlicensed purpose; that is, the indication, formulation, age range or route being used differs from that in the licensed product information provided by the manufacturer. In paediatrics, this is usually because the manufacturer had insufficient research evidence to support a licensing application for the use of the medication in children. However, the use of the medication in children can still be considered to be appropriate if there is still good quality clinical evidence to support its use, if there are exceptional circumstances or alternative options are not appropriate, and where the patient and carers have been given appropriate information and have then made an informed decision whether or not to accept treatment (Sinha & Cranswick 2007).

---

[1]Definitions from the *Australian Pharmaceutical Formulary and Handbook*, 23rd Ed., 2015, published by the Pharmaceutical Society of Australia.

Pharmacokinetic differences in the younger person

When a medication is administered to a patient, the medication may undergo four pharmacokinetic processes in the body (absorption, distribution, metabolism and elimination). Whether it undergoes all of these processes, and the extent to which the medication is ultimately affected, is dependent on a number of variables including the properties of the medication itself and also its route of administration (see Chapter 1). In addition, in children, these pharmacokinetic processes may not be fully developed and so each pharmacokinetic stage may be affected; however, some changes are more clinically significant than others.

Absorption

There are a number of physiological changes in children that may impact on the absorption of drugs administered by the oral route. At different ages, young children exhibit reduced gastric acid production, reduced gastric motility, a relatively immature intestinal mucosa and immature enzymatic activity and bile acid production compared to older children and adults (Funk, Brown & Abdel-Rahman 2012; Sansom 2015; Sinha & Cranswick 2007). Children have been shown to have reduced gastric acid production and raised gastric pH until about 20 months of age, which may decrease the absorption of weakly acidic drugs (e.g. phenytoin) and enhance the absorption of drugs that are weak bases (e.g. penicillins) (Funk, Brown & Abdel-Rahman 2012). There may also be reduced gastric decomposition of some acid-labile drugs (e.g. some penicillins) (Funk, Brown & Abdel-Rahman 2012). Delayed gastric emptying and reduced intestinal motility have been reported in children below the age of 6–8 months and this appears to have a variable effect on drug absorption, potentially slowing the rate of absorption and the time to reach peak plasma concentrations, but it does not appear to alter the total amount of drug absorbed in neonates (Funk, Brown & Abdel-Rahman 2012). In contrast, the immature production of pancreatic enzymes and bile may affect the absorption of some fat-soluble medications (Funk, Brown & Abdel-Rahman 2012; Sinha & Cranswick 2007).

Distribution

Body composition varies with age, with neonatal body composition being 70–80% total body water and 10–15% body fat (Funk, Brown & Abdel-Rahman 2012). The proportion of body water decreases with age, with body composition at 1 year of age being approximately 60% total body water and 20–25% total body fat, and by adolescence and into adulthood the total body water content has decreased to approximately 50% (Funk, Brown & Abdel-Rahman 2012). Hydrophilic drugs (e.g. gentamicin) will predominantly reside in the water compartment of the body and, as a result, have a larger volume of distribution and relatively larger dosage requirements in neonates than older children or adults (Funk, Brown & Abdel-Rahman 2012). Infants and neonates also have relatively low plasma albumin concentrations, which may result in reduced protein binding and an increase in the unbound fraction of highly protein bound drugs (Funk, Brown & Abdel-Rahman 2012).

Metabolism

Children have relatively immature liver function compared to adults. The metabolic pathways for drugs in the liver are generally divided into two phases. Phase 1 enzyme systems are responsible for the oxidation of drugs and many of these reactions are catalysed by the cytochrome P-450 (CYP450) group of enzymes. Some CYP450 enzyme systems are not present at birth and other systems are immature. These systems mature at different rates and reach maturity at different times. Most mature within 1–3 years; however, some, such as CYP2D6, do not reach maturity until adolescence (Funk, Brown & Abdel-Rahman 2012). Phase 2 enzyme systems are responsible for the conjugation of drug molecules with other molecules. This makes drug molecules more water-soluble and, as a result, enhances their elimination. Phase 2 reactions are involved in the metabolism of paracetamol, ibuprofen and warfarin. When a drug's primary route of metabolism is immature, if possible, the drug is then metabolised by alternative pathways. For example, in adults, paracetamol is primarily metabolised by glucuronidation, whereas in infants it is primarily metabolised by sulfonation, as this pathway is more active in this age group. This is thought to be the main reason why lower levels of paracetamol toxicity are seen in infants, as the sulfonated metabolite is less toxic than the glucuronide metabolite (Funk, Brown & Abdel-Rahman 2012).

In summary, it must be noted that, because of the differences in liver physiology between different age groups, the first-pass metabolism of some drugs will be variable and the clearance and half-life of some drugs can be adversely affected. This must be considered when dosing different age groups of patients (Funk, Brown & Abdel-Rahman 2012).

Elimination

The functional capacity of the kidney in a term infant is approximately 20–40% that of an adult and renal blood flow and glomerular filtration rate (GFR)[2] are also lower (Funk, Brown & Abdel-Rahman 2012). In the first weeks of life, renal perfusion and GFR increase markedly and normalise 4–5 weeks after birth reaching maximum capacity at 6–12 months of age. These differences in renal physiology need to be taken into consideration when dosing patients with very water-soluble, renally-cleared drugs such as gentamicin and other aminoglycosides (Funk, Brown & Abdel-Rahman 2012; Sinha & Cranswick 2007).

Pharmacodynamic differences in the younger person

It is thought that pharmacodynamic differences also exist between children and adults. However, limited research has been performed in this area. As a result, it is sometimes difficult to discern the difference between drug actions attributable to pharmacokinetic factors and those caused by pharmacodynamic factors. For example, any differences in response to beta-adrenoceptor agonists

---

[2]The glomerular filtration rate (GFR), which is the rate at which fluid is filtered through the kidneys, is an indication of renal function.

(e.g. salbutamol) between neonates and older children may be due to the relative stage of development of the respiratory system in the neonate as well as any potential difference in the density of beta-adrenoceptors in the respiratory tissue (Funk, Brown & Abdel-Rahman 2012; Sansom 2015; Sinha & Cranswick 2007).

Dosage calculations

Weight-based dosing

This is the most common method of calculating an accurate dose for a child (Sansom 2015) and, where possible, a recent accurate measurement of the child's weight should be used. Ideal body weight (IBW) should also be used for oedematous or obese children as it takes into account changes in body composition that may affect drug distribution. For children aged 1–18 years, IBW can be calculated using the following equation (Sansom 2015):

$$\text{Ideal body weight (kg)} = \frac{[\text{Height (cm)}]^2 \times 1.65}{1000}$$

Body surface area-based dosing

Body surface area (BSA) dosing is generally considered more accurate than body weight for calculating doses in children (Sansom 2015); however, in practice it is limited due to the difficulty in accurately calculating or estimating the BSA of the child. In practice, BSA may be estimated either with an approved nomogram or by using Mosteller's equation (Sansom 2015):

$$\text{Body surface area (m}^2) = \sqrt{\frac{\text{Height (cm)} \times \text{Weight (kg)}}{3600}}$$

Medication administration considerations in the younger person

The oral route is the most commonly used route of drug administration in paediatrics, as with adults and the elderly. Oral liquid dosage forms are preferred in children younger than 5 years of age; liquid preparations are readily and commercially available for medications commonly used in this age group (e.g. antibiotics); however, they are not so readily available for many other drugs. Therefore, solid dosage forms may have to be considered. It is generally accepted that children below the age of 5 years are unable to swallow tablets or capsules whole. Hence these may have to be altered, either by halving or dividing adult tablets to give the required dose and/or by crushing the solid dosage form and mixing it with food, infant formula or drink to administer it to the child. It has to be remembered that dividing a solid dosage form introduces some level of inaccuracy into the dosing process and the crushing process may alter the release properties of the medication from the dosage form and also the rate and extent of absorption of the medication, thereby increasing the risk of adverse effects to the patient. Ideally, commercially available or approved or official formulations of extemporaneously prepared liquid preparations should be used when dosing young children, and dosages should be measured with relatively accurate devices such as oral syringes.

Medication issues in the elderly

Introduction

It is well recognised that, in the 'older person/elderly', as the body ages certain age-related physiological changes occur that can potentially alter the way in which the body handles medications compared to younger adults. These pharmacokinetic and pharmacodynamic differences, combined with the fact that many older persons also have multiple co-morbidities and, as a result, may be taking multiple medications, makes them at greater risk of medication-related problems. This section will examine some of these age-related pharmacokinetic and pharmacodynamic differences and highlight some of medication groups that may be more problematic for older patients. However, firstly it is necessary to define the patient group we will be discussing. Traditionally, the term 'elderly' or 'older person' is used to describe someone who is over 65 years of age. However, there is no accepted definition with some clinicians only using the term 'elderly' to describe persons over 75 years of age, whereas others also recognise that age-related pharmacokinetic changes can become significant in some individuals younger than 65 years of age. Therefore, a more individualised approach is now recommended with older people not being categorised solely based on age so that some younger individuals should also be assessed for age-related physiological changes, multiple diseases and medications and appropriate action may be taken when necessary.

Pharmacokinetic changes associated with ageing

When a medication is administered to a patient, the medication can undergo four pharmacokinetic processes in the body (absorption, distribution, metabolism and elimination) – see Chapter 1. Age-related changes can occur at each stage; however, some changes are more clinically significant than others.

Absorption

Reported age-related physiological changes in the gastrointestinal tract include elevations in gastric pH, delayed gastric emptying and decreased gastrointestinal motility and blood flow. However, there appears to be little effect on active transport mechanisms (Mangoni & Jackson 2004; Turnheim 2003). As a result, although physiological changes may potentially delay drug absorption, the extent of drug absorption is usually unaffected and therefore effects are rarely clinically significant. However, these effects may contribute to the malabsorption of some dietary nutrients reliant on gastric acid for their absorption such as iron and vitamin B12 (Mangoni & Jackson 2004; Turnheim 2003). Medication-induced changes in gastric pH can lead to similar effects (i.e. prolonged use of proton pump inhibitors or H_2-receptor antagonists can cause reduced B12 absorption).

Distribution

Reported age-related changes in body composition in the elderly include a progressive decline in lean body mass and total and percentage body water content and an increase in total body fat (Mangoni & Jackson 2004). In addition, frail elderly people often have lower serum albumin concentrations compared to younger people (Mangoni & Jackson 2004). As a result, the volume of distribution of hydrophilic drugs (e.g. gentamicin or digoxin) may decrease; whereas that of lipophilic drugs (e.g. diazepam) will increase (Mangoni & Jackson 2004). Changes in serum albumin concentrations will also affect the distribution and excretion of medications that are highly protein bound (Mangoni & Jackson 2004).

Metabolism

Reported age-related physiological changes that may affect drug metabolism include reductions in liver mass, liver blood flow and enzyme activity that may, in turn, affect the hepatic biotransformation, metabolism and response to some medications in elderly people. The first-pass metabolism of drugs may decrease in older people; this may result in an increase in the bioavailability of drugs, which may then undergo extensive first-pass metabolism (e.g. amitriptyline and metoprolol) and a reduction in the hepatic activation of some prodrugs (e.g. perindopril) (Mangoni & Jackson 2004; McLachlan & Pont 2012). Likewise, the hepatic clearance of drugs with high hepatic extraction ratios (e.g. diltiazem, levodopa and morphine) may be reduced. However, the effect of these age-related hepatic changes on the clearance of drugs with low hepatic extraction ratios (e.g. naproxen, ibuprofen, temazepam and sodium valproate) is more variable. As a result, with some agents, individualised drug regimens are required to reduce the potential impact of increased serum levels and increased risk of adverse effects associated with these age-related changes in hepatic function (Mangoni & Jackson 2004; McLachlan & Pont 2012).

Elimination

As the kidney is the most important organ in the body for the clearance of many drugs, the age-related decline in kidney function seen in many older people may have a major impact on drug therapy. The glomerular filtration rate (GFR) of an elderly person may be half that of an equivalent younger person (Sansom 2015). In turn, this may affect the elimination of drugs that are predominantly cleared by the kidneys (e.g. digoxin) or drugs with active metabolites predominantly cleared by the kidneys (e.g. morphine, allopurinol and its metabolite oxypurinol), thereby resulting in raised serum drug concentrations and increased risk of adverse effects. This would be particularly important when the older person is prescribed drugs with a narrow therapeutic index (Sansom 2015). The GFR in the elderly may be decreased due to age-related reductions in renal mass, nephron number and function and renal blood flow. Common co-morbidities in the elderly, such as diabetes and hypertension, may also contribute to the renal impairment (Sansom 2015). It cannot, however, be assumed that all elderly people have clinically significant renal impairment, and therefore estimations of each patient's GFR should be made and dosage adjustments should be made only if appropriate. Dosage adjustments are most commonly made in patients with significant renal impairment and with medications that are principally eliminated by the kidneys, especially those with a narrow therapeutic index (e.g. digoxin, gentamicin, lithium and vancomycin). Due to reduced muscle mass in the elderly, serum creatinine levels may appear normal and it is therefore important to estimate the patient's creatinine clearance with an appropriate algorithm. The Cockcroft-Gault equation is a commonly used equation to estimate creatinine clearance (Cl_{CR}) and the GFR based on the patient's age, body weight and serum creatinine (Sansom 2015):

$$\text{Estimated creatinine clearance } Cl_{CR} \text{ (mL/min)(male)}$$

$$= \frac{(140 - \text{Age (years)}) \times \text{Ideal body weight (kg)}}{0.815 \times \text{Serum creatinine (micromol/L)}}$$

For females, multiply the answer by 0.85:

* Ideal body weight males = 50 kg + 0.9 kg for every cm above 152 cm
* Ideal body weight females = 45.5 kg + 0.9 kg for every cm above 152 cm

(Use actual body weight if the person's actual body weight is below ideal body weight.)

Pharmacodynamic changes associated with ageing

Older patients appear to be more sensitive or intolerant to certain medications than younger patients, suggesting some form of altered pharmacodynamic response, as well as some changes in receptor properties. These include reductions in the number, sensitivity or responsiveness of some receptors (e.g. reduced responsiveness in beta-adrenergic receptors), depletion in neurotransmitters (e.g. acetylcholine, dopamine or serotonin) or some other physiological changes. However, it is also recognised that some homeostatic responses are also reduced or blunted in older people, which contributes towards any perceived increase in medication sensitivity (Mangoni & Jackson 2004; McLachlan & Pont 2012; Sansom 2015; Turnheim 2003). An example of how homeostatic systems and mechanisms may be affected is the age-related changes to the baroreceptor reflex. In elderly patients, the baroreceptor reflex involved in blood pressure control is impaired and becomes sluggish, as is the mechanism that causes a reflex tachycardia in response to vasodilation on standing. As a result, older patients tend to be more prone to orthostatic hypotension and are therefore at increased risk of falls. These effects may be exacerbated by the co-administration of medications that reduce blood pressure, either intentionally (e.g. antihypertensive medications, especially those with alpha-adrenoceptor blocking actions, e.g. prazosin) or as adverse effects (e.g. tricyclic antidepressants and some antipsychotics) or by co-morbidities such as diabetes and Parkinson's disease (Mangoni & Jackson 2004; McLachlan & Pont 2012; Sansom 2015; Turnheim 2003).

Medications of concern in the elderly

Due to some of the pharmacokinetic and pharmacodynamic changes described above, some medications are more problematic in the elderly because they cause significant adverse effects and others should be used with caution or avoided in this age group (Sansom 2015; Mangoni & Jackson 2004; McLachlan & Pont 2012; Turnheim 2003). Some examples are discussed in the following sections.

Medications acting on the central nervous system (CNS)

Sedatives/hypnotics

The half-lives of many benzodiazepines (e.g. diazepam, nitrazepam and temazepam) and some active metabolites increase in older people making them more prone to adverse effects such as over-sedation, ataxia, confusion, respiratory depression and short-term memory impairment. The presence of renal and hepatic impairment exacerbates these effects (Mangoni & Jackson 2004; McLachlan & Pont 2012; Sansom 2015; Turnheim 2003).

Antidepressants and antipsychotics
Care is required in using antipsychotic agents in the elderly, as their use has been associated with increased risk of stroke and death. With both antipsychotics and antidepressants, if used, they should initially be administered at low dose with slow, gradual incremental dose increases if needed. The elderly are more prone to the side effects associated with these agents, in particular orthostatic hypotension and confusion and their extrapyramidal and anticholinergic effects (Mangoni & Jackson 2004; McLachlan & Pont 2012; Sansom 2015; Turnheim 2003).

Analgesics
The opioid analgesics show variable age-related changes in pharmacokinetics. However, opioid dose requirement decreases with age and the elderly are at increased risk of cognitive impairment, sedation, respiratory depression and falls. Initially, lower doses should be used and the dose titrated against analgesic response. The elderly are also more prone to heart failure, gastrointestinal irritation and renal impairment with the non-steroidal anti-inflammatory drugs (NSAIDs) (Mangoni & Jackson 2004; McLachlan & Pont 2012; Sansom 2015; Turnheim 2003).

Anticholinergic agents
Elderly people are particularly prone to the central effects (e.g. drowsiness, memory impairment, restlessness and confusion) and peripheral effects (e.g. constipation, dry mouth, blurred vision, urinary retention) of anticholinergic agents. These adverse effects may be caused by agents used principally for their anticholinergic effects (e.g. oxybutynin, used in the management of incontinence) but also other agents prone to cause anticholinergic side effects (e.g. tricyclic antidepressants, antihistamines and antipsychotics) (Mangoni & Jackson 2004; McLachlan & Pont 2012; Sansom 2015; Turnheim 2003).

Multiple diseases and medicines (polypharmacy)
Older people often suffer from multiple medical conditions and co-morbidities. This often results in elderly people taking multiple medications, multiple doses of medications and/or using a range of pharmaceutical products and formulations. It is estimated that almost all Australians older than 65 years of age have at least one chronic medical condition and that at least 25% of older Australians are subject to polypharmacy (taking five or more medications) and are, as a result, at increased risk of adverse effects and drug interactions. These medical conditions and co-morbidities can also further modify the pharmacokinetic and pharmacodynamic changes normally associated with increasing age and the patient's response to their medication. Finally, each medical condition may also require multiple medications, and as a result, many elderly people take very complex medication regimens and have a significant 'pill burden' with an associated risk of poor adherence or confusion. This may be further complicated by the person also taking a range of over-the-counter medications and complementary medications and, subsequently, as the medication regimen

grows, further medications may also be added to combat the side effects associated with previously prescribed agents (Mangoni & Jackson 2004; McLachlan & Pont 2012; Sansom 2015; Turnheim 2003). Therefore, it is recommended that a thorough medication review is performed on each elderly person on a regular basis. This involves assessing the person's drug burden and reviewing their medications for evidence of efficacy or harm. In particular, the need for medications with anticholinergic and/or sedative properties should be evaluated. A careful de-prescribing process can then be followed. This involves reviewing all of the person's current medications, identifying medications that need to be reduced, substituted or ceased and planning a gradual change to the new medication regimen. The medication review can also identify any difficulties that the person may have regarding the handling, storage and use of their medications (Mangoni & Jackson 2004; McLachlan & Pont 2012; Sansom 2015; Turnheim 2003).

Route and administration

Medications are traditionally given by the oral route if possible, usually in the form of solid dosage forms (e.g. tablets and capsules). However, many older people have difficulty swallowing and, as a result, need liquid dosage forms (e.g. suspensions or syrups) or require their tablets to be crushed and administered in food, drinks or via a nasogastric tube. This crushing process may alter the release properties of the medication from the dosage form and also the rate and extent of absorption of the medication, thereby increasing the risk of adverse effects to the patient. Therefore, generally, extended- or sustained-release products, enteric-coated or sublingual products should not be crushed before administration. Health professionals should use only commercially-available or approved or official formulations of extemporaneously prepared liquid preparations when liquid formulations are required. Solid dosage forms should only be crushed and administered to patients if there is evidence to suggest that crushing will not affect the integrity, stability or absorption characteristics of the medication itself, and ultimately risk harming the patient.

Adherence/compliance

Non-adherence is a commonly reported problem in the elderly and a multitude of factors have been identified as contributing to, or increasing the risk of, non-adherence. These include: multiple medications, brands and doses; multiple chronic diseases and long-term therapy; the use of multiple doctors and pharmacies; psychiatric illness; cognitive impairment; ineffective communication between health professionals and between health professionals and the patient; and impaired physical dexterity, sight and hearing. The patient's perceptions of the effectiveness of their medication regimen may also play a significant role, as can their trust and confidence in their own health professionals. However, irrespective of the cause, non-adherence may result in poor clinical outcomes and/or an increased risk of adverse effects. Therefore, in the medication review process, the person's medication regimen should also be altered to aid adherence by ideally reducing the number and doses of medication. The person should also be empowered and educated about the importance of adherence and their medications in general and, if necessary, compliance aids or dosage administration aids (DAAs) may also be used to aid adherence. However, some dosage forms and medications may not be suitable for repackaging into DAAs, including dosage forms that are effervescent, dispersible and chewable or designed for sublingual administration and medications that are hygroscopic or sensitive to light, moisture and heat (Sansom 2015).

■ References

Funk, R.S., Brown, J.T., Abdel-Rahman, S.M., 2012. Pediatric pharmacokinetics: human development and drug disposition. Pediatric Clinics of North America 59 (5), 1001–1016.

Mangoni, A.A., Jackson, S.H., 2004. Age-related changes in pharmacokinetics and pharmacodynamics: basic principles and practical applications. British Journal of Clinical Pharmacology 57 (1), 6–14.

McLachlan, A.J., Pont, L.G., 2012. Drug metabolism in older people: a key consideration in achieving optimal outcomes with medicines. Journals of Gerontology, Series A, Biological Sciences and Medical Sciences 67A (2), 175–180.

Sansom, L.N. (Ed.), 2015. Australian Pharmaceutical Formulary and Handbook, twenty-third ed. Pharmaceutical Society of Australia, Canberra.

Sinha, Y., Cranswick, N.E., 2007. How to use medicines in children: principles of paediatric clinical pharmacology. Journal of Paediatrics and Child Health 43 (3), 107–111.

Turnheim, K., 2003. When drug therapy gets old: pharmacokinetics and pharmacodynamics in the elderly. Experimental Gerontology 38 (8), 843–853.

Index

Page numbers followed by '*f*' indicate figures, '*t*' indicate tables, and '*b*' indicate boxes.